Recent Results in Cancer Research 179

Managing Editors
P. M. Schlag, Berlin   H.-J. Senn, St. Gallen

Associate Editors
P. Kleihues, Zürich   F. Stiefel, Lausanne
B. Groner, Frankfurt   A. Wallgren, Göteborg

Founding Editor
P. Rentchnick, Geneva

Per-Ulf Tunn (Ed.)

Treatment of Bone and Soft Tissue Sarcomas

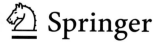

Editors
Dr. Per-Ulf Tunn
Leiter Department Tumororthopädie
Klinik für Orthopädie und
Orthopädische Rheumatologie
HELIOS-Klinikum Berlin
Schwanebecker Chaussee 50
13125 Berlin
per-ulf.tunn@helios-kliniken.de

ISBN: 978-3-540-77959-9   e-ISBN: 978-3-540-77960-5

DOI: 10.1007/978-3-540-77960-5

Library of Congress Control Number: 2008930161

© 2009 Springer-Verlag Berlin Heidelberg

This work is subject to copyright. All rights are reserved, whether the whole or part of the material is concerned, specifically the rights of translation, reprinting, reuse of illustrations, recitation, broadcasting, reproduction on microfilm or in any other way, and storage in data banks. Duplication of this publication or parts thereof is permitted only under the provisions of the German Copyright Law of September 9, 1965, in its current version, and permission for use must always be obtained from Springer. Violations are liable to prosecution under the German Copyright Law.

The use of general descriptive names, registered names, trademarks, etc. in this publication does not imply, even in the absence of a specific statement, that such names are exempt from the relevant protective laws and regulations and therefore free for general use.

Product liability: The publishers cannot guarantee the accuracy of any information about dosage and application contained in this book. In every individual case the user must check such information by consulting the relevant literature.

Cover design: Frido Steimen-Broo, eStudio Calamar, Spain

Printed on acid-free paper

9 8 7 6 5 4 3 2 1

springer.com

Contents

Part I Diagnostics

**1 Biopsy of Bone and Soft Tissue Tumours:
   Hints and Hazards**... 3
   Andreas Leithner, Werner Maurer-Ertl, and Reinhard Windhager

   1.1   Introduction 3
   1.2   Diagnostic Algorithm 3
   1.3   Biopsy 5
   1.3.1 Biopsy Technique 6
   1.4   Hints 7
   1.5   Hazards 7
   1.6   Definitive Diagnosis 9
         References 10

**2 The Role of Intra-operative Pathological Evaluation
   in the Management of Musculoskeletal Tumours** 11
   Robert U. Ashford, Richard A. Scolyer, Stanley W. McCarthy,
   S. Fiona Bonar, Rooshdiya Z. Karim, and Paul D. Stalley

   2.1   Introduction: Indications for Intra-operative Pathological
         Evaluation in Musculoskeletal Surgical Oncology 11
   2.2   Pathological Options for Intra-operative Evaluation 12
   2.2.1 Frozen Section 12
   2.2.2 Fine Needle Aspiration Cytology 14
   2.2.3 Touch Imprint Cytology 16
   2.3   Uses of Frozen Section in Musculoskeletal Tumours 16
   2.3.1 Operative Core Biopsy of Presumed Sarcoma 17
   2.3.2 Surgical Margin Biopsy/Imprint 18
   2.3.3 Confirmation of Diagnosis Prior to Definitive Treatment 19
   2.3.4 Evaluation of Tumour Spread 20
   2.3.5 Intramedullary Nailing of Presumed Metastasis 20

2.3.6	Frozen Section for Everyone?		20
2.3.7	Beware the Pitfalls of Frozen Section		20
2.4	Cost-Effectiveness		21
2.5	Discussion		22
	References		23

3 Sentinel Node Biopsy in Soft Tissue Sarcoma 25
Dimosthenis Andreou and Per-Ulf Tunn

3.1	Introduction	25
3.2	Technique of Lymphatic Mapping and Sentinel Lymph Node Biopsy	26
3.2.1	Preoperative Lymphoscintigraphy	26
3.2.2	Intraoperative Lymphatic Mapping	28
3.2.3	Histopathological Examination	30
3.3	Sentinel Node Biopsy in the Management of Soft Tissue Sarcoma	31
3.3.1	Clear Cell Sarcoma	31
3.3.2	Synovial Sarcoma	31
3.3.3	Rhabdomyosarcoma	32
3.3.4	Epithelioid Sarcoma	32
3.4	Discussion	33
	References	34

Part II Bone Sarcomas

4 Modular Endoprosthetic Reconstruction in Malignant Bone Tumors: Indications and Limits 39
Maurice Balke, Helmut Ahrens, Arne Streitbürger, Georg Gosheger, and Jendrik Hardes

4.1	Introduction	39
4.2	Surgical Technique	40
4.3	Postoperative Management	42
4.4	Complications	42
4.5	Indications and Limits	44
4.5.1	Tumor Prostheses in Children	45
4.6	Functional Results	46
	Summary	47
	References	48

5	**Allograft Reconstruction in Malignant Bone Tumors: Indications and Limits**	51

Kevin A. Raskin and Francis Hornicek

5.1	Introduction	51
5.1.1	Biology	52
5.2	Indications and Types	52
5.2.1	Intercalary Allografts	52
5.2.2	Osteoarticular Allografts	53
5.2.3	Allograft Arthrodesis	53
5.2.4	Allograft–Prosthetic Composites	55
5.3	Limits	55
	Summary	57
	References	57

6	**Expandable Endoprostheses in Malignant Bone Tumors in Children: Indications and Limitations**	59

Rainer Baumgart and Ulrich Lenze

6.1	Introduction	59
6.2	Principles of Expandable Tumor Endoprosthesis	60
6.3	The Expandable Tumor Endoprosthesis MUTARS Xpand	61
6.4	The "Bioexpandable" Tumor Endoprosthesis MUTARS Bio-Xpand	62
6.5	Indications	64
6.5.1	Step 1	64
6.5.2	Step 2	64
6.6	Limitations	65
6.7	Clinical Cases	66
6.8	Conclusion	68
	References	72

7	**The Long-Term Risks of Infection and Amputation with Limb Salvage Surgery Using Endoprostheses**	75

Lee Jeys and Robert Grimer

7.1	Introduction	75
7.2	Long-Term Limb Salvage	76
7.3	Infection and Endoprostheses	77
7.4	New Techniques to Combat Infection	81
7.4.1	Surface Treatments	81
7.4.2	Antibiotic Prophylaxis	82
7.5	Conclusions	82
	References	82

8	**Reconstruction of the Pelvis After Resection of Malignant Bone Tumours in Children and Adolescents**	85

Martin Dominkus, Eslam Darwish, and Philipp Funovics

8.1	Introduction	85
8.2	Diagnosis	86
8.3	Biopsy	86
8.4	Preoperative Staging and Therapy	86
8.5	Resection Type I: Os Ilium	88
8.5.1	Partial Resection of the Ilium Without Discontinuity of the Pelvic Ring	88
8.5.2	Complete Resection of the Os Ilium with Discontinuity of the Pelvic Ring	88
8.6	Resection Type II: Acetabulum	89
8.6.1	Biological Reconstruction Methods	92
8.6.2	Endoprosthetic Reconstruction Methods	96
8.7	Resection Type I–II +/− IV	101
8.7.1	Allograft	101
8.7.2	Autograft	102
8.7.3	Flail Hip	102
8.7.4	Hip Transpositionplasty	102
8.8	Resection Type III	103
8.9	Resection Type II, III	104
8.10	Resection Type I–III/IV	104
8.10.1	Flail Hip: No Reconstruction	105
8.10.2	Hemipelvis Allograft	106
8.11	Future Aspects	108
	Summary	108
	References	109

9	**Methods of Biological Reconstruction for Bone Sarcoma: Indications and Limits**	113

Pierre Kunz and Ludger Bernd

9.1	Introduction	113
9.2	Biological Reconstruction Procedures and Outcome	114
9.2.1	Transplantation of Vital Autografts	114
9.2.2	Implantation of Avital Bone: Extracorporeal Devitalized Autografts	119
9.2.3	De Novo Bone Formation: Distraction Osteogenesis	123
9.3	Discussion	127
9.3.1	Vital Bone Grafts: Vascularization	128
9.3.2	Biomechanical Aspects in Free Bone Grafts: Union, Hypertrophy, Fracture	130
9.3.3	Complications and Functional Outcome in Vital Grafts	131
9.3.4	Extracorporeal Devitalized Grafts	131

9.3.5	Distraction Osteogenesis	132
9.3.6	Indications and Limitations	133
9.4	Conclusion	134
	References	135

10 Bone Sarcoma of the Spine ... 141
Klaus-Dieter Schaser, I. Melcher, A. Luzzati, and A. C. Disch

10.1	Introduction and Epidemiology	141
10.2	Clinical Presentation	142
10.3	Diagnostics and Radiographic Imaging	143
10.4	Role and Technique of Biopsy	143
10.5	Oncosurgical Staging Systems of Primary Vertebral Tumors	144
10.6	Surgical Approaches	146
10.6.1	Posterior/Posterolateral Approach	146
10.6.2	Anterior Approaches	146
10.7	Surgical Strategies, Patient Selection, Treatment Decisions and Surgical Techniques	149
10.8	Surgical Technique of En Bloc Spondylectomy/Total En Bloc Vertebrectomy	150
10.8.1	Resection Technique	151
10.8.2	Technique: Spinal Reconstruction	152
10.9	Current Management of Individual Primary Malignant Vertebral Column Tumors	152
10.9.1	Osteosarcoma	152
10.9.2	Ewing Sarcoma	155
10.9.3	Chondrosarcoma	158
10.9.4	Chordoma	158
10.10	Nonsurgical Treatment Options	159
10.10.1	Radiation	159
10.10.2	Chemotherapy	161
10.10.3	Embolization	161
10.10.4	Pain Management	161
10.11	Complications	161
10.12	Prognosis	162
	References	162

11 Computer-Assisted Pelvic Tumor Resection: Fields of Application, Limits, and Perspectives ... 169
Sebastian Fehlberg, Sebastian Eulenstein, Thomas Lange, Dimosthenis Andreou, and Per-Ulf Tunn

11.1	Introduction	169
11.2	Navigation Procedures	171
11.2.1	Preoperative Imaging and Segmentation	171

	11.2.2	Tracking Systems	172
	11.2.3	Intraoperative Patient-to-Image Registration	173
	11.2.4	Intraoperative Visualization	176
	11.3	Fields of Application	176
	11.4	Clinical Results	178
	11.5	Limits and Perspectives	179
		Summary	180
		References	180
12	**Pulmonary Metastasectomy for Osteosarcoma: Is It Justified?**		**183**
	Klaus-Dieter Diemel, Heinz-Jürgen Klippe, and Detlev Branscheid		
	12.1	History of Osteosarcoma and Pulmonary Metastasectomy	183
	12.2	Thoracic Surgery Becomes Important Part of Interdisciplinary Concepts	185
	12.2.1	From Single-Centre Experience to Large Databases	187
	12.3	Evaluating the Patient with Pulmonary Metastases	187
	12.3.1	Computed Tomography of the Lung	188
	12.3.2	SPECT and PET Scans	188
	12.4	Prognostic Factors and Their Impact for Pulmonary Metastasectomy	189
	12.4.1	Factors Correlating to Modalities and Therapies of the Primary Tumour	189
	12.4.2	Factors Concerning the Time of Presentation of Metastases	190
	12.4.3	Factors Concerning Properties of Metastases and Surgical Remission	190
	12.5	Techniques in Pulmonary Metastasectomy	190
	12.5.1	Operative Approach to the Metastatic Lung	190
	12.5.2	Techniques in Pulmonary Resection	193
	12.6	Our Own Results	196
	12.7	Discussion	200
	12.7.1	The Reviewed Studies	200
	12.7.2	Risk Factors Affecting Survival After Pulmonary Metastasectomy	202
	12.7.3	Surgical Approach for Pulmonary Metastasectomy	203
	12.7.4	A Place for Minimally Invasive Surgery (VATS)?	204
	12.8	Conclusions	204
		References	205

Part III Soft Tissue Sarcomas

13 Standardized Approach to the Treatment of Adult Soft Tissue Sarcoma of the Extremities 211
Per-Ulf Tunn, Christoph Kettelhack, and Hans Roland Dürr

Abbreviations 211
13.1 Introduction 212
13.2 Biopsy Techniques 212
13.3 Surgical Therapy in Soft Tissue Sarcoma: General Principles 213
13.3.1 The Influence of Surgical Margins 215
13.3.2 The Influence of an Unplanned Excision 216
13.3.3 The Influence of Local Recurrence 218
13.4 Neoadjuvant and Adjuvant Treatment Modalities in Soft Tissue Sarcoma 218
13.4.1 The Role of Systemic Chemotherapy 219
13.4.2 The Role of Isolated Limb Perfusion 220
13.4.3 The Role of Radiotherapy 220
13.4.4 Response Assessment After Neoadjuvant Treatment in Soft Tissue Sarcoma 222
Summary 224
References 224

14 Evaluating Surgery Quality in Soft Tissue Sarcoma 229
Eberhard Stoeckle, Jean-Michel Coindre, Michèle Kind, Guy Kantor, and Binh N. Bui

14.1 Introduction 229
14.2 What End-Points for Assessing Local Tumour Control? 230
14.3 Local Recurrence Rates 231
14.4 Margins and Their Impact on Local Control 232
14.4.1 Margin Determination and Local Outcome 232
14.4.2 Co-factors Influencing Margin Quality 235
14.4.3 Impact of Margin and Other Factors on Local Recurrence 237
14.5 Long-Term Follow-Up with Actuarial Estimates in Homogeneous Patient Groups 238
14.6 Recapitulation: Criteria for Evaluating Surgery Quality with STS 238
References 238

15 Peripheral Nerve Considerations in the Management of Extremity Soft Tissue Sarcomas 243
Peter C. Ferguson, Anna A. Kulidjian, Kevin B. Jones, Benjamin M. Deheshi, and Jay S. Wunder

15.1 Introduction 243
15.2 Diagnosis of Peripheral Nerve Involvement 244

15.2.1	History and Physical Examination	244
15.2.2	Imaging	245
15.2.3	Other Diagnostic Considerations	246
15.3	Management of Peripheral Nerve Involvement	246
15.3.1	General Approach	246
15.3.2	Epineural Dissection	246
15.3.3	Nerve Resection Without Reconstruction	249
15.3.4	Nerve Resection and Reconstruction	252
15.3.5	Distal Functional Restoration: Tendon Transfers	253
15.3.6	Distal Functional Restoration: Distal Nerve Transfers	254
15.3.7	Amputation	254
15.4	Conclusions	255
	References	255

16 Isolated Limb Perfusion with TNF-α and Melphalan in Locally Advanced Soft Tissue Sarcomas of the Extremities ... 257
Dirk J. Grünhagen, Johannes H.W. de Wilt, Albertus N. Van Geel, Cornelis Verhoef, and Alexander M.M. Eggermont

16.1	Introduction	257
16.2	Isolated Limb Perfusion	258
16.3	The Rationale for Using Tumour Necrosis Factor-α in ILP	259
16.4	TNF-Based Isolated Limb Perfusion for STS	261
16.5	Results with TNF Plus Doxorubicin	262
16.6	Toxicity of a TNF-Based ILP	262
16.7	Special Patient Categories	265
16.7.1	Patients with Overt Metastatic Disease	265
16.7.2	Patients with Multiple Tumours in the Extremity	265
16.7.3	Patients with Recurrent Tumours in an Irradiated Field	265
16.7.4	Elderly Patients (>75 Years Old)	265
16.7.5	TNF-Based ILP Activity in Other Histologies	265
16.8	Future Perspectives	266
16.9	Conclusions	266
	References	266

17 Management of Locally Recurrent Soft Tissue Sarcoma after Prior Surgery and Radiation Therapy ... 271
Peter Hohenberger and Matthias H.M. Schwarzbach

17.1	Introduction	271
17.2	Treatment Options	272
17.3	Problems for Surgery Encountered with Previous Radiotherapy	273
17.4	Practical Management of In-Field Sarcoma Recurrence	275
17.5	Treatment Decisions in Surgical Re-intervention	276
17.6	Indication for Multimodal Re-treatment	277
17.7	Conclusion	281
	References	281

18	**Management of Vascular Involvement in Extremity Soft Tissue Sarcoma**		285
	Ashish Mahendra, Yair Gortzak, Peter C. Ferguson, Benjamin M. Deheshi, Thomas F. Lindsay, and Jay S. Wunder		
	18.1	Introduction	285
	18.2	Indications for Vascular Resection and Reconstruction in Extremity Soft Tissue Sarcoma	286
	18.3	Patient Workup	287
	18.4	Surgical and Functional Outcome	289
	18.4.1	Amputation Risk	290
	18.4.2	Use of Muscle Flaps	290
	18.4.3	Wound Complications	290
	18.4.4	Postoperative Limb Edema and DVT	290
	18.4.5	Risk of Local Recurrence	291
	18.4.6	Risk of Systemic Disease	291
	18.4.7	Functional Outcome	291
	18.5	Vascular Outcome	293
	18.5.1	Arterial Reconstruction	293
	18.5.2	Venous Reconstruction	293
	18.5.3	Type of Vascular Graft	294
	18.6	Effects of Radiotherapy	296
		Summary	298
		References	298
19	**Current Concepts in the Management of Retroperitoneal Soft Tissue Sarcoma**		301
	Matthias H.M. Schwarzbach and Peter Hohenberger		
	19.1	Introduction	301
	19.2	Definitions Referring to Retroperitoneal Sarcomas	302
	19.3	Diagnostic Requirements in Retroperitoneal Sarcomas	302
	19.4	Vascular Involvement	303
	19.5	Surgical Therapy in Localized Soft Tissue Sarcomas of the Retroperitoneum	305
	19.6	Surgical Therapy in Metastasized Soft Tissue Sarcomas of the Retroperitoneum	314
	19.7	Prognosis	315
	19.8	Chemotherapy and Radiation Therapy	315
		Summary	317
		References	317

20	**Pulmonary Metastasectomy for Soft Tissue Sarcomas: Is It Justified?**	321

Joachim Pfannschmidt, Hans Hoffmann, Thomas Schneider, and Hendrik Dienemann

20.1	Introduction	321
20.2	Clinical Features	323
20.3	Radiology	323
20.4	Patient Selection	324
20.5	Surgery	325
20.6	Video-Assisted Thoracic Surgery	326
20.7	Prognostic Factors	327
20.7.1	Overall Survival	327
20.7.2	Recurrent Pulmonary Metastases	331
20.7.3	Perioperative Chemotherapy	331
20.8	Future Directions	332
20.9	Conclusions	333
	References	333

Part IV Quality of Life Assessment

21	**Quality of Life (QOL) in Patients with Osteosarcoma**	339

Rajaram Nagarajan

21.1	Osteosarcoma	339
21.2	Treatment and Survival	340
21.3	Quality of Life	340
21.4	Outcomes Model	341
	References	343

22	**Clinical Trials in Osteosarcoma Treatment: Patients' Perspective Through Art**	345

Lizzie Burns and Martha Perisoglou

22.1	Introduction	345
22.2	Patients with Osteosarcoma and the EURAMOS 1 Clinical Trial	346
22.3	Bringing Medicine to Life	346
22.4	The Patients' Perspective	347
22.4.1	Syed	347
22.4.2	Omar	350
22.4.3	Shane	350
22.4.4	Laura	351
22.4.5	Meg	352
22.4.6	Simon	353

22.4.7	Bhavin	355
22.4.8	Sam	357
22.4.9	Charlie	357
22.5	Art and Cancer	359
22.6	Conclusion	360
	Acknowledgements	360
	References	360

List of Contributors

Helmut Ahrens, MD
Department of Orthopedics
University of Münster
Albert-Schweitzer-Str. 33
48149 Münster
Germany

Dimosthenis Andreou, MD
Department of Orthopedic Oncology
Sarkomzentrum Berlin-Brandenburg
Helios Klinikum Berlin-Buch
Schwanebecker Chaussee 50
13125 Berlin
Germany

Robert U. Ashford, MD
East Midlands Sarcoma Service
Leicester Royal Infirmary
Infirmary Square
Leicester LE1 5WW, UK

Maurice Balke, MD
Department of Orthopedics
University of Münster
Albert-Schweitzer-Str. 33
48149 Münster
Germany

Rainer Baumgart, MD, PhD
Zentrum für korrigierende und rekonstruktive
Extremitätenchirurgie München (ZEM)
Limb Lengthening Center Munich/Germany
Nymphenburgerstr. 1
80335 Munich
Germany

Ludger Bernd, MD, PhD
Städtisches Krankenhaus Bielefeld
Teutoburger Str. 50
33604 Bielefeld
Germany

S. Fiona Bonar, FRCPath, FRCPA
New South Wales Bone and Soft Tissue
Tumour Service
Royal Prince Alfred Hospital
Missenden Road
Camperdown
NSW 2050
Australia

Detlev Branscheid, MD, PhD
Department of General Thoracic Surgery
Krankenhaus Grosshansdorf, Hamburg
Wöhrendamm 80
22927 Großhansdorf
Germany

Binh N. Bui, MD
Department of Surgery
Institut Bergonie
Regional Cancer Centre
229 Cours de I'Argonne
33076 Bordeaux Cedex
France

Lizzie Burns, PhD
Artist-in-residence
The London Sarcoma Service
University College Hospital
Complementary Therapy Group
1st Floor Rosenheim Building
25 Grafton Way
London WC1E 6AU UK

Jean-Michel Coindre, MD, PhD
Department of Surgery
Institut Bergonie
Regional Cancer Centre
229 Cours de I'Argonne
33076 Bordeaux Cedex
France

Eslam Darwish, MD
Medical University of Vienna
University Clinic of Orthopaedics
Waehringer Guertel 18-20
1090 Vienna
Austria

Benjamin M. Deheshi, MD, FRCSC
University Musculoskeletal Oncology Unit
Mount Sinai Hospital
476-600 University Avenue
Toronto, ON M5G 1X5
Canada

Klaus D. Diemel, MD
Department of General Thoracic Surgery
Krankenhaus Grosshansdorf, Hamburg
Wöhrendamm 80
22927 Großhansdorf
Germany

Hendrik Dienemann, MD, PhD
Department of Surgery
Thoraxklinik Heidelberg
Amalienstr. 5
69126 Heidelberg
Germany

A.C. Disch, MD
Section for Musculoskeletal
Tumor Surgery
Center for Musculoskeletal Surgery
Charité University Medicine Berlin
Augustenburger Platz 1
13353 Berlin, Germany

Martin Dominkus, MD, PhD
Medical University of Vienna
University Clinic of Orthopaedics
Waehringer Guertel 18-20
1090 Vienna, Austria

Hans Roland Dürr, MD, PhD
Orthopaedic Oncology, Department of
Orthopaedic Surgery
Ludwig-Maximilians-University Munich
Marchioninistr. 15
81377 Munich
Germany

Alexander M.M. Eggermont, MD, PhD
Department of Surgical Oncology
Erasmus MC
Daniel den Hoed Cancer Center
P.O. Box 5201
3008 AE Rotterdam
The Netherlands

Sebastian Eulenstein
Clinic for Surgery and Surgical Oncology
Charité Campus Buch
Robert-Rössle-Klinik
Lindenberger Weg 80
13125 Berlin
Germany

List of Contributors

Sebastian Fehlberg, MD
Department of Orthopedic Oncology
Sarkomzentrum Berlin-Brandenburg
Helios Klinikum Berlin-Buch
Schwanebecker Chaussee 50
13125 Berlin
Germany

Peter C. Ferguson, MD, MSc, FRCSC
University Musculoskeletal Oncology Unit
Mount Sinai Hospital
476-600 University Avenue
Toronto,
ON M5G 1X5
Canada

Philipp Funovics, MD
Medical University of Vienna
University Clinic of Orthopaedics
Waehringer Guertel 18-20
1090 Vienna
Austria

Albertus N. van Geel, MD, PhD
Department of Surgical Oncology
Erasmus MC
Daniel den Hoed Cancer Center
P.O. Box 5201
3008 AE Rotterdam
The Netherlands

Yair Gortzak, MD, MSc
University Musculoskeletal
Oncology Unit
Mount Sinai Hospital
476-600 University Avenue
Toronto,
ON M5G 1X5
Canada

Georg Gosheger, MD, PhD
Department of Orthopedics
University of Münster
Albert-Schweitzer-Str. 33
48149 Münster
Germany

Rob Grimer, FRCS, MD, PhD
Oncology Service
Royal Orthopaedic Hospital
Bristol Road South
Northfield, Birmingham B31 2AP
UK

Dirk J. Grünhagen, MD, PhD
Department of Surgical Oncology
Erasmus MC
Daniel den Hoed Cancer Center
P.O. Box 5201
3008 AE Rotterdam
The Netherlands

Jendrik Hardes, MD
Department of Orthopedics
University of Münster
Albert-Schweitzer-Str. 33
48149 Münster
Germany

Hans Hoffmann, MD, PhD
Department of Surgery
Thoraxklinik Heidelberg
Amalienstr. 5
69126 Heidelberg
Germany

Peter Hohenberger, MD, PhD
Divison of Surgical Oncology
and Thoracic Surgery
Department of Surgery
University Hospital Mannheim
Theodor Kutzer Ufer 1-3
68167 Mannheim
Germany

Francis Hornicek, MD, PhD
Orthopaedic Oncology
Massachusetts General Hospital
55 Fruit Street, GRB 607
Boston
MA 02114-2696
USA

Lee Jeys, MSc, FRCS
School House Farm
Purshull Green
Droitwich
Worcestershire WR90NL
UK

Kevin B. Jones, MD
Mount Sinai Hospital
600 University Ave., Suite 476G
Toronto
ON M5G 1X5
Canada

Guy Kantor, MD, PhD
Department of Surgery
Institut Bergonie
Regional Cancer Centre
229 Cours de I'Argonne
33076 Bordeaux Cedex
France

Rooshdiya Z. Karim, FRCPA
New South Wales Bone and Soft Tissue
Tumour Service
Royal Prince Alfred Hospital
Missenden Road
Camperdown
NSW 2050
Australia

Christoph Kettelhack, MD
Department of Surgery
University Hospital Basel
Spitalstr. 21
4031 Basel
Switzerland

Michèle Kind, MD
Department of Surgery
Institut Bergonie
Regional Cancer Centre
229 Cours de I'Argonne
33076 Bordeaux Cedex
France

Heinz-Jürgen Klippe, MD
Department of Anaesthesiology
Krankenhaus Grosshansdorf, Hamburg
Wöhrendamm 80
22927 Grosshansdorf
Germany

Anna A. Kulidjian, MD, FRCSC
Mount Sinai Hospital
600 University Ave. Suite 476G
Toronto
ON M5G 1X5
Canada

Pierre Kunz, MD
Stiftung Orthopädische Universitätsklinik
Heidelberg
Schlierbacher Landstrasse 200a
69118 Heidelberg
Germany

Thomas Lange
Clinic for Surgery and Surgical Oncology
Charité Campus Buch
Robert-Rössle-Klinik
Lindenberger Weg 80
13125 Berlin
Germany
e-mail: thomas.lange@charite.de

Andreas Leithner, MD, PhD
Universitätsklinik für Orthopädie
Medizinische Universität Graz
Auenbruggerplatz 5
8036 Graz
Austria

Ulrich Lenze, MD
Zentrum für korrigierende und rekonstruktive
Extremitätenchirurgie München
Nymphenburgerstr. 1
80335 Munich
Germany

List of Contributors

Thomas F. Lindsay, MDCM, MSc, FRCS, FACS
Division of Vascular Surgery
University Health Network
190 Elizabeth St.
Toronto
ON M5G 2C4
Canada

A. Luzzati, MD
Div. Ortopedia e Traumatologia
Istituto Ospitalieri Cremona
Italy

Ashish Mahendra, FRCS, MS, MCh
Department of Orthopaedics
Glasgow Royal Infirmary
Glasgow, UK

Werner Maurer-Ertl, MD
Universitätsklinik für Orthopädie
Medizinische Universität Graz
Auenbruggerplatz 5
8036 Graz, Austria

Stanley W. McCarthy, AO, FRCPA
New South Wales Bone and Soft Tissue Tumour Service
Royal Prince Alfred Hospital
Missenden Road, Camperdown
NSW 2050, Australia

I. Melcher, MD
Section for Musculoskeletal Tumor Surgery
Center for Musculoskeletal Surgery
Charité University Medicine Berlin
Augustenburger Platz 1
13353 Berlin
Germany

Rajaram Nagarajan, MD, MS
Cincinnati Children's Hospital Medical Center
Division of Hematology/Oncology
3333 Burnet Ave
MLC 7015, Cincinnati
OH 45229
USA

Martha Perisoglou, MD
Department of Oncology
University College Hospital
1st Floor East, 250 Euston Road
London NW1 2PG
UK

Joachim Pfannschmidt, MD, PhD
Department of Surgery
Thoraxklinik Heidelberg
Amalienstr. 5
69126 Heidelberg
Germany

Kevin A. Raskin, MD
Instructor, Orthopaedic Surgery
Harvard Medical School
Orthopaedic Oncology Service
Massachusetts General Hospital
55 Fruit Street
Yawkey Outpatient Center Suite 3B
Boston, MA 02114
USA

Klaus-Dieter Schaser, MD
Section for Musculoskeletal Tumor Surgery
Center for Musculoskeletal Surgery
Charité University Medicine Berlin
Augustenburger Platz 1
13353 Berlin
Germany

Thomas Schneider, MD
Department of Surgery
Thoraxklinik Heidelberg
Amalienstr. 5
69126 Heidelberg
Germany

Matthias H.M. Schwarzbach, MD, PhD
Department of Surgery
University Clinic of Mannheim
University of Heidelberg
Theodor Kutzer Ufer 1-3
68167 Mannheim
Germany

Richard A. Scolyer, FRCPA, FRCPath
New South Wales Bone and Soft Tissue
Tumour Service
Royal Prince Alfred Hospital
Missenden Road
Camperdown
NSW 2050
Australia

Paul D. Stalley, FRACS
New South Wales Bone and Soft Tissue
Tumour Service
Royal Prince Alfred Hospital
Missenden Road
Camperdown, NSW 2050
Australia

Eberhard Stoeckle, MD
Department of Surgery
Institut Bergonie
Regional Cancer Centre
229 Cours de l'Argonne
33076 Bordeaux Cedex, France

Arne Streitbürger, MD
Department of Orthopedics
University of Münster
Albert-Schweitzer-Str. 33
48149 Münster
Germany

Per-Ulf Tunn, MD
Department of Orthopaedic Oncology
Sarkomzentrum Berlin-Brandenburg
Helios Klinikum Berlin-Buch
Schwanebecker Chaussee 50
13125 Berlin, Germany

Cornelis Verhoef, MD, PhD
Department of Surgical Oncology
Erasmus MC
Daniel den Hoed Cancer Center
P.O. Box 5201
3008 AE Rotterdam
The Netherlands

Johannes H.W. de Wilt, MD, PhD
Department of Surgical Oncology
Erasmus MC
Daniel den Hoed Cancer Center
P.O. Box 5201
3008 AE Rotterdam
The Netherlands

Reinhard Windhager, MD
Universitätsklinik für Orthopädie
Medizinische Universität Graz
Auenbruggerplatz 5
8036 Graz
Austria

Jay S. Wunder, MD, MSc, FRCSC
University Musculoskeletal Oncology Unit
Mount Sinai Hospital
476-600 University Avenue
Toronto, ON M5G 1X5, Canada

Part I
Diagnostics

Biopsy of Bone and Soft Tissue Tumours: Hints and Hazards

Andreas Leithner, Werner Maurer-Ertl, and Reinhard Windhager

Abstract Although the diagnostic algorithm of a suspected bone or soft tissue tumour, as well as the biopsy itself, are well defined, avoidable errors still happen. Major flaws might lead to unnecessary tissue contamination resulting in amputations or recurrences. In the current review we will focus in particular on biopsy guidelines and possible biopsy-related problems such as haematomas, sampling errors, and postoperative fractures. Finally, we will provide ten simple rules for a successful biopsy.

1.1 Introduction

In suspicion of a bone or soft tissue sarcoma, biopsy is the key procedure in a well-defined diagnostic algorithm. Although the primary goal of a biopsy (from old Greek: *bíos*, "life", and *ópsis*, "look/appearance") is to provide enough and representative tumour tissue for a histological diagnosis,

Andreas Leithner (✉)
Univ. Clinic of Orthopaedic Surgery
Medical University of Graz
Auenbruggerplatz 5
8036 Graz
Austria
E-mail: andreas.leithner@meduni-graz.at

the performing surgeons should remember that avoidable errors could compromise subsequent surgery. Major flaws might lead to unnecessary tissue contamination possibly resulting in amputations or recurrences (Mankin et al. 1982, 1996).

Some people may regard biopsies as the simplest procedures that could easily be handed over to the youngest and most inexperienced surgeons. These people are partly right in that biopsies are technically easy to perform, considering national or international guidelines (Bickels et al. 1999; Leithner and Windhager 2007a, b; Mankin et al. 1996). However, simple mistakes can lead to an increased morbidity rate (Bhangu et al. 2004; Mankin et al. 1982; Mankin et al. 1996; Zacherl et al. 2006). In the 1982 study by Mankin et al., biopsy-related problems occurred three to five times more frequently when the biopsy was performed at a referring rather than in a specialised centre (Mankin et al. 1982).

1.2 Diagnostic Algorithm

Jaffe stated in a book published in 1958 that a biopsy should be regarded as the final diagnostic procedure, not as a mere shortcut to diagnosis

(Jaffe 1958). Therefore, biopsies should always be preceded by primary diagnostics such as medical history, clinical examination, primary imaging studies such as X-rays and simple blood tests, and special diagnostic studies such as magnetic resonance imaging (MRI) and case-dependent computed tomography (CT), whole body bone scintigraphy, positron emission tomography (PET) and angiography (for a simplified diagram see Fig. 1.1).

A useful medical history should include start, kind, and duration of symptoms. A possible familial predisposition should be questioned (e.g. in hereditary osteochondromatosis or neurofibromatosis). Clinical examination consists of inspection and palpation to get an idea of the extent and the consistency of the swelling (solid/elastic/bony/...) and its relation to neighbouring structures. The size of the palpable mass should be documented in centimetres or millimetres and not in terms with great variability such as fruits, fists or children's heads (Gray et al. 2003). If the swelling is located near a joint, its function and a possible intraarticular effusion should be noted. Sensomotoric deficiencies have to be documented in detail in order to facilitate the early diagnosis of changes. In addition, the patient should be inspected undressed as, for example, café-au-lait spots would help to lead to the diagnosis of neurofibromatosis.

Primary imaging studies of a suspected bone tumour comprise X-rays of the affected region in two planes. Nearly all bone tumours have their characteristic radiological features (Lodwick et al. 1980). Even for suspected soft tissue tumours X-rays might be useful, as calcifications might be shown. Unfortunately there are no reliable blood screening tests for musculoskeletal tumours available. Some general blood parameters, however, could be helpful in determining local bone resorption and signs of infection (e.g. red and white blood cell count, C-reactive protein (CRP), calcium, alkaline phosphatase, etc.).

When these primary diagnostic procedures still leave the suspicion of a musculoskeletal tumour, secondary or special diagnostic procedures are indicated. Especially the importance of MRI for bone and soft tissue tumours is unchallenged. Prior to definitive surgery a contrast-enhanced MRI of the affected region and its neighbouring compartments is mandatory to detect possible skip lesions or regional metastases. The advantage of CT, in contrast to MRI, lies in the better visualisation of bony structures, for example in order to detect cortical destruction. Knowing its limitations (sometimes false-negative for chondromatous tumours),

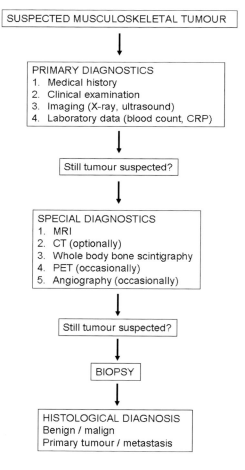

Fig. 1.1 Diagram of the simplified diagnostic algorithm recommended. (Translated from Leithner et al. 2007)

whole body bone scintigraphy demonstrates the biological activity of a bone process and might detect a systemic spread (e.g. bone metastases) or a multifocal disease (e.g. enchondromatosis). Sensitivity, specificity, and accuracy of PET for the detection of sarcomas are still considered controversial (Bastiaannet et al. 2004).

1.3 Biopsy

After undertaking the diagnostic tasks mentioned above, one has to decide whether or not a biopsy is indicated. If the tumour is clinically and radiologically unmistakably identified as a benign lesion one could omit a biopsy (Windhager et al. 2006). For example, some benign tumours could be observed (e.g. non-ossifying fibroma) or treated without prior biopsy (e.g. osteoid osteoma). When a bone metastasis is suspected in a case of a known systemic spread of a primary disease a biopsy is indicated only as an exception. However, one should be aware that pathological fractures in older patients are not always due to osteoporosis or metastatic disease—if the cause of the fracture or the imaging of the area are unclear, a biopsy should be performed to exclude a primary malignant tumour like a chondrosarcoma.

Again, when it is still not possible to exclude a primary malignant tumour as a potential differential diagnosis after all the previous steps of the diagnostic algorithm are complete, one has to perform a biopsy. The goal of a biopsy is to acquire enough representative tissue for histological examination and contaminate as little as possible of the neighbouring tissue with the biopsy tract. If the presence of a malign tumour is confirmed, one has to excise the tumour including the biopsy tract with, in most instances, a surrounding cuff of normal tissue (Fig. 1.2; Enneking et al. 1980). If the biopsy tract is not resected, local recurrences might occur (Schwartz and Spengler 1997). If an inadequate biopsy led to the contamination of a joint and/or main neurovascular structures even an amputation might be indicated in some cases (Mankin et al. 1982, 1996). It is internationally

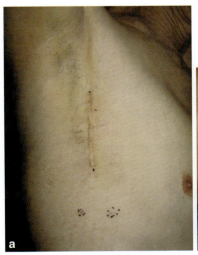
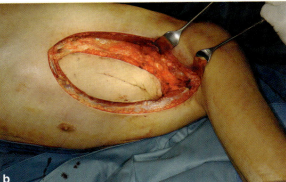

Fig. 1.2 a Photograph after an inadequate intralesional resection ("whoops procedure") of a fibromyxoid sarcoma G1 of the right axilla of a 49-year-old man. Note the two distant drainage exits resulting in an even larger re-resection **b** and the need for reconstruction with a musculocutaneous flap

accepted that primary malignant musculoskeletal tumours have to be resected with wide or radical margins according to the Enneking classification, while intralesional or marginal resections are associated with higher recurrence/mortality rates and are therefore indicated only in exceptional circumstances (Enneking et al. 1980).

To perform a representative and technically adequate biopsy, the following preconditions are necessary:

1. Exact preoperative imaging. "Whoops procedures" (e.g. when a so-called ganglion intraoperatively turns out to be a highly malignant soft tissue sarcoma) are in most instances the result of no or inadequate preoperative imaging and are therefore avoidable (Davies et al. 2004). X-rays in two planes, an MRI (and sometimes a CT), a whole body bone scintigraphy or a PET should help to preoperatively define one main suspected entity and two to three potential differential diagnoses. Preoperative imaging studies should not be older than 4 weeks.
2. Preoperative planning. The shortest/simplest way to a tumour is not always the wisest. Before performing a biopsy one should think about how to resect the tumour when it would turn out to be malignant. According to these resection lines the biopsy has to be planned, as the biopsy tract is assumed to be contaminated with tumour cells and has therefore to be resected with wide margins, as with the primary tumour itself. This implies that the surgeon doing the biopsy should be well acquainted with how the definitive surgery will proceed. For these reasons it is required that even the biopsy should be performed by an orthopaedic oncologist, or at least after consultation with one and following his recommendations. Springfield and Rosenberg put all this in a simple "take home message": "Do not biopsy what you are not going to treat" (Springfield and Rosenberg 1996).

1.3.1
Biopsy Technique

Generally, two types of biopsies exist—closed biopsies (e.g. core needle biopsies) and open biopsies (excisional or incisional biopsies).

1. Core needle biopsies (CNB), using a 14-gauge needle, and fine needle aspiration biopsies (FNAB), using 22- to 25-gauge needles, have been shown to be reliable techniques for bone and soft tissue tumours (Kilpatrick et al. 2001; Mitsuyoshi et al. 2006). Especially when the tumour is homogeneous, diagnostic accuracy is high. Even cytogenetic analyses have been shown to be possible in FNAB specimens from bone and soft tissue sarcomas (Kilpatrick et al. 2006). Both techniques are faster, simpler and cheaper compared to open biopsies and present less of infection and haematoma that can delay or compromise further treatment. Although sensitivity and specificity have been reported to be similar to open biopsy (Kilpatrick et al. 2001; Mitsuyoshi et al. 2006), other authors reported high rates of diagnostic errors for closed biopsies (den Heeten et al. 1985; Mankin et al. 1996). We are of the opinion that one should individually decide whether to perform a closed or an open biopsy based on individual patient factors, including location, suspected tumour type and homogeneity of the tumour, and according to the pathologist's need. Guidance by fluoroscope or CT for bony lesions or MRI in soft tissue cases is recommended to ensure that the area most suspicious of malignancy is chosen. With a closed biopsy one should never forget to exactly document and/or mark the biopsy canal entry point, as in case of malignancy this biopsy tract has to be resected and it is sometimes hard to detect the skin perforation after healing. For the same reason, if the closed biopsy is performed by a radiologist, the orthopaedic oncologist has to define the path of the needle/trocar.

2. With an incisional biopsy a representative tumour specimen is taken at the extremities through the smallest possible longitudinal incision. This technique is preferably chosen when a closed biopsy is impossible or the result of a closed biopsy was inconclusive or did not correlate with the clinical presentation and/or radiological finding. Other advantages are associated with the large amount of tumour tissue available for sometimes necessary additional pathological studies. When at the end of the diagnostic algorithm the diagnosis of a benign tumour is evident, an excisional biopsy may be performed. In these cases the whole tumour is resected—e.g. an osteochondroma or an insuspect subcutaneous tumour of less than 5 cm in diameter.

1.4 Hints

We propose ten rules for a successful biopsy:

1. Do not hurry
2. Do not contaminate nerves, vessels or joints
3. Do not operate without adequate preoperative imaging
4. Send the biopsy specimen to a bone-/soft tissue pathologist
5. Take the shortest way through one compartment only
6. Plan your biopsy according to later resections
7. Gain enough and representative tissue
8. Operate as atraumatically as possible
9. Avoid a postoperative haematoma by all possible means
10. Insert a drain, and lead it out through your biopsy tract

An *intraoperative frozen section* is necessary when it is not certain if only the reactive zone or tumour itself was hit. In highly malignant tumours it is sometimes hard to macroscopically divide between vital tumour tissue and the predominantly present necrotic tissue. Here again an instant frozen section should be waited for.

If a potential differential diagnosis is a bacterial infection, an *intraoperative swab* should be gained prior to the administration of a perioperative antibiotic prophylaxis.

When performing an open biopsy of a bony lesion, the *shape of the cortical window* should be oblong with rounded ends, as it has been shown to provide greater residual strength when compared to rectangular holes with round or square corners (Clark et al. 1977).

1.5 Hazards

With some surgical procedures *haematomas* are regarded as unwelcome but acceptable side products. A haematoma at biopsy, however, could lead to an amputation (Mankin et al. 1982; Mankin et al. 1996). Especially with open biopsies it is therefore mandatory to insert a drain and lead it out through the biopsy tract or in proximity and continuation with the skin incision, as the drain path is considered contaminated. Using a tourniquet during biopsy may be helpful in highly vascularised lesions; it should be opened, however, before wound closure to ensure exact haemostasis. In case of an iatrogenic cortical window and massive bleeding through it, one could close the hole using polymethylmethacrylate. If a haematoma already exists before biopsy one should photograph it to document its existence and its extent to enable an adequate resection of the tumour and the area that contained the haematoma (Fig. 1.3).

The risk of having a "sampling error" is minimised by sticking to the guidelines described above, but unfortunately such an error can never be totally excluded. As presented in Fig. 1.4, the malignant part of a heterogeneous and otherwise benign tumour is missed by 1 mm only.

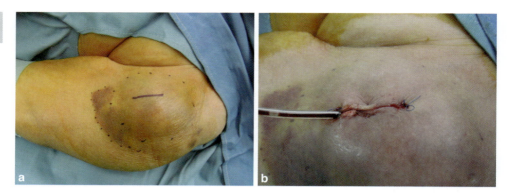

Fig. 1.3 a Perioperative photograph of the left proximal arm of a 59-year-old male patient with a suspected soft tissue sarcoma; note the existing haematoma. **b** The drain leaves directly through the biopsy canal

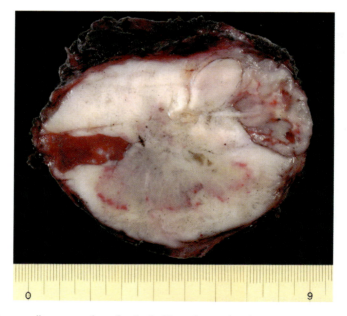

Fig. 1.4 "Sampling error": cross-section of a 6×5×11-cm large sclerosing epithelioid fibrosarcoma G3 of a 69-year-old female patient. Although the biopsy tract (*red area left*) is 3 cm deep, it did not reach the highly malignant (*violet*) central part. Therefore the histological diagnosis of a (benign) desmoplastic fibroblastoma was given

Therefore, multiple samples from different parts of the tumour should be obtained.

Especially incisional and excisional biopsies should keep incorrect histological diagnoses to a minimum. In a retrospective analysis of 602 patients that had been operated on due to a soft tissue tumour at our institution, histological diagnoses of referring centres were reviewed as

Table 1.1 Incorrect histological diagnosis[a]

		Histological errors	
Study	Centre performing biopsy	Total	Major[b]
Mankin et al. 1982	Referring centre (n=143)	56 (39%)	43 (30%)
	Specialised centre (n=186)	26 (14%)	17 (9%)
Mankin et al. 1996	Referring centre (n=282)	-	52 (18%)
	Specialised centre (n=315)	-	29 (9%)
A. Leithner, W. Maurer-Ertl,	Referring centre (n=187)	41 (22%)	17 (9%)
R. Windhager, unpublished	Specialised centre (n=249)	16 (6%)	13 (5%)

[a] Number of patients, with percentages in parentheses
[b] "Major" means of therapeutic relevance

well as diagnoses based on open biopsies at our own institution. The histological diagnoses made by referring pathologists had to be corrected by the specialised pathologist in 41 of 187 cases (22%), and the histological change was of therapeutic relevance (e.g. benign to malign) in 17 cases (9%). At our centre the histological diagnosis at biopsy had to be changed after obtaining the whole specimen at definitive surgery in 16 of 249 cases (6%). Thirteen changes were of therapeutic relevance (5%) (Leithner et al. 2007). These results are slightly better compared to two other reports (Mankin et al. 1982, 1996; Table 1.1). The improvement may be attributed to a higher awareness of possible flaws due to articles such as Mankin's. The histological diagnosis of a soft tissue tumour should therefore always be made or at least controlled by a specialised pathologist at a tumour centre. Both surgeon and pathologist are responsible for a correct diagnosis.

Using local anaesthesia in tumour biopsy is sometimes risky as the area could be easily contaminated with tumour cells.

Post-biopsy, care with mobilisation is recommended. Immobilisation and local compression should minimise the risk of a postoperative haematoma. Due to the same dangers after incisional or excisional biopsies, drains should be left for at least 2 days. Especially after a bone biopsy at an extremity, the limb should be mobilised without load to reduce the risk of a postoperative fracture.

To the best of our knowledge it has not been sufficiently proved that a initial, technically poor biopsy decreases a patient's chance of survival. However, it has been shown extensively that mistakes at biopsy might lead to higher morbidity due to unnecessarily large resections, re-resections, extensive reconstructions, postoperative radiation and eventually amputations.

1.6
Definitive Diagnosis

The final diagnosis of a musculoskeletal tumour should never be based on histological findings alone. Only the synopsis drawn from all findings—imaging studies, histology, age, location and medical history—will lead to a reliable diagnosis. A tight co-operation between all specialists of a multidisciplinary team is therefore mandatory.

References

Bastiaannet E, Groen H, Jager PL, Cobben DC, van der Graaf WT, Vaalburg W, Hoekstra HJ (2004) The value of FDG-PET in the detection, grading and response to therapy of soft tissue and bone sarcomas; a systematic review and meta-analysis. Cancer Treat Rev 30:83–101

Bhangu AA, Beard JS, Grimer RJ (2004) Should soft tissue sarcomas be treated at a specialist centre? Sarcoma 8:1–6

Bickels J, Jelinek JS, Shmookler BM, Neff RS, Malawer MM (1999) Biopsy of musculoskeletal tumors. Current concepts. Clin Orthop Relat Res 368:212–219

Clark CR, Morgan C, Sonstegard DA, Matthews LS (1977) The effect of biopsy-hole shape and size on bone strength. J Bone Joint Surg Am 59:213–217

Davies AM, Mehr A, Parsonage S, Evans N, Grimer RJ, Pynsent PB (2004) MR imaging in the assessment of residual tumour following inadequate primary excision of soft tissue sarcomas. Eur Radiol 14:506–513

den Heeten GJ, Oldhoff J, Oosterhuis JW, Schraffordt KH (1985) Biopsy of bone tumours. J Surg Oncol 28:247–251

Enneking WF, Spanier SS, Goodman MA (1980) A system for the surgical staging of musculoskeletal sarcoma. Clin Orthop 153:106–120

Gray JM, Khan MT, Grimer RJ, Pynsent PB (2003) Is fruit a useful indicator of the size of an object? Bull R Coll Surg Engl 85:18–19;33

Jaffe HL (1958) Introduction: problems of classification and diagnosis. In: Jaffe HL (ed) Tumors and tumorous conditions of the bones and joints. Lea and Febiger, Philadelphia, pp 9–17

Kilpatrick SE, Cappellari JO, Bos G, Gold SH, Ward WG (2001) Is fine-needle aspiration biopsy a practical alternative to open biopsy for the primary diagnosis of sarcoma? Experience with 140 patients. Am J Clin Pathol 115:59–68

Kilpatrick SE, Bergman S, Pettenati MJ, Gulley ML (2006) The usefulness of cytogenetic analysis in fine needle aspirates for the histologic subtyping of sarcomas. Mod Pathol 19:815–819

Leithner A, Windhager R (2007a) Diagnostik von Tumoren des Stütz- und Bewegungsapparates. Wien Med Wochenschr 157:21–26

Leithner A, Windhager R (2007b) Guidelines for the biopsy of bone and soft tissue tumours. Orthopade 36:167–175

Leithner A, Maurer-Ertl W, Glehr M, Beham A, Windhager R (2007) Sampling error at biopsy! Does it still happen? Abstract book of the 20th EMSOS meeting 99

Lodwick GS, Wilson AJ, Farrell C, Virtama P, Dittrich F (1980) Determining growth rates of focal lesions of bone from radiographs. Radiology 134:577–583

Mankin HJ, Lange TA, Spanier SS (1982) The hazards of biopsy in patients with malignant primary bone and soft-tissue tumors. J Bone Joint Surg Am 64:1121–1127

Mankin HJ, Mankin CJ, Simon MA (1996) The hazards of the biopsy, revisited. Members of the Musculoskeletal Tumor Society. J Bone Joint Surg Am 78:656–663

Mitsuyoshi G, Naito N, Kawai A, Kunisada T, Yoshida A, Yanai H, Dendo S, Yoshino T, Kanazawa S, Ozaki T (2006) Accurate diagnosis of musculoskeletal lesions by core needle biopsy. J Surg Oncol 94:21–27

Schwartz HS, Spengler DM (1997) Needle tract recurrences after closed biopsy for sarcoma: three cases and review of the literature. Ann Surg Oncol 4:228–236

Springfield DS, Rosenberg A (1996) Biopsy: complicated and risky. J Bone Joint Surg Am 78:639–643

Windhager R, Kastner N, Leithner A (2006) Benigne Knochentumoren und tumorähnliche Läsionen. Monatsschr Kinderhlkd 154:20–31

Zacherl M, Leithner A, Koch H, Windhager R (2006) Weichteilsarkome—jeder zweite Patient primär inadäquat therapiert. Wiener Klin Magazin 1:22–28

The Role of Intra-operative Pathological Evaluation in the Management of Musculoskeletal Tumours

Robert U. Ashford, Richard A. Scolyer, Stanley W. McCarthy, S. Fiona Bonar, Rooshdiya Z. Karim, and Paul D. Stalley

Abstract A tissue biopsy is usually a critical aspect in guiding appropriate initial management in patients with musculoskeletal tumours. We have previously outlined the role of intra-operative frozen section in both the determination of adequacy of a biopsy and for its diagnostic utility. In this article, the options and techniques for intra-operative pathological evaluation, namely frozen section, fine needle aspiration cytology and touch imprint cytology are reviewed. Frozen section examination may be applicable in the following Sections, including (1) at core biopsy, (2) at surgical margins, (3) at confirming diagnosis prior to definitive treatment or to evaluate tumour spread, and (4) at establishing a diagnosis of a metastasis prior to intramedullary nailing. There are also situations in which frozen section is inappropriate. Pitfalls associated with frozen sections are also highlighted. There are also cost implications, which we have quantified, of performing frozen sections.

Robert U. Ashford (✉)
East Midlands Sarcoma Service
Leicester Royal Infirmary
Infirmary Square
Leicester LE1 5WW, UK
E-mail: Robert.ashford@sky.com

In our experience that the use of intra-operative pathological evaluation reduces the non-diagnostic rate of bone and soft tissue sarcoma biopsies, eliminates the need for re-biopsy hence alleviating stress, and is a useful addition to the armamentarium in evaluating musculoskeletal tumours.

2.1 Introduction: Indications for Intra-operative Pathological Evaluation in Musculoskeletal Surgical Oncology

The optimal management of musculoskeletal tumours requires a multidisciplinary team approach that includes input from surgical, medical and radiation oncologists, radiologists and pathologists. Because it usually establishes a definite pathological diagnosis, a tissue biopsy is a critical aspect in guiding appropriate initial patient management. However, it is very important that the biopsy is carefully planned. This usually requires assessment with appropriate radiological imaging [18, 23] which is necessary to assess the anatomical extent of the tumour prior to biopsy. There are a number of principles that apply to performing a tissue biopsy of sarcomas. In order to avoid compromising subsequent treatment, the biopsy should be in a site that can be included en bloc within the definitive tumour resection and ideally should be performed following consultation with the surgeon who will be performing the definitive surgical procedure. The previous author has already outlined the potential consequences of poorly performed biopsies. These include pathological misdiagnosis (as a consequence of non-representative sampling), functional impairment, amputation and death. The types of biopsy that may be performed include core biopsy, fine needle biopsy (FNB), and incisional or excisional biopsies. For a number of years in our clinical practice at the Royal Prince Alfred Hospital (RPAH), Sydney, Australia, we have been performing biopsies (usually core biopsies) under general anaesthetic, with intra-operative frozen section to confirm that representative and diagnostic tissue has been obtained [2]. There are a number of reasons for using this biopsy protocol in our clinical practice. First, it has been shown that the technique is highly accurate, with a zero non-diagnostic biopsy rate [2], and the infrastructure is in place to support it. Second, many of the patients who are referred to our unit for management reside in excess of 1,000 km away and it is therefore particularly important that a diagnosis be established with a single biopsy procedure because it is not practicable for them to return at a later date for a second biopsy if the initial biopsy is inadequate or non-diagnostic. While our initial diagnostic protocol may not be suitable for every patient in all units, it can be utilised for some or all patients depending on local logistical arrangements of the multidisciplinary sarcoma service and individual patient circumstances.

Apart from determining whether an adequate tissue biopsy has been obtained, intraoperative pathological examination in soft tissue sarcoma surgical oncology may occasionally be indicated for other reasons. Determination of whether or not tumour is present at the margins of excision specimens can be determined pathologically (including by frozen section examination) and this may influence the extent of tissue removed during the surgical procedure. Intraoperative pathological evaluation may also be used for confirmation of the diagnosis of some benign tumours such as aneurysmal bone cyst, giant cell tumour of bone and chondroblastoma. Many such cases with typical clinical and radiological features can be treated definitively with curettage, which can be performed relatively easily and safely as a single operative procedure.

2.2 Pathological Options for Intra-operative Evaluation

2.2.1 Frozen Section

Microscopic examination of frozen tissue sections is the most commonly used technique for intraoperative pathological evaluation. The procedure is performed as follows. Representative fresh, unfixed tissue is selected for examination. The quantity and type of tissue frozen will vary depending on the indication and the amount and appearance of the tissue obtained. The pieces of tissue are placed on a "chuck" (which is about 50% of the size of a standard paraffin block) in a mounting medium such as OCT (optimal cutting temperature; Fig. 2.1A). The tissue is then rapidly frozen in liquid nitrogen (Fig. 2.1B). The chuck is placed in a cryostat and progressively trimmed with a microtome blade until "full face" sections (i.e. sections including all areas of the tissue) are obtained (Fig. 2.1C). Frozen tissue sections that are 5 μm thick are cut and placed onto glass slides. The slides are stained with haematoxylin and eosin (H&E) using the progressive method. The latter can be performed

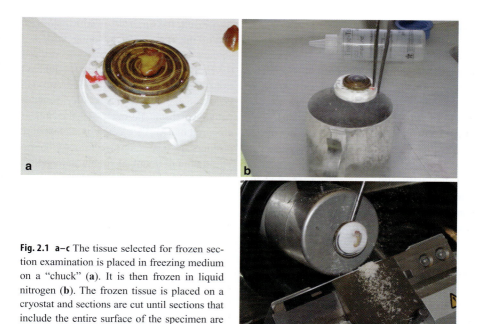

Fig. 2.1 a–c The tissue selected for frozen section examination is placed in freezing medium on a "chuck" (**a**). It is then frozen in liquid nitrogen (**b**). The frozen tissue is placed on a cryostat and sections are cut until sections that include the entire surface of the specimen are obtained (**c**)

considerably more quickly than the regressive method of H&E staining used for permanent sections but generally results in inferior staining quality. Usually two sections from each frozen section block are examined microscopically. It usually takes about 10–15 min to dissect, freeze, cut, stain and evaluate frozen sections.

In the case of multiple core biopsies from a suspected soft tissue sarcoma where the primary purpose of frozen section assessment is to determine whether diagnostic tissue has been obtained, only a portion of the procured tissue sample should be frozen. Ideally the selection of the tissue submitted for frozen section examination should involve input from both the surgeon and the pathologist. Depending on the frozen section appearances, portions of the unfrozen fresh tissue should remain available for any appropriate ancillary investigations such as flow cytometry (in the case of suspected haemopoietic malignancies), cytogenetics (which is particularly useful in soft tissue sarcomas that harbour specific balanced chromosomal translocations), electron microscopy and immunohistochemistry (which may be suboptimal when performed on tissue that has previously been frozen).

At the Royal Prince Alfred Hospital, Sydney, Australia, patients with suspected sarcomas admitted for a core needle biopsy (CNB) attend our day case unit. Under general anaesthetic the CNB is performed, through a stab incision, using a 14G Trucut (Allegiance Healthcare, McGaw Park, IL) needle. Multiple specimens are taken. For purely intra-osseous lesions, the medullary cavity is opened with a 3.5-mm drill prior to CNBs being taken. The specimen is taken fresh to the pathology laboratory by the surgeon along with the imaging. Typically two representative cores selected by the pathologist in conjunction with the surgeon are chosen for frozen section examination. The frozen sections are then evaluated by a musculoskeletal pathologist (in the presence of the surgeon) and the features correlated with the clinical and radiological findings.

2.2.2 Fine Needle Aspiration Cytology

Fine needle aspiration cytology (FNAC) is a rapid, minimally invasive and cost-effective technique employed in the diagnostic workup of mass lesions occurring in a wide variety of organs. FNAC is reported to have high sensitivity and specificity in the diagnosis of musculoskeletal sarcomas when performed by experienced cytopathologists and is commonly used as the primary diagnostic modality in Scandinavian countries [5, 25]. It can be performed and interpreted in a short period of time (about 10 min) and hence is a technique suitable for intraoperative pathological evaluation. FNAC requires minimal specialised equipment. In some instances, particularly hypocellular lesions or tumours associated with a prominent fibrous stroma or reticulin network, it may be impossible to obtain sufficient material for definitive diagnosis. Furthermore, limited sampling may also make it problematic to perform and interpret appropriate ancillary investigations such as immunochemistry (usually performed on a cell block preparation), cytogenetics or electron microscopy. Because the preparation of a cell block takes a number of hours, it is not possible to determine with certainty at the time of the FNAC procedure whether satisfactory material has been obtained. For these reasons, FNAC is not the preferred method for intraoperative pathological evaluation, except perhaps in some specialised centres staffed by individuals with excellent skills and appropriate experience with this technique who have awareness of its limitations and potential pitfalls.

FNAC may be performed using the needle-only technique or the aspiration technique on palpable or impalpable lesions, the latter under radiological guidance. Palpable lesions are localised and stabilised with the fingers of the non-dominant hand. A hollow bore needle (generally 25 gauges) is inserted directly into the mass and the needle is moved swiftly back and forth within the mass for approximately 10 s. As a result, the tip of the needle dislodges cells within the mass, which, along with a small amount of fluid (blood and interstitial fluid) travel up the needle by capillary action. When a small amount of material (blood and cells) is visible in the hub of the needle, the needle is withdrawn from the mass and the bulk of the procured material is ejected onto glass slides by pushing air from a syringe through the needle. The material is spread evenly across the slide using another glass slide. In some cases, where insufficient material is obtained using the 'needle-only' technique, a syringe may be attached to the needle, and while the needle is being moved within the lesion, suction is applied to the syringe in an attempt to aspirate the cellular components of the lesion. The former technique is preferred for several reasons. First, it affords better control of the needle. Second, it allows for a better 'feel' of where the needle tip is located, and experienced operators can judge from the 'feel' whether the needle is well within the mass. Third, unlike the 'aspiration' technique, it is less likely to result in excessive blood dilution of the sample or in the formation of blood clots, within which the cellular material is often entrapped (and is therefore very difficult to interpret under the microscope). Non-palpable lesions are generally localised by a radiologist using imaging modalities such as ultrasound or computed tomography (CT). The radiologist inserts the needle into the mass under radiological guidance and follows a similar procedure to that described above.

The slides may be air-dried and stained immediately with a rapid Romanowsky stain such as Diff Quik (Lab AIDS Pty, Narrabeen, NSW, Australia) or fixed in alcohol and later stained with the Papanicolaou method (Fig. 2.2). While the bulk of the procured material in the needle is expelled onto slides as described above, the small amount of residual material in the needle is washed into Hank's balanced salt solution for later preparation of cell blocks using the serum/prothrombin method or cytocentrifuge preparations. Immunochemical stains

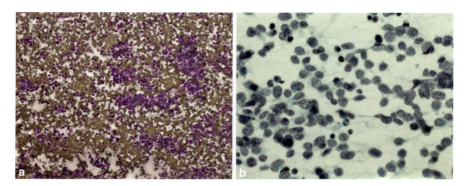

Fig. 2.2 a, b Cytology slides from a fine needle biopsy specimen stained with a Romanowsky stain (**a**) and by the Papanicolaou method (**b**)

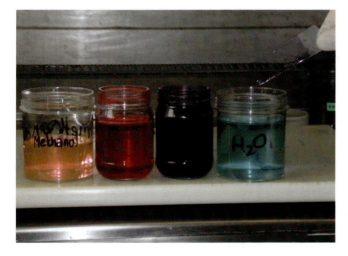

Fig. 2.3 At the time of the fine needle biopsy procedure the material can be stained with the Romanowsky method and interpreted in real time. The staining method involves placing the slide sequentially in a series of solutions

may be applied to the cell block and cytocentrifuge preparations later. The air-dried, rapid Romanowsky-stained slides are examined by the cytopathologist at the time of the procedure (Fig. 2.3). Depending on the amount, type and morphological features of the cellular material obtained, additional passes are performed if necessary to obtain material for further smears or ancillary tests such as immunochemistry. An immediate provisional result, based on the interpretation of the air-dried, rapid Romanowsky-stained slides, may be communicated to the clinician. The puncture tract can be tattooed immediately after performing the biopsy to enable removal of the tract at definitive surgery. Once again consultation with the sarcoma surgeon is advisable to ascertain the surgical approach for the definitive resection.

When used as a combined approach, Domanski reported an accuracy of 97.7% (127 of 130 cases);

however, there were diagnostic discrepancies between FNAC and CNB in another 10 cases (usually one or another specimen being insufficient or inconclusive) [5]. When used as an isolated biopsy procedure, FNAC performs well for metastatic disease, myeloma and lymphoma [25]. With an experienced cytopathologist, Wedin et al. were able with FNAC to determine the site and type of malignancy in two-thirds of patients with skeletal metastases [25]. Dupuy et al. compared CT-guided FNAC and CT-guided CNB in the same connective tissue oncology unit and the accuracy was 80% for FNAC compared with 97% for CNB [6]. Jelinek et al. used FNAC to confirm adequacy of specimen quality [11].

2.2.3
Touch Imprint Cytology

Imprint cytology is a technique in which slides are placed directly onto fresh tissue and some of the tissue is transferred onto slides (Fig. 2.4). The latter are usually stained by a Romanowsky method (as described above for FNAC) and examined microscopically, and the appearances are similar to those seen cytologically in FNAC specimens. The technique allows for rapid assessment of the presence of viable tissue, and can often distinguish between benign and malignant tissue. Because it requires fresh tissue, it is often used in conjunction with frozen section evaluation of fresh tissue. It can be particularly helpful in diagnosing haemopoietic tumours, including lymphomas and leukaemias, or in difficult-to-interpret frozen sections in which imprint cytology may provide supportive evidence of a particular diagnosis.

2.3
Uses of Frozen Section in Musculoskeletal Tumours

Simon and Biermann in their Instructional Course Lecture [22] stated that "wherever possible, the surgeon should obtain a specimen for frozen section at biopsy", in order to determine whether enough viable and representative tissue has been obtained. It is our experience that frozen section rarely takes more than 15 min to perform. By notifying the pathologist in advance of the list, and then give them a further warning

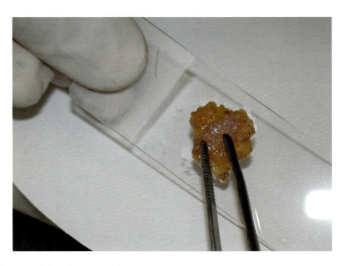

Fig. 2.4 Performing a touch imprint preparation

at the start of the case, delays are less likely to occur. The mean length of operating time, including frozen section, in our series was 34 min (range 25 to 45) [2]. Over a much larger series involving 700 hospitals in seven countries, 90% of frozen sections were turned around in 20 min in one study [17].

2.3.1
Operative Core Biopsy of Presumed Sarcoma

There are two aspects to the use of frozen section for presumed sarcoma. It is our opinion that confirmation that the sample is adequate for diagnosis is the primary reason for using frozen section. Achieving the final diagnosis at the time of frozen section should be seen as a bonus.

Our protocol at RPAH, Sydney for management of presumed sarcomas has been described previously (Fig. 2.5) [2]. A biopsy is performed in accordance with standard sarcoma practice and then a frozen section performed whilst the patient remains anaesthetised. It is our practice to ensure that sufficient cores of tissue (at least four) are taken to allow both frozen section examination to be performed and keeping some unfrozen tissue available for permanent paraffin sections and any necessary ancillary investigations such as immunochemistry or elcectron microscopy. If the frozen section either establishes the diagnosis or clearly demonstrates that electron representative tissue has been obtained, on which a definitive diagnosis can be made, then the protocol is complete and the patient is recovered from their general anaesthetic. If there is no representative tissue then either a repeat CNB or an open biopsy is performed and a further frozen section analysis undertaken to determine whether representative tissue has been obtained. The procedure is repeated until adequate tissue is obtained to enable a diagnosis to be made. The presence of extensive necrosis or cyst formation may make it difficult to obtain a diagnostic specimen and are common reasons for multiple biopsies [15].

We reviewed 104 patients who were put through this protocol over a two-year period at RPAH, Sydney. These were compared with 24 patients who had CT-guided biopsies of musculo-skeletal. The latter were principally performed because the tumours were located at sites inaccessible to surgical biopsy. There were 71 malignant bone lesions, 20 malignant soft tissue lesions and 37 benign lesions (24 bone, 13 soft-tissue). Using the biopsy and frozen section protocol there were no non-diagnostic biopsies.

In our series the chance of needing to convert to an open biopsy was 23% for soft-tissue lesions and 4% for bone lesions. In 96% of malignant lesions the diagnosis was established on CNB, but this figure was lower 73% in ultimately benign lesions. This may represent the fact that it is easier for a pathologist to establish that something is malignant than to be certain that it is not.

There was one minor diagnostic error in the group attributable to misinterpretation at frozen section. This case involved a 62-year-old female who had a thigh mass with non-specific clinical and radiological features. A core biopsy was non-diagnostic. A decision was made to proceed to open biopsy rather than repeat the CNB. Frozen section analysis of the open biopsy revealed atypical lymphoid tissue possibly Hodgkin lymphoma. The definitive tissue diagnosis was B cell non-Hodgkin lymphoma. Surgical management of this patient was not affected.

Whilst a biopsy, if performed with poor technique, can have immediate complications, if performed well, they are unlikely. We had no infections, haematomas or unplanned return to theatres in any of the patients in our series.

Whilst we have emphasised the role of frozen section in biopsy, subsequent review of clinical, pathological and radiological data is performed at the weekly multidisciplinary Bone and Soft Tissue Tumour Meeting at our institution and a final

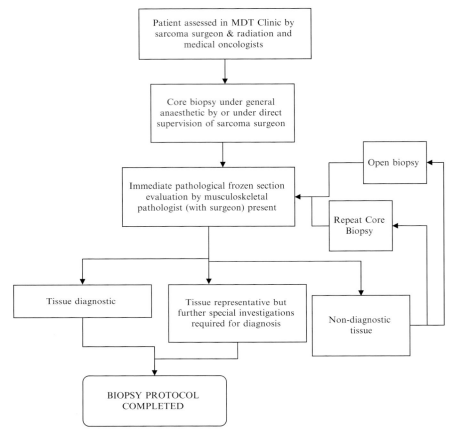

Fig. 2.5 Surgeon-led operative core biopsy with frozen section evaluation protocol of the NSW Sarcoma Service. (Reproduced with permission and copyright of the British Editorial Society of Bone and Joint Surgery [2])

diagnosis is only established upon review of all of the data [2].

We are not the only authors to report on the use of frozen section analysis in musculoskeletal tumours. Dupuy and colleagues at Massachusetts General Hospital have utilised frozen section on CNB samples taken under CT guidance. The accuracy of those where frozen section was utilised was 94% compared with 88% where it was not [6].

If there are any doubts on frozen section diagnosis, definitive surgery should be delayed pending full pathological analysis [22].

The majority of this article has been concerned with diagnosis of bone and soft tissue sarcomas, however there are other circumstances in our practice where we utilise intra-operative frozen section.

2.3.2
Surgical Margin Biopsy/Imprint

When resecting a primary bone sarcoma where there is residual long bone, the medullary contents may be curetted as a margin biopsy. A frozen section can be performed on the specimen to determine whether or not tumour is present. If there is malignant or even questionable tissue at that margin, then re-resection of that margin and re-biopsy of the new margin and repeat the frozen section is indicated. Once the all clear has been given for the margins, one can proceed with the reconstruction [15].

2.3.3
Confirmation of Diagnosis Prior to Definitive Treatment

Frozen section evaluation may be used in the definitive management of some benign lesions. Aneurysmal bone cyst, giant cell tumour of bone and chondroblastoma (Fig. 2.6) all have characteristic radiological appearances. Definitive management is usually curettage for all three of these pathologies. In cases with typical clinical and radiological in features, frozen section examination can be used to confirm the diagnosis allowing the definitive management to be safely performed.

Frozen section evaluation may also be useful in patients with metastases. In patients with known primary tumours and a solitary lesion, then it is wise to confirm the diagnosis with a biopsy and exclude the possibility of a primary bone tumour. In the event of a pathological fracture this can be undertaken immediately prior to intra-medullary nailing.

Intraoperative pathological examination can also be used to avoid a "whoops procedure" such as the shelling out of a lump only to find that it is a sarcoma a few days later when the results of routine pathological analysis become available [3, 16]. A frozen section performed on a CNB or open biopsy will most likely reveal malignancy if present.

Heslin et al reported results of frozen section biopsies as part of their series of biopsies in soft tissue sarcoma [8]. They defined a frozen section biopsy as "a tumour resection without prior biopsy and a frozen section diagnosis given at time of operation". They had two false-negatives (both reported as benign adipose tumours that were subsequently revealed as liposarcomas) and two false-positives (a desmoid tumour that was

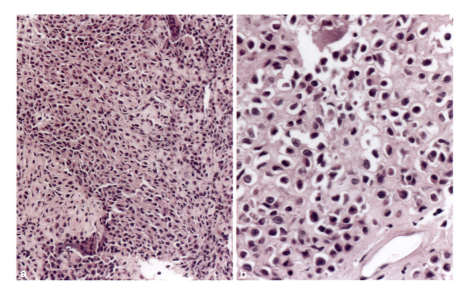

Fig. 2.6 a, b Histological features of a chondroblastoma

in fact an atypical lipoma and a skin tumour that was finally classified as hidradenoma). Distinguishing atypical lipomatous tumour (low-grade liposarcoma) from lipomas can be notoriously difficult and the former may include large areas indistinguishable from the latter on microscopic examination. For these reasons, we recommend marginal excision (without frozen section evaluation) for all low grade fatty tumours and establishing the diagnosis by routine pathology.

There are other circumstances where one should be wary of using frozen section for confirmation of diagnosis. While, for example in high grade chondrosarcoma and giant cell tumour, only a small amount of tumour may be necessary to establish the diagnosis, in low-grade chondroid tumous it often difficult or impossible to determine the diagnosis on frozen section [15].

2.3.4
Evaluation of Tumour Spread

Whilst performing musculoskeletal tumour surgery, one sometimes encounters a questionable or suspicious area separate from the main tumour. Frozen section can help determine the nature of such a focus. For example, frozen section may establish that the focus is a satellite deposit of tumour or that the area is an enlarged lymph node, and furthermore frozen section can determine if it is involved by an inflammatory or malignant process. Alternatively FNAC of a suspicious lymph node could be performed before surgery (if it is detected preoperatively) or during the operative procedure. The results of such investigations can aid surgical decision making intra-operatively.

2.3.5
Intramedullary Nailing of Presumed Metastasis

In patients with known primary tumours and radiological evidence of disseminated skeletal metastases it is probably not necessary to perform a biopsy. However, if the skeletal metastasis is isolated or there is a pathological fracture then utilising frozen section is probably appropriate. In the instance of an isolated skeletal metastasis, in our institution the biopsy would usually be as a separate diagnostic procedure along the lines of our sarcoma biopsy protocol [2]. In the second, as outlined earlier, we would perform a biopsy and if it proves metastatic malignancy, immediately proceed to intramedullary nailing.

2.3.6
Frozen Section for Everyone?

There are situations where frozen section evaluation is inappropriate. The main one is in the diagnosis of low grade fatty tumours. The discrimination between benign lipoma and atypical lipomatous tumour (formerly known as low-grade liposarcoma) is notoriously difficult. We would treat both by marginal excision (without biopsy or frozen section), enabling the pathologist to receive the whole specimen and so make a final diagnosis upon pathological examination of entire specimen.

The other situation that does not avail itself to frozen section is the pure bone lesion. Well mineralised tissue cannot be cut for frozen section, however, almost all malignant tumours of bone have soft areas suitable for frozen section analysis [21].

2.3.7
Beware the Pitfalls of Frozen Section

We have outlined the pros and cons of frozen section throughout this article. It is important to clarify the pitfalls, so that one can avoid them. The first is inadequate tissue, both for frozen and permanent section analysis. It is beholden on the surgeon to provide the pathologist with sufficient representative tissue and the pathologist indicate when the biopsy contains insufficient tissue or is non-diagnostic so that the surgeon can return to the operating theatre to collect a further biopsy if it is appropriate. The second and third pitfall relate to the tissue provided. If the tissue is not representative of the entire lesion then the diagnosis ventured may be wrong. This highlights the importance of tying together clinical, radiological and pathological data. Tissues that are heavily calcified are difficult to section and therefore difficult to provide an intra-operative diagnosis upon. Another pitfall is artefact. These can be surgical caused by technique (crushing of the specimen, for example by removing the CNB from the biopsy needle with forceps) or pathological caused by poor freezing technique. Because frozen sections are almost always of inferior quality to permanent paraffin embedded sections (Fig. 2.7), misinterpretation of frozen sections is another potential hazard.

2.4 Cost-Effectiveness

There is obviously a cost implication to performing frozen sections on biopsies. Based on our biopsy strategy we estimated costs to be approximately €1,119 (AU $1,804) per case. In his further opinion, Grimer proposed a compromise strategy, upon which we also have included costings [7]. Whilst we maintain that our strategy is the gold standard, we do accept that it may not be reproducible in some healthcare situations.

The compromise suggested is as follows (Table 2.1):

We estimated costs based on the Australian Medicare rebate system and have converted to

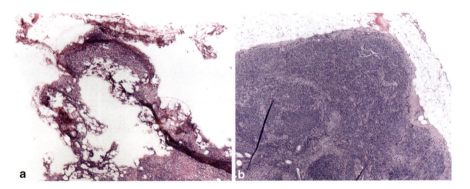

Fig. 2.7 a, b Frozen sections (**a**) are generally of inferior quality to those of paraffin sections (**b**)

Table 2.1 Different biopsy strategies for various musculoskeletal tumour scenarios, based on Grimer [7]

	Outpatient (LA)	Frozen Section	Image Guidance	GA
Accessible soft-tissue lesion	✓			
In-accessible soft tissue lesion		✓	✓	✓
"Worrying" bone tumours	✓		✓	
"Worrying" deep tumours/children		✓	✓	✓

Euros based on a mean exchange rate for the latter half of 2005 of AU $1:€0.62. Theatre and scan time have been estimated at 1 h per procedure. Full details of the remainder or the estimates are documented in our original article [2]. We have also estimated costs for the other scenarios mentioned earlier (Table 2.2).

Core needle biopsy with frozen section is more expensive than outpatient biopsy as one would expect. CT-guided biopsy is approximately three-quarters of the cost of our protocol biopsy. If one considers there is up to a 20% re-biopsy rate, which makes the true cost of each CT-guided biopsy €1,035. Outpatient CNB remains a valuable and cost-effective technique.

Furthermore, when we utilise intra-operative frozen section for confirmation of a benign diagnosis, rather than doing a separate biopsy procedure, if one allows an extra €800 for the additional theatre time, surgical and anaesthetic charges, there are significant cost savings over two separate procedures.

2.5 Discussion

Simon and Biermann have stated that biopsy "frequently demands relatively few technical skills" but that the "decisions related to the performance of the biopsy requires considerable thought and expertise" [22].

A poorly performed biopsy may result in inappropriate treatment and have a negative impact on patient survival [4]. CNB has been shown to be accurate in diagnosing musculoskeletal tumours, with reported accuracies of 93%–99% in soft-tissue sarcomas [8, 9] and between 97% and 98% in bone tumours [20, 24] when performed in some specialist centres. However, low rates of accuracy, even in specialist centres, have also been reported. For image-guided CNB there are reports of error rates (incorrect diagnosis) of between 6% and 12% [13, 14].

Table 2.2 Approximate cost (€) for core needle biopsies performed with and without image guidance or frozen section

Service	CNB with frozen section (protocol)	Outpatient CNB	Image-guided (CT) CNB	Image-guided CNB with F/S and GA
MDT assessment	320	320	320	320
Pre-op assessment	112	0	0	112
Anaesthesia	117	20	62	117
Surgeon/radiologist	99	0	62	62
Operating theatre cost	146	0	0	0
Scanner cost	0	0	211	211
Consumables	37	37	62	62
In-patient bed	131	0	0	131
Pathology cost				
Frozen section	63	0	0	63
Definitive section	94	94	94	94
Total	1,119	471	811	1,172

CNB, core needle biopsy; F/S, frozen section; GA, general anaesthetic

When the biopsy has been performed in the referring centre, incorrect diagnosis can be a problem as can adverse consequences of the biopsy. In a series reported from our unit, errors related to the biopsy significantly altered definitive treatment in 38% of cases where the biopsy had been performed in the referring centre [19]. Of the patients in this series, 15% required an amputation where limb-salvage would have been appropriate had the biopsy been performed in a satisfactory manner. When directly comparing referring and treating centres the complication rate of biopsy was 29.1% in referring centres and 4.1% in treating centres [14]. In the same article, from referring centre biopsies there was a diagnostic error rate of 27.4% and a non-representative rate of 5.7%. It was necessary to alter treatment in 36.3% and amputate in 4.3% [14]. These two series add to the evidence on why biopsies should be performed in specialist centres.

Non-representative biopsies are another problem in musculoskeletal tumour surgery. There is no question that the time spent waiting for a biopsy result is difficult for the patient. In a number of studies, image-guided biopsies have been demonstrated to fail to determine the diagnosis between 5% and 20% of the time [1, 6, 10, 11, 12, 20].

By incorporating frozen section into our biopsy protocol at the Royal Prince Alfred Hospital in Sydney, Australia, it has been possible to eradicate the problem of the non-diagnostic protocol. This is in part necessary because of the geographical distribution of our patients. It is unreasonable to expect patients to travel in excess of 1,000 km for a biopsy and to return that same distance for a repeat biopsy when the initial biopsy is non-diagnostic. Simon suggested back in 1982 that "wherever possible a specimen for frozen section should be obtained at all biopsies" [21] and reiterated the message a decade later [22].

There may be infrastructure reasons why frozen sections are inappropriate in some units and the cost may appear prohibitive, but at the very least, any patient undergoing a biopsy under general anaesthetic should have a frozen section performed.

References

1. Altuntas AO, Slavin J, Smith PJ, Schlict SM, Powell GJ, Ngan S, Toner G, Choong PF (2005) Accuracy of computed tomography guided core needle biopsy of musculoskeletal tumours. ANZ J Surg 75:187–191
2. Ashford RU, McCarthy SW, Scolyer RA, Bonar SF, Karim RZ, Stalley PD (2006) Surgical biopsy with intra-operative frozen section. An accurate and cost-effective method for diagnosis of musculoskeletal sarcomas. J Bone Joint Surg 88:1207–1211
3. Bhangu AA, Beard JAS, Grimer RJ (2003) Should soft tissue sarcomas be treated at a specialist centre? Sarcoma 8:1–6
4. Bickels J, Jelinek JS, Shmookler BM, Neff RS, Malawer MM (1999) Biopsy of musculoskeletal tumors. Current concepts. Clin Orthop Relat Res 368:212–219
5. Domanski HA, Akerman M, Carlen B, Engellau J, Gustafson P, Jonsson K, Mertens F, Rydholm A (2005) Core-needle biopsy performed by the cytopathologist: a technique to complement fine-needle aspiration of soft tissue and bone lesions. Cancer 105:229–239
6. Dupuy DE, Rosenberg AE, Punyaratabandhu T, Tan MH, Mankin HJ (1998) Accuracy of CT-guided needle biopsy of musculoskeletal neoplasms. Am J Roentgenol 171:759–762
7. Grimer RJ (2006) Further opinion. J Bone Joint Surg 88:1–2
8. Heslin MJ, Lewis JJ, Woodruff JM, Brennan MF (1997) Core needle biopsy for diagnosis of extremity soft tissue sarcoma. Ann Surg Oncol 4:425–431
9. Hoeber I, Spillane AJ, Fisher C, Thomas JM (2001) Accuracy of biopsy techniques for limb and limb girdle soft tissue tumors. Ann Surg Oncol 8:80–87
10. Issakov J, Flusser G, Kollender Y, Merimsky O, Lifschitz-Mercer B, Meller I (2003) Computed tomography-guided core needle biopsy for bone and soft tissue tumors. Isr Med Assoc J 5:28–30
11. Jelinek JS, Murphey MD, Welker JA, Henshaw RM, Kransdorf MJ, Shmookler BM, Malawer MM (2002) Diagnosis of primary bone tumors

with image-guided percutaneous biopsy: experience with 110 tumors. Radiology 223:731–737
12. Kruyt RH, Oudkerk M, van Sluis D (1998) CT-guided bone biopsy in a cancer center: experience with a new apple corer-shaped device. J Comput Assist Tomogr 22:276–281
13. Mankin HJ, Lange TA, Spanier SS (1982) The hazards of biopsy in patients with malignant primary bone and soft-tissue tumors. J Bone Joint Surg Am 64:1121–1127
14. Mankin HJ, Mankin CJ, Simon MA (1996) The hazards of the biopsy, revisited. Members of the Musculoskeletal Tumor Society. J Bone Joint Surg Am 78:656–663
15. McCarthy EF, Frassica FJ (1998) Management of orthopaedic pathology specimens from the operating room to the microscope. In: McCarthy EF, Frassica FJ (eds) Pathology of bone and joint disorders. WB Saunders, Philadelphia, pp 365–371
16. Nijhuis PH, Schaapveld M, Otter R, Hoekstra HJ (2001) Soft tissue sarcoma-compliance with guidelines. Cancer 91:2186–2195
17. Novis DA, Zarbo RJ (1997) Interinstitutional comparison of frozen section turnaround time. A College of American Pathologists Q-Probes study of 32868 frozen sections in 700 hospitals. Arch Pathol Lab Med 121:559–567
18. Peabody TD, Gibbs CP, Simon MA (1998) Current concepts review—evaluation and staging of musculoskeletal neoplasms. J Bone Joint Surg 80:1204–1218
19. Pollock RC, Stalley PD (2004) Biopsy of musculoskeletal tumours-beware. ANZ J Surg 74:516–519
20. Saifuddin A, Mitchell R, Burnett SJ, Sandison A, Pringle JA (2000) Ultrasound-guided needle biopsy of primary bone tumours. J Bone Joint Surg Br 82:50–54
21. Simon MA (1982) Biopsy of musculoskeletal tumors. J Bone Joint Surg Am 64:1253–1257
22. Simon MA, Biermann JS (1993) Biopsy of bone and soft-tissue lesions. J Bone Joint Surg Am 75:616–621
23. Simon MA, Finn HA (1993) Diagnostic strategy for bone and soft-tissue tumors. J Bone Joint Surg Am 75:622–631
24. Stoker DJ, Cobb JP, Pringle JA (1991) Needle biopsy of musculoskeletal lesions. A review of 208 procedures. J Bone Joint Surg Br 73:498–500
25. Wedin R, Bauer HC, Skoog L, Soderlund V, Tani E (2000) Cytological diagnosis of skeletal lesions. Fine-needle aspiration biopsy in 110 tumours. J Bone Joint Surg Br 82:673–678

Sentinel Node Biopsy in Soft Tissue Sarcoma

Dimosthenis Andreou and Per-Ulf Tunn

Abstract While regional lymphatic spread develops in only 3%–4% of all patients with soft tissue sarcoma, there are several histological subtypes associated with a significantly higher propensity for regional lymph node metastasis. These include clear cell sarcoma, synovial sarcoma, rhabdomyosarcoma, and epithelioid sarcoma. To date there is no validated, noninvasive method to assess regional lymph node status. A potentially useful diagnostic tool is lymphatic mapping with sentinel lymph node biopsy, a concept that has revolutionized the treatment of patients with intermediate thickness melanoma and early stage breast cancer. The purpose of this study is to provide an overview of the procedure of sentinel lymph node biopsy and the data available on its application in patients with soft tissue sarcomas.

3.1 Introduction

The most common site of metastatic disease for soft tissue sarcomas is the lung, with approximately 20% of all patients presenting with or developing pulmonary metastases (Billingsley et al. 1999; Potter et al. 1985; Gadd et al. 1993). In general, regional lymph node metastasis develops in 3%–4% of all patients with soft tissue sarcoma (Fong et al. 1993; Behranwala et al. 2004; Riad et al. 2004). However, there are several histological subtypes associated with a significantly higher incidence of regional lymphatic spread; these include clear cell sarcoma, synovial sarcoma, rhabdomyosarcoma, and epithelioid sarcoma (Fong et al. 1993; Ham et al. 1998; Behranwala et al. 2004). The evaluation of the regional lymph node status is of great significance for these entities, since early detection and aggressive surgical resection of nodal metastases has proved to be a requisite for long-term survival (Fong et al. 1993; Behranwala et al. 2004; Riad et al. 2004). Nevertheless there is currently no validated, noninvasive method to assess regional lymph node status, especially considering that regional nodes may be histologically positive even when they are clinically negative (Ruka et al. 1988; Neville et al. 2000b; Morton et al. 2005).

A potentially useful diagnostic tool for detecting lymph node metastases in patients with soft tissue sarcoma is lymphatic mapping with sentinel node biopsy, a technique first described in its present form by Morton et al. (1990) for patients with malignant melanoma. The concept of this

Dimosthenis Andreou (✉)
Department of Orthopedic Oncology
Sarkomzentrum Berlin-Brandenburg
Helios Klinikum Berlin-Buch
Schwanebecker Chaussee 50
13125 Berlin, Germany
E-mail: dimosthenis.andreou@helios-kliniken.de

procedure is that the sentinel represents the first node to receive lymphatic drainage from a tumor; it thereby follows that an involvement of this lymph node could indicate a potential tumor spread in the entire regional basin, whereas a tumor-free sentinel would render nodal involvement unlikely (Morton et al. 1992).

Sentinel node biopsy has been established over the years in the treatment of intermediate thickness malignant melanoma (Morton et al. 2005) and early stage breast cancer (Naik et al. 2004), while its role is being currently explored in cancers of the gastrointestinal tract (Bilchik et al. 2006) and numerous other carcinomas (Leong et al. 2006). This appears to be reasonable, as up to 20% of patients with early stage breast cancer (McMasters et al. 2000), 20% of patients with intermediate thickness melanoma (Morton et al. 2005), and approximately 50% of patients with cancer of the gastrointestinal tract (Leong et al. 2006) will develop lymph node metastasis. The relatively high incidence of these malignancies in the general population (Jemal et al. 2007; Micheli et al. 2002) provides an excellent setting for researchers to investigate the feasibility, results, and potential benefits of sentinel node biopsy in these patients. The low incidence of soft tissue sarcomas (Jemal et al. 2007), and particularly of the entities with a high propensity for regional lymphatic spread (Rydholm et al. 1984), could account for the fact that, to date, only 31 cases of sentinel node biopsy in patients with soft tissue sarcoma have been reported in the literature. So far all cases refer to tumors localized in the extremities.

The purpose of this study is to provide an overview of the procedure of sentinel lymph node (SLN) biopsy and the data available on its application in patients with soft tissue sarcomas.

3.2
Technique of Lymphatic Mapping and Sentinel Lymph Node Biopsy

Vital blue dye (patent blue or isosulfan blue) was initially utilized for intraoperative lymphatic mapping in the setting of sentinel node biopsy (Morton et al. 1992). The employment of the dye alone required the visualization of blue-stained lymphatics from the edge of the wound, which were then followed by means of dissection to the sentinel node. Though the false-negative rate of this method was low, the ability to successfully identify the SLNs was directly correlated with the surgeon's prior experience with the technique (Albertini et al. 1996; Bostick et al. 1999). Technical difficulties resulting in unsuccessful explorations occurred in up to 20% of the cases (Albertini et al. 1996). Other researches employed preoperative lymphoscintigraphy, allowing for improved localization of the regional basin as well as the sentinel node itself with less dissection (Alex et al. 1993; van der Veen et al. 1994). The combined application of both techniques produced the best results in identifying the sentinel node with a low false-negative rate, so that it was soon included in most protocols (Morton et al. 1999; Cochran et al. 2000; McMasters et al. 2000).

3.2.1
Preoperative Lymphoscintigraphy

The preoperative lymphoscintigraphy involves the injection of a radioisotope around the primary tumor or its excision site (Cochran et al. 2000). ^{99m}Tc-labeled albumin nanocolloid is most commonly used in Europe; ^{99m}Tc sulfur colloid, ^{99m}Tc human serum albumin, or ^{99m}Tc albumin colloid is usually applied in the United States (Morton et al. 1999). A large field scintillation camera documents the drainage pattern to the regional lymph nodes (Bostick et al. 1999). Continuous monitoring with dynamic imaging is recommended after the injection of the radiopharmaceutical agent until the first nodes are visualized, which is followed, if necessary, by delayed static images (Albertini et al. 1996; Bostick et al. 1999; Cochran et al. 2000). The sentinel node is defined as the first node that receives afferent lymphatic drainage from the primary injection site (Nieweg et al. 2001).

Occasionally more than one lymph node are identified simultaneously, and in some cases two or more separate afferent lymphatic channels are depicted, leading to different lymph nodes. Each of these nodes is considered to be a sentinel node (Nieweg et al. 2001). The body image is then outlined to create the radiograph, and the skin surface overlying the identified sentinel nodes is marked with indelible ink (Bostick et al. 1999; Figs. 3.1, 3.2, and 3.3).

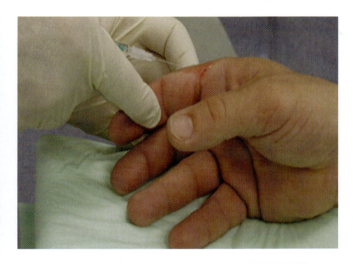

Fig. 3.1 Injection of ^{99m}Tc-labeled albumin nanocolloid around the excision site of a soft tissue sarcoma in the right index finger

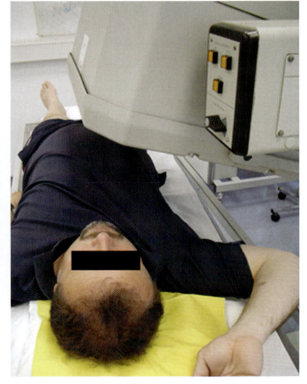

Fig. 3.2 Large field scintillation camera

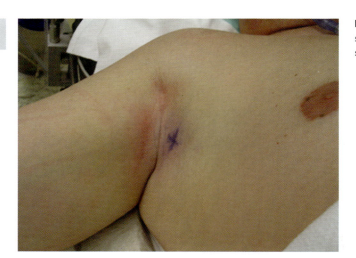

Fig. 3.3 Marking on the skin surface overlying the identified sentinel node

3.2.2 Intraoperative Lymphatic Mapping

After induction of general or local anesthesia, vital blue dye is injected around the primary site, which is then gently massaged to facilitate the passage of the dye in the lymphatics (Bostick et al. 1999). The areas that have been marked during the lymphoscintigraphy are examined with a handheld γ-probe to affirm the presence of radioactivity. Subsequently a small incision is made at the marked site (Albertini et al. 1996; Bostick et al. 1999). Some surgeons choose to identify and follow the lymphatics to the blue-stained lymph nodes, which are then excised and controlled with the probe (Albertini et al. 1996; Bostick et al. 1999; Morton et al. 1999), while others use the probe primarily as a localizer for the radioactive nodes in the wound, with the dye serving as an additional visual aid (Cochran et al. 2000; Estourgie et al. 2003; van Akkooi et al. 2006; Figs. 3.4, 3.5, 3.6, and 3.7).

Determining which of the identified nodes is indeed a sentinel node is a further point of controversy, seeing as how difficult it is to ascertain during the operation which node is truly the first node to receive afferent lymphatic drainage from the primary site (Nieweg et al. 2001). The findings of a large multicenter trial in the United States and Canada for melanoma patients led to the so-called "10% rule" (McMasters et al. 2004), according to which all blue-stained lymph nodes, all palpable lymph nodes, and all nodes with a radioactivity exceeding 10% of that of the hottest node should be regarded as sentinel nodes and thereupon excised. The same study demonstrated that, following these guidelines, an average of two nodes per lymphatic basin are removed.

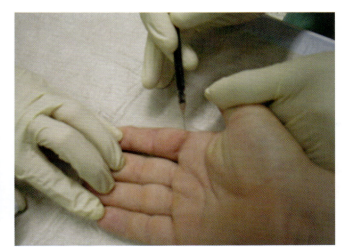

Fig. 3.4 Injection of blue dye around the primary site

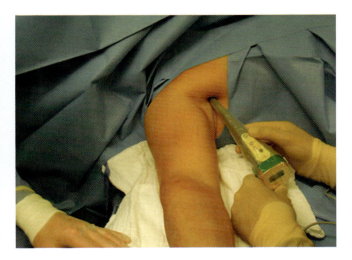

Fig. 3.5 The handheld γ-probe confirms the presence of radioactivity

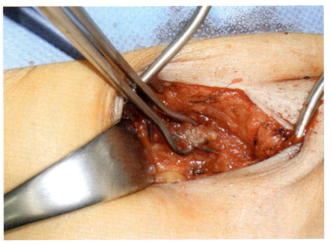

Fig. 3.6 A blue-stained lymphatic channel leading to a sentinel node

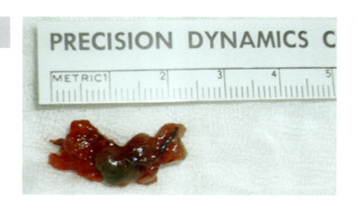

Fig. 3.7 The excised blue-stained sentinel node

3.2.3 Histopathological Examination

Theoretically, an optimal histopathological analysis of the excised sentinel nodes would include serial sectioning of each sentinel node to extinction (Morton et al. 1999), a method which is too expensive and time-consuming, and therefore impractical. Several approaches have been suggested as an attempt at a compromise between the ideal and the possible, with the goal being to keep the false-negative rate to a minimum. The exact methodology of each protocol depends on the type of the primary tumor; as such, there are currently no validated data regarding the optimal pathological assessment of sentinel lymph nodes for soft tissue sarcomas. The guidelines proposed from the EORTC Melanoma Group (Cook et al. 2003) include fixing the excised nodes in buffered formalin for 24 h and then cutting through the hilum and the longest dimension of the nodes, embedding them in paraffin. Twenty sections with five 50-μm steps up to a depth of 250 μm are cut from each face of the sentinel and subjected to hematoxylin and eosin (H&E) and immunohistochemical staining, with unstained sections retained at each level to be used for further stains in problematic cases. The combination of H&E and immunohistochemical staining is also proposed for breast cancer patients (Cserni et al. 2003).

Immunohistochemistry is considered to be essential, since evaluation of lymph nodes by H&E alone misses up to 12% of positive nodes (Morton et al. 2005). Furthermore, Takeuchi et al. recently showed that melanoma-associated markers were detected in multiple-marker reverse transcriptase polymerase chain reaction assays in 30% of patients with histopathologically negative sentinel nodes and that these patients had a significantly higher risk for developing long-term disease recurrence (Takeuchi et al. 2004), raising further questions regarding the best possible examination of sentinel nodes.

A further issue concerns intraoperative frozen-section analysis. Despite the obvious advantage of sparing the patient a second operating procedure, several authors now recommend the use of permanent sections alone (Morton et al. 1999; Cochran et al. 2000; Estourgie et al. 2003), which minimizes the loss of diagnostic material during "facing up." Given the inexperience in applying the sentinel node technique in patients with soft tissue sarcomas, our group recently advised against frozen sections for these patients (Tunn et al. 2007).

3.3
Sentinel Node Biopsy in the Management of Soft Tissue Sarcoma

To date, a total of 31 cases of sentinel node biopsy in patients with soft tissue sarcomas have been described in the literature (Neville et al. 2000a; McMulkin et al. 2003; Al-Refaie et al. 2004; Picciotto et al. 2005; Seal et al. 2005; Nishida et al. 2005; van Akkooi et al. 2006; Albores-Zuniga et al. 2006; Tunn et al. 2007; Fantini et al. 2007). With the exception of two patients with malignant schwannoma and alveolar soft tissue sarcoma in a series of pediatric patients (Neville et al. 2000a), all cases involved entities with a high propensity for regional nodal metastasis, namely clear cell sarcoma, synovial sarcoma, rhabdomyosarcoma, and epithelioid sarcoma. The only other histological subtype with a high rate of regional nodal metastases (Mazeron and Suit 1987; Fong et al. 1993; Mark et al. 1996) is angiosarcoma. Blazer et al. have already debated the possibility of applying sentinel node biopsy in these tumors, yet their distinctly different biological behavior with a predilection for disseminated disease—also reflected in the fact that angiosarcomas are excluded from the American Joint Committee on Cancer (AJCC) staging system (Kotilingam et al. 2006)—render the potential utility of the technique difficult to support (Blazer et al. 2003).

two large retrospective studies (Eckardt et al. 1983; Deenik et al. 1999) distant metastases appeared within 2 years in all instances, once the regional lymph nodes had become clinically positive. As such, the possible benefits of applying sentinel node biopsy were quickly proposed (Deenik et al. 1999).

So far 13 cases of sentinel node biopsy in clear cell sarcoma have been reported (Neville et al. 2000a; Al-Refaie et al. 2004; Picciotto et al. 2005; Nishida et al. 2005; van Akkooi et al. 2006; Albores-Zuniga et al. 2006; Fantini et al. 2007), including a series of 5 patients (van Akkooi et al. 2006). In total, 28 nodes were identified, with 9 nodes in 7 patients being positive for metastasis. A regional lymph node dissection was performed in 6 patients, 5 of whom had evidence of nodal metastasis in at least one further, nonsentinel lymph node. Of those patients, 3 developed multiple metastases shortly after the procedure; 2 of them died of disease, and the third was transferred to a palliative care unit. Another patient developed a local recurrence and underwent an isolated limb perfusion of the lower limb. After surgical re-excision, he remained disease-free for 3.5 years in follow-up.

Two patients developed regional nodal metastases 12 and 13 months after a negative sentinel node biopsy. Distant metastases were reported for both patients. The remaining four patients showed no evidence of recurrent disease in follow-up.

3.3.1
Clear Cell Sarcoma

Clear cell sarcoma, also known as malignant melanoma of soft parts, is a rare tumor, representing 1% of all soft tissue sarcomas (Kuiper et al. 2003; Blazer et al. 2003). It has one of the highest documented rates of regional lymph node metastases, developing in approximately one-third of the patients (Eckardt et al. 1983; Mazeron and Suit 1987; Deenik et al. 1999). In

3.3.2
Synovial Sarcoma

Synovial sarcoma is a highly aggressive tumor, representing approximately 5%–10% of all soft tissue sarcomas (Rydholm et al. 1984; Ferrari et al. 2004; Spurrell et al. 2005). The median age of patients at the time of diagnosis lies in the third decade of life, with approximately 30% of the cases being children and adolescents younger than 20 years of age (Andrassy et al.

2001; Okcu et al. 2003). Regional lymphatic spread has been reported in 2%–17% of all patients (Weingrad and Rosenberg 1978; Ruka et al. 1988; Fong et al. 1993; Andrassy et al. 2001), rendering synovial sarcoma the most common form of soft tissue sarcomas for which nodal recurrence is a potential clinical concern (Ariel 1988; Blazer et al. 2003).

Our group recently published preliminary results from applying sentinel node biopsy in a series of 11 consecutive patients with synovial sarcoma (Tunn et al. 2007). Of them, four patients presented at the time of initial diagnosis, one with a local recurrence, one with a subcutaneous metastasis in the lower limb, and five patients were referred to us from other centers after marginal resection of a synovial sarcoma. The patient presenting with the subcutaneous metastasis had received adjuvant radiochemotherapy during the treatment of the primary tumor, while a further patient presenting with a primary tumor received neoadjuvant chemotherapy prior to wide resection and sentinel node biopsy; the remaining patients had received neither radiation nor chemotherapy at the time of the sentinel node biopsy.

Of the 15 sentinels identified, 1 was positive and 14 negative for metastasis. The regional lymph node dissection performed in the patient with the positive sentinel revealed no evidence of further nodal involvement; 17 months after surgery the patient remained disease-free in follow-up.

One patient developed regional nodal metastases, despite negative sentinel node biopsy, as well as pulmonary metastases 7 months after surgery. She died of sepsis and respiratory failure, after receiving five cycles of systemic chemotherapy. Another patient developed pulmonary metastases 31 months after negative sentinel node biopsy, so that third-line chemotherapy was initiated. The clinical and sonographic examination showed no evidence of tumor spread in the regional lymph nodes. The remaining patients developed neither local recurrences nor regional or systemic metastases.

3.3.3
Rhabdomyosarcoma

Rhabdomyosarcoma is the most common soft tissue sarcoma in children and adolescents, comprising 50% of the cases and 4%–8% of all pediatric malignancies (Neville et al. 2000c; Esnaola et al. 2001). It is far less common in adults, representing 2%–5% of adult soft tissue sarcomas (Hawkins et al. 2001). The incidence of regional lymph node involvement varies; at least 14% of all children with localized disease and approximately 40% of adult patients are believed to be positive for regional lymphatic spread (Lawrence et al. 1987; Hawkins et al. 2001; Little et al. 2002; Wharam et al. 2004). Lymph node involvement at diagnosis in children and adolescents has been reported to be the single factor most predictive of increased total failure risk (Wharam et al. 2004).

A series of 13 pediatric patients who underwent lymphatic mapping with sentinel node biopsy (Neville et al. 2000a) included 3 patients with rhabdomyosarcoma. Sampled were nine lymph nodes, two of which in one patient were positive for metastatic disease. Regional lymph node dissection was not performed. The details of the therapy were not described; however, no recurrences were reported for all three patients. In a further pediatric patient, 13 sentinel nodes from two lymph basins were examined (McMulkin et al. 2003) and found to be negative for malignancy. The patient was disease-free in follow-up, 32 months after excisional biopsy and adjuvant radiochemotherapy.

3.3.4
Epithelioid Sarcoma

Epithelioid sarcoma is rare malignancy, constituting less than 1% of all soft tissue sarcomas (de Visscher et al. 2006); it primarily affects the distal upper extremity and young male adults (Spillane et al. 2000; Baratti et al. 2007) and exhibits typical clinical features, such as a tendency to be multifocal and a high relapse rate. Regional lymph node metastasis occurs in 20%–30% of all patients and has been identified as an independent negative prognostic factor (Bos et al. 1988; Spillane et al. 2000; Baratti et al. 2007).

Although sentinel node biopsy for epithelioid sarcoma has been suggested by several authors (Blazer et al. 2003; de Visscher et al. 2006; Baratti et al. 2007), only one case has been described in the literature so far (Seal et al. 2005). The method was applied in a patient following marginal excision of an epithelioid sarcoma of the hand and local radiation of 50 Gy. The patient remained disease-free 16 months after negative sentinel biopsy and wide re-excision.

3.4
Discussion

The data presented above demonstrate how the rarity of soft tissue sarcomas, especially of the subtypes associated with a high rate of regional lymph node metastasis, renders assessing the possible benefits of applying sentinel node biopsy in these entities difficult. So far there have been reports of 31 cases from 10 different institutions over a period of 7 years. On the other hand, in order to participate in the large, multi-institutional trials designed to evaluate the use, accuracy, and morbidity of sentinel node biopsy in early-stage melanoma, all centers were required to complete a learning phase performing a minimum of 30 consecutive cases with a sentinel identification rate of at least 85%. For each individual surgeon the minimum was 15 consecutive cases (Morton et al. 2005), while similar recommendations apply for sentinel node biopsy in breast cancer (McMasters et al. 2000).

A further problem lies in the fact that, both in malignant melanoma and in breast cancer, the technique was introduced as an alternative to elective lymph node dissection, which was, until then, performed regularly in selected groups of patients. Therefore, the accuracy of the technique itself in early stages (and later on of the individual surgeon applying it) in predicting the tumor status of the regional basin could be easily evaluated by performing regional node dissections even in cases of negative sentinel nodes, thus histopathologically confirming the absence of tumor cells in the nonsentinel nodes. A similar approach cannot be justified for soft tissue sarcoma, since regional lymph node dissection is not recommended for patients with clinically negative nodes (Fong et al. 1993; Skinner and Eilber 1996; Behranwala et al. 2004).

A review of the published cases reveals that sentinel node biopsy can be performed successfully and safely in patients with soft tissue sarcomas of the extremities; at least one sentinel was identified in every patient, while no biopsy-related complications have been reported. The highest rate of patients with positive sentinel nodes was described in clear cell sarcoma, while false-negative biopsies have already been reported in clear cell sarcoma and synovial sarcoma. Several possible reasons have been proposed for false-negatives; insufficient experience with the technique, suboptimal pathological evaluation, obstruction of the lymphatics by tumor emboli or by a sentinel node grossly invaded by tumor, and prior operation or radiation (Neville et al. 2000c; Estourgie et al. 2003; Morton et al. 2005).

The limited number of patients, the inhomogeneity of patient status at presentation and of the therapeutic strategies that were followed, and the rather short recorded follow-up preclude definitive conclusions regarding the utility and prognostic significance of sentinel node biopsy in the subtypes of soft tissue sarcomas with a high propensity for regional lymphatic spread. In our opinion, these issues should be addressed in prospective multicenter trials.

References

Al-Refaie WB, Ali MW, Chu DZ, Paz IB, Blair SL (2004) Clear cell sarcoma in the era of sentinel lymph node mapping. J Surg Oncol 87:126–129

Albertini JJ, Cruse CW, Rapaport D, Wells K, Ross M, DeConti R, Berman CG, Jared K, Messina J, Lyman G, Glass F, Fenske N, Reintgen DS (1996) Intraoperative radio-lympho-scintigraphy improves sentinel lymph node identification for patients with melanoma. Ann Surg 223:217–224

Albores-Zúñiga O, Padilla-Rosciano AE, Martínez-Said H, Cuéllar-Hubbe M, Ramírez-Bollas J (2006) Clear cell sarcoma and sentinel lymph node biopsy. Case report and literature review. Cir Cir 74:121–125

Alex JC, Weaver DL, Fairbank JT, Rankin BS, Krag DN (1993) Gamma-probe-guided lymph node localization in malignant melanoma. Surg Oncol 2:303–308

Andrassy RJ, Okcu MF, Despa S, Raney RB (2001) Synovial sarcoma in children: surgical lessons from a single institution and review of the literature. J Am Coll Surg 192:305–313

Ariel IM (1988) Incidence of metastases to lymph nodes from soft-tissue sarcomas. Semin Surg Oncol 4:27–29

Baratti D, Pennacchioli E, Casali PG, Bertulli R, Lozza L, Olmi P, Collini P, Radaelli S, Fiore M, Gronchi A (2007) Epithelioid sarcoma: prognostic factors and survival in a series of patients treated at a single institution. Ann Surg Oncol 14:3542–3551

Behranwala KA, A'Hern R, Omar AM, Thomas JM (2004) Prognosis of lymph node metastasis in soft tissue sarcoma. Ann Surg Oncol 11:714–719

Bilchik AJ, DiNome M, Saha S, Turner RR, Wiese D, McCarter M, Hoon DS, Morton DL (2006) Prospective multicenter trial of staging adequacy in colon cancer: preliminary results. Arch Surg 141:527–533

Billingsley KG, Burt ME, Jara E, Ginsberg RJ, Woodruff JM, Leung DH, Brennan MF (1999) Pulmonary metastases from soft tissue sarcoma: analysis of patterns of diseases and postmetastasis survival. Ann Surg 229:602–610

Blazer DG 3rd, Sabel MS, Sondak VK (2003) Is there a role for sentinel lymph node biopsy in the management of sarcoma? Surg Oncol 12:201–206

Bos GD, Pritchard DJ, Reiman HM, Dobyns JH, Ilstrup DM, Landon GC (1988) Epithelioid sarcoma. An analysis of fifty-one cases. J Bone Joint Surg Am 70:862–870

Bostick P, Essner R, Glass E, Kelley M, Sarantou T, Foshag LJ, Qi K, Morton D (1999) Comparison of blue dye and probe-assisted intraoperative lymphatic mapping in melanoma to identify sentinel nodes in 100 lymphatic basins. Arch Surg 134:43–49

Cochran AJ, Balda BR, Starz H, Bachter D, Krag DN, Cruse CW, Pijpers R, Morton DL (2000) The Augsburg Consensus. Techniques of lymphatic mapping, sentinel lymphadenectomy, and completion lymphadenectomy in cutaneous malignancies. Cancer 89:236–241

Cook MG, Green MA, Anderson B, et al (2003) The development of optimal pathological assessment of sentinel lymph nodes for melanoma. J Pathol 200:314–319

Cserni G, Amendoeira I, Apostolikas N, et al (2003) Pathological work-up of sentinel lymph nodes in breast cancer. Review of current data to be considered for the formulation of guidelines. Eur J Cancer 39:1654–1667

de Visscher SA, van Ginkel RJ, Wobbes T, Veth RP, Ten Heuvel SE, Suurmeijer AJ, Hoekstra HJ (2006) Epithelioid sarcoma: still an only surgically curable disease. Cancer 107:606–612

Deenik W, Mooi WJ, Rutgers EJ, Peterse JL, Hart AA, Kroon BB (1999) Clear cell sarcoma (malignant melanoma) of soft parts: a clinicopathologic study of 30 cases. Cancer 86:969–975

Eckardt JJ, Pritchard DJ, Soule EH (1983) Clear cell sarcoma. A clinicopathologic study of 27 cases. Cancer 52:1482–1488

Esnaola NF, Rubin BP, Baldini EH, Vasudevan N, Demetri GD, Fletcher CD, Singer S (2001) Response to chemotherapy and predictors of survival in adult rhabdomyosarcoma. Ann Surg 234:215–223

Estourgie SH, Nieweg OE, Valdés Olmos RA, Hoefnagel CA, Kroon BB (2003) Review and evaluation of sentinel node procedures in 250 melanoma patients with a median follow-up of 6 years. Ann Surg Oncol 10:681–688

Fantini F, Monari P, Bassissi S, Maiorana A, Cesinaro A (2007) Sentinel lymph node biopsy in clear cell sarcoma. J Eur Acad Dermatol Venereol 21:1271–1272

Ferrari A, Gronchi A, Casanova M, Meazza C, Gandola L, Collini P, Lozza L, Bertulli R, Olmi P, Casali PG (2004) Synovial sarcoma: a retrospective analysis of 271 patients of all ages treated at a single institution. Cancer 101:627–634

Fong Y, Coit DG, Woodruff JM, Brennan MF (1993) Lymph node metastasis from soft tissue sarcoma in adults. Analysis of data from a prospective database of 1772 sarcoma patients. Ann Surg 217:72–77

Gadd MA, Casper ES, Woodruff JM, McCormack PM, Brennan MF (1993) Development and treatment of pulmonary metastases in adult patients with extremity soft tissue sarcoma. Ann Surg 218:705–712

Ham SJ, van der Graaf WT, Pras E, Molenaar WM, van den Berg E, Hoekstra HJ (1998) Soft tissue sarcoma of the extremities. A multimodality diagnostic and therapeutic approach. Cancer Treat Rev 24:373–391

Hawkins WG, Hoos A, Antonescu CR, Urist MJ, Leung DH, Gold JS, Woodruff JM, Lewis JJ, Brennan MF (2001) Clinicopathologic analysis of patients with adult rhabdomyosarcoma. Cancer 91:794–803

Jemal A, Siegel R, Ward E, Murray T, Xu J, Thun MJ (2007) Cancer statistics, 2007. CA Cancer J Clin 57:43–66

Kotilingam D, Lev DC, Lazar AJ, Pollock RE (2006) Staging soft tissue sarcoma: evolution and change. CA Cancer J Clin 56:282–291

Kuiper DR, Hoekstra HJ, Veth RP, Wobbes T (2003) The management of clear cell sarcoma. Eur J Surg Oncol 29:568–570

Lawrence W Jr, Hays DM, Heyn R, Tefft M, Crist W, Beltangady M, Newton W Jr, Wharam M (1987) Lymphatic metastases with childhood rhabdomyosarcoma. A report from the Intergroup Rhabdomyosarcoma Study. Cancer 60:910–915

Leong SP, Cady B, Jablons DM, Garcia-Aguilar J, Reintgen D, Jakub J, Pendas S, Duhaime L, Cassell R, Gardner M, Giuliano R, Archie V, Calvin D, Mensha L, Shivers S, Cox C, Werner JA, Kitagawa Y, Kitajima M (2006) Clinical patterns of metastasis. Cancer Metastasis Rev 25:221–232

Little DJ, Ballo MT, Zagars GK, Pisters PW, Patel SR, El-Naggar AK, Garden AS, Benjamin RS (2002) Adult rhabdomyosarcoma: outcome following multimodality treatment. Cancer 95:377–388

Mark RJ, Poen JC, Tran LM, Fu YS, Juillard GF (1996) Angiosarcoma. A report of 67 patients and a review of the literature. Cancer 77:2400–2406

Mazeron JJ, Suit HD (1987) Lymph nodes as sites of metastases from sarcomas of soft tissue. Cancer 60:1800–1808

McMasters KM, Tuttle TM, Carlson DJ, Brown CM, Noyes RD, Glaser RL, Vennekotter DJ, Turk PS, Tate PS, Sardi A, Cerrito PB, Edwards MJ (2000) Sentinel lymph node biopsy for breast cancer: a suitable alternative to routine axillary dissection in multi-institutional practice when optimal technique is used. J Clin Oncol 18:2560–2566

McMasters KM, Noyes RD, Reintgen DS, et al (2004) Lessons learned from the Sunbelt Melanoma Trial. J Surg Oncol 86:212–223

McMulkin HM, Yanchar NL, Fernandez CV, Giacomantonio C (2003) Sentinel lymph node mapping and biopsy: a potentially valuable tool in the management of childhood extremity rhabdomyosarcoma. Pediatr Surg Int 19:453–456

Micheli A, Mugno E, Krogh V, et al (2002) Cancer prevalence in European registry areas. Ann Oncol 13:840–865

Morton D, Cagle L, Wong J, et al (1990) Intraoperative lymphatic mapping and selective lymphadenectomy: technical details of a new procedure for clinical stage I melanoma. Presented at the Annual Meeting of the Society of Surgical Oncology. Washington DC

Morton DL, Wen DR, Wong JH, Economou JS, Cagle LA, Storm FK, Foshag LJ, Cochran AJ (1992) Technical details of intraoperative lymphatic mapping for early stage melanoma. Arch Surg 127:392–399

Morton DL, Thompson JF, Essner R, Elashoff R, Stern SL, Nieweg OE, Roses DF, Karakousis CP, Mozzillo N, Reintgen D, Wang HJ, Glass EC, Cochran AJ (1999) Validation of the accuracy of intraoperative lymphatic mapping and sentinel lymphadenectomy for early-stage melanoma: a multicenter trial. Multicenter Selective Lymphadenectomy Trial Group. Ann Surg 230:453–463

Morton DL, Cochran AJ, Thompson JF, et al (2005) Sentinel node biopsy for early-stage melanoma: accuracy and morbidity in MSLT-I, an international multicenter trial. Ann Surg 242:302–311

Naik AM, Fey J, Gemignani M, Heerdt A, Montgomery L, Petrek J, Port E, Sacchini V, Sclafani L, VanZee K,

Wagman R, Borgen PI, Cody HS 3rd (2004) The risk of axillary relapse after sentinel lymph node biopsy for breast cancer is comparable with that of axillary lymph node dissection: a follow-up study of 4008 procedures. Ann Surg 240:462–468

Neville HL, Andrassy RJ, Lally KP, Corpron C, Ross MI (2000a) Lymphatic mapping with sentinel node biopsy in pediatric patients. J Pediatr Surg 35:961–964

Neville HL, Andrassy RJ, Lobe TE, Bagwell CE, Anderson JR, Womer RB, Crist WM, Wiener ES (2000b) Preoperative staging, prognostic factors, and outcome for extremity rhabdomyosarcoma: a preliminary report from the Intergroup Rhabdomyosarcoma Study IV (1991–1997). J Pediatr Surg 35:317–321

Neville HL, Raney RB, Andrassy RJ, Cooley DA (2000c) Multidisciplinary management of pediatric soft-tissue sarcoma. Oncology 14:1471–1481

Nieweg OE, Tanis PJ, Kroon BB (2001) The definition of a sentinel node. Ann Surg Oncol 8:538–541

Nishida Y, Yamada Y, Tsukushi S, Shibata S, Ishiguro N (2005) Sentinel lymph node biopsy reveals a positive popliteal node in clear cell sarcoma. Anticancer Res 25:4413–4416

Okcu MF, Munsell M, Treuner J, Mattke A, Pappo A, Cain A, Ferrari A, Casanova M, Ozkan A, Raney B (2003) Synovial sarcoma of childhood and adolescence: a multicenter, multivariate analysis of outcome. J Clin Oncol 21:1602–1611

Picciotto F, Zaccagna A, Derosa G, Pisacane A, Puiatti P, Colombo E, Dardano F, Ottinetti A (2005) Clear cell sarcoma (malignant melanoma of soft parts) and sentinel lymph node biopsy. Eur J Dermatol 15:46–48

Potter DA, Glenn J, Kinsella T, Glatstein E, Lack EE, Restrepo C, White DE, Seipp CA, Wesley R, Rosenberg SA (1985) Patterns of recurrence in patients with high-grade soft-tissue sarcomas. J Clin Oncol 3:353–366

Riad S, Griffin AM, Liberman B, Blackstein ME, Catton CN, Kandel RA, O'Sullivan B, White LM, Bell RS, Ferguson PC, Wunder JS (2004) Lymph node metastasis in soft tissue sarcoma in an extremity. Clin Orthop Relat Res 129–134

Ruka W, Emrich LJ, Driscoll DL, Karakousis CP (1988) Prognostic significance of lymph node metastasis and bone, major vessel, or nerve involvement in adults with high-grade soft tissue sarcomas. Cancer 62:999–1006

Rydholm A, Berg NO, Gullberg B, Thorngren KG, Persson BM (1984) Epidemiology of soft-tissue sarcoma in the locomotor system. A retrospective population-based study of the inter-relationships between clinical and morphologic variables. Acta Pathol Microbiol Immunol Scand 92:363–374

Seal A, Tse R, Wehrli B, Hammond A, Temple CL (2005) Sentinel node biopsy as an adjunct to limb salvage surgery for epithelioid sarcoma of the hand. World J Surg Oncol 3:41

Skinner KA, Eilber FR (1996) Soft tissue sarcoma nodal metastases: biologic significance and therapeutic considerations. Surg Oncol Clin N Am 5:121–127

Spillane AJ, Thomas JM, Fisher C (2000) Epithelioid sarcoma: the clinicopathological complexities of this rare soft tissue sarcoma. Ann Surg Oncol 7:218–225

Spurrell EL, Fisher C, Thomas JM, Judson IR (2005) Prognostic factors in advanced synovial sarcoma: an analysis of 104 patients treated at the Royal Marsden Hospital. Ann Oncol 16:437–444

Takeuchi H, Morton DL, Kuo C, Turner RR, Elashoff D, Elashoff R, Taback B, Fujimoto A, Hoon DS (2004) Prognostic significance of molecular upstaging of paraffin-embedded sentinel lymph nodes in melanoma patients. J Clin Oncol 22:2671–2680

Tunn PU, Andreou D, Illing H, Fleige B, Dresel S, Schlag PM (2007) Sentinel node biopsy in synovial sarcoma. Eur J Surg Oncol doi:10.1016/j.ejso.2007.07.014

van Akkooi AC, Verhoef C, van Geel AN, Kliffen M, Eggermont AM, de Wilt JH (2006) Sentinel node biopsy for clear cell sarcoma. Eur J Surg Oncol 32:996–999

van der Veen H, Hoekstra OS, Paul MA, Cuesta MA, Meijer S (1994) Gamma probe-guided sentinel node biopsy to select patients with melanoma for lymphadenectomy. Br J Surg 81:1769–1770

Weingrad DN, Rosenberg SA (1978) Early lymphatic spread of osteogenic and soft-tissue sarcomas. Surgery 84:231–240

Wharam MD, Meza J, Anderson J, Breneman JC, Donaldson SS, Fitzgerald TJ, Michalski J, Teot LA, Wiener ES, Meyer WH (2004) Failure pattern and factors predictive of local failure in rhabdomyosarcoma: a report of group III patients on the third Intergroup Rhabdomyosarcoma Study. J Clin Oncol 22:1902–1908

Part II
Bone Sarcomas

Modular Endoprosthetic Reconstruction in Malignant Bone Tumors: Indications and Limits

Maurice Balke, Helmut Ahrens, Arne Streitbürger, Georg Gosheger, and Jendrik Hardes

Abstract Modular tumor prostheses are well established today for the reconstruction of osseous defects after resection of malignant bone tumors. Almost every joint and even total bones (e.g., total femur or humerus) can be replaced with promising functional results, dramatically reducing the need for ablative procedures. Although the complication rate with the use of modern modular endoprostheses is constantly decreasing, the need for revision surgery is still significantly higher than in primary joint arthroplasty. In this review we present the modular endoprosthesis system developed in our institution, summarize the postoperative management, and discuss the indications, limits, and complications as well as the functional results.

Maurice Balke (✉)
Department of Orthopedics
University of Muenster
Albert-Schweitzer-Str. 33
48149 Müenster, Germany
E-mail: maurice.balke@web.de

4.1 Introduction

Nowadays the majority of patients with malignant bone tumors can be treated with limb salvage procedures whenever wide margins are achievable (Mittermayer et al. 2001; Sluga et al. 1999). If reasonable from an oncological point of view ablative measures such as amputations or rotationplasty almost never become necessary. The use of tumor prostheses for reconstruction has gained more and more acceptance over the past few decades and has not shown any adverse effect on local recurrence and survival (Gosheger et al. 2006; Ruggieri et al. 1993). While custom-made material was used in the beginning of the era of tumor prostheses, surgeons now accept the modern modular replacement systems as state-of-the-art (Wirganowicz et al. 1999; Zeegen et al. 2004).

Custom-made implants were expensive and time-consuming in fabrication, which sometimes led to a reduced outcome due to delayed optimal therapy. With modern modular endoprostheses, defects of some of the most extreme cases can be reconstructed individually, achieving excellent functional results while saving time and resources (Tunn et al. 2004).

During the last 30 years the 5-year survival rate of megaendoprostheses has increased dramatically from 20% to 85%, despite patients being generally young and physically active and putting high demands on the material (Mittermayer et al. 2001). Nevertheless, the complication rate cannot compete with primary joint arthroplasty (Donati et al. 2001; Eckardt et al. 1985; Safran et al. 1994).

In the following we will give an overview of the modular endoprosthesis system used in our department, provide advice for postoperative management, and summarize its indications, typical complications, and limits as well as functional outcome.

4.2 Surgical Technique

With the use of the Modular Universal Tumor and Revision System (MUTARS—Implantcast, Buxtehude), major osseous defects of the upper and lower extremities can be successfully reconstructed (Gosheger et al. 2006).

The modular design allows individual reconstruction of defects in 2-cm steps and torsion adjustments in 5° increments (Fig. 4.1). The different modular components are fixed with screws.

Frequently, tumor prostheses are used for reconstruction of the proximal and distal femur, the proximal tibia, and proximal humerus. Even replacements of total bones, such as the total femur or humerus including the adjacent joints, are becoming increasingly common (Gosheger et al. 2006; Ward et al. 1995).

Nowadays stem-anchorage of most tumor prostheses can be accomplished without bone cement. We use hydroxyapatite-coated titanium stems with a hexagonal shape that provide excellent primary rotation stability (Fig. 4.1). The usual stems have a length of 12 cm whereas the diameter is planned individually on digital X-rays (usually not measuring below the 12-mm core diameter).

Cemented anchorage in tumor prostheses is mostly indicated in (1) older patients (over 60 years of age), (2) those with advanced osteopenia, prolonged preoperative immobilization, or neoadjuvant chemotherapy, and (3) cases in which press-fit anchorage in the meta-diaphyseal region is impossible.

The articulating parts are usually connected with a rotating hinge and a polyethylene inlay. In cases in which extraordinary forces occur, such as total or distal femoral replacement or after extraarticular knee-joint resections, the new PEEK-Optima lock shows excellent properties for femoro-tibial locking. It has been available since 2003 and shows a fatigue strength that is five times higher than in polyethylene.

Refixation of muscles and tendons (e.g., gluteal muscles in proximal femur, patellar

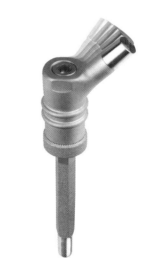

Fig. 4.1 MUTARS proximal femur with hydroxyapatite-coated titanium stem. The hexagonal shape provides excellent primary rotation stability. The modular design allows torsion adjustments in 5° increments

ligament in proximal tibia, or rotator-cuff in proximal humerus) is usually accomplished by sewing to a MUTARS attachment tube (Implantcast, Buxtehude) tied around the prosthesis (Gosheger et al. 2001; Fig. 4.2). Moreover, this strong and durable yet flexible material (polyethylene terephthalate—PET) is routinely used for refixation of the gastrocnemius flap for defect-coverage, especially in the proximal tibia. In these cases, where tension-free primary wound closure is hardly possible, an additional mesh-graft often becomes unavoidable.

Besides its use for refixation of soft tissue and tendons, the MUTARS attachment tube provides excellent results in reconstruction of capsular structures (Fig. 4.2) in proximal femur replacement (Gosheger et al. 2001). In combination with a bipolar cup we were able to completely prevent postoperative dislocation in our patient collective (Bickels et al. 2000; Gosheger et al. 2001; Morris et al. 1995).

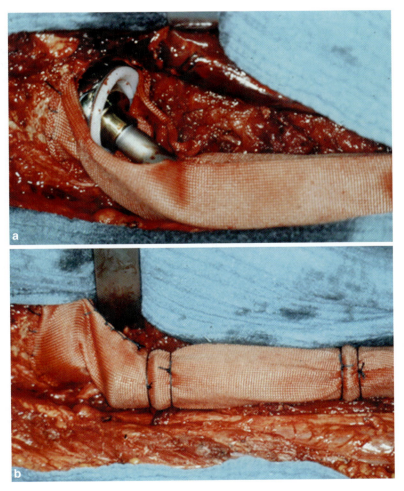

Fig. 4.2 MUTARS attachment tube in proximal femur reconstruction in combination with a bipolar cup **a** before and **b** after closure and fixation of the neo-capsule

4.3 Postoperative Management

Postoperatively all patients are treated with intravenous antibiotics (e.g., cephalosporin of third generation) for 3–7 days, followed by oral medication until completion of wound healing. Moreover, patients are informed about the necessity of prophylactic intake of antibiotics in cases of possible bacteremia (e.g., systemic/local infections or dental treatment) preventing the danger of hematogenous seeding and late endoprosthetic infections.

Patients with proximal humerus reconstruction are immobilized for 4–6 weeks in a Gilchrist-bandage in which training of the elbow, wrist, and fingers usually remains unrestricted.

We follow a relatively strict immobilization regimen after cementless implantation of tumor prostheses in the lower extremities: 6 weeks of 10 kg weight bearing followed by a stepwise increase of 5–10 kg per week (depending on the patient's weight) until achievement of full weight bearing. In patients with proximal femur replacement in combination with a bipolar cup and MUTARS attachment tube, range of motion of the hip joint is unrestricted, even immediately after the operation. When an acetabular cup is implanted additionally, bed rest of 4 weeks is necessary to prevent possible dislocation until the full stability of the scar tissue of the "new" capsule is developed. Range of motion in patients with distal femur replacement is only limited (4 weeks immobilization in extension) when a gastrocnemius muscle flap is performed for better coverage of the prosthesis. In proximal tibia replacement, immobilization of the extended knee joint is essential due to the reattachment of the patellar ligament to the attachment tube. This is usually accomplished by wearing a knee immobilizer for 4 weeks. From the fifth week, post-operative mobilization has to be started but should be restricted to a maximal flexion of 90°. Otherwise an accelerated wear of the polyethylene bushing is at risk.

When a mesh graft is necessary to allow tension-free skin closure (especially in distal femur or proximal tibia) we usually achieve excellent results with an additional vacuum-sealing of the graft for the first 5 days.

After resection of tumors involving the knee joint, eminent attention has to be turned to weakness or paralysis of the anterior and lateral compartment muscles, resulting in foot drop.

The common fibular nerve with its terminal branches is explored routinely and may be affected by hooks as well as edema or hematoma. Mild pressure or stretching of the nerve can produce a temporary impairment of local circulation that interrupts normal nerve conduction. If foot drop is apparent, a prophylaxis of plantar flexion contracture should be started immediately and an ankle–foot orthosis (AFO) should be prescribed. The lesion is usually incomplete, and in most cases the function recovers within a few months.

4.4 Complications

Local recurrence is the worst possible complication, accompanied as it is by a dismal prognosis (Picci et al. 1994). The rate of local recurrence after limb salvage with tumor prostheses in the literature ranges from 1% to 9% (Table 4.1), which is comparable to ablative procedures (Eckardt et al. 1985; Tunn et al. 2004). To avoid this result at least a wide resection according to Enneking (1988) is required.

The 5- to 10-year survival rate for modern megaendoprostheses averages from 69% to 90% (Table 4.2; Gosheger et al. 2006; Horowitz et al. 1991; Kumar et al. 2003). Due to their lower general exposure, reconstructions of the upper extremities and hip have higher survival rates than reconstructions around the knee joint (Gosheger et al. 2006; Horowitz et al. 1991,

1993; Malawer and Chou 1995; Morris et al. 1995; Roberts et al. 1991; Zeegen et al. 2004).

The most common complications leading to explantation of the prosthesis are aseptical loosening, periprosthetic infection, and fracture of the stem or adjacent bone (Table 4.1; Ham et al. 1998; Mittermayer et al. 2001; Shin et al. 1999; Unwin et al. 1996; Wirganowicz et al. 1999; Zeegen et al. 2004). The literature indicates infection rates from 1% to 36% with the lowest rates for upper extremity and the highest rates for reconstruction of the proximal tibia (Grimer et al. 1999; Kumar et al. 2003). In case of infection, a two-stage approach with a temporary static cement spacer charged with antibiotics prior to reimplantation of the prosthesis usually becomes unavoidable (Grimer et al. 2002; Hardes et al. 2006). Only in early infections is a one-stage procedure with debridement, pulse lavage, and replacement of the polyethylene bushing possibly sufficient (Hardes et al. 2006). Deep infection constitutes the most serious complication at which, when uncontrollable, secondary amputation frequently

Table 4.1 Average complication rates in endoprosthetic reconstructions

Complication	Average rate	Literature
Local recurrence	1%–9%	Asavamongkolkul et al. 1999; Bickels et al. 2000; Bos et al. 1987; Eckardt et al. 1985; Gosheger et al. 2006; Ilyas et al. 2002; Morris et al. 1995; Plotz et al. 2002; Tunn et al. 2004
Aseptical loosening	5%–27%	Bickels et al. 2000; Gosheger et al. 2006; Ilyas et al. 2002; Mittermayer et al. 2001; Plotz et al. 2002; Unwin et al. 1996
Periprosthetic infection	1%–36%	Gosheger et al. 2006; Grimer et al. 1999; Ilyas et al. 2002; Kabukcuoglu et al. 1999; Kumar et al. 2003; Mittermayer et al. 2001; Morris et al. 1995
Fracture of the stem or adjacent bone	1%–22%	Gosheger et al. 2006; Grimer et al. 1999; Mittermayer et al. 2001; Plotz et al. 2002
Dislocation (proximal humerus)	11%–56%	Asavamongkolkul et al. 1999; Bos et al. 1987; Kumar et al. 2003; Ross et al. 1987
Dislocation (proximal femur)	0%–20%	Bickels et al. 2000; Donati et al. 2001; Gosheger et al. 2001; Ilyas et al. 2002; Kabukcuoglu et al. 1999; Morris et al. 1995; Ward et al. 1995

Table 4.2 Average 5- to 10-year prosthetic survival rates

Prosthetic survival	Average rate	Literature
5-year survival	69%–90%	
Upper extremity	89%–90%	Asavamongkolkul et al. 1999; Gosheger et al. 2006
Lower extremity	69%–87%	Gosheger et al. 2006; Ham et al. 1998; Kabukcuoglu et al. 1999; Mittermayer et al. 2001; Plotz et al. 2002; Zeegen et al. 2004
10-year survival	69%–87%	
Upper extremity	87%	Kumar et al. 2003
Lower extremity	69%–80%	Ham et al. 1998; Mittermayer et al. 2001; Plotz et al. 2002

(19%–46%) becomes necessary (Jeys et al. 2003; Malawer and Chou 1995). It increasingly seems as if the routine use of an antibacterial silver coating in MUTARS tumor prostheses is able to reduce the rate of infection without any toxicological side effects (Gosheger et al. 2004; Hardes et al. 2007).

Aseptical loosening of the stem occurs in up to 27% in the lower extremity (Table 4.1). In these cases revision surgery is almost always feasible (Mittermayer et al. 2001; Plotz et al. 2002). Even stem fractures with an incidence of 1%–22% are usually reparable (Grimer et al. 1999; Hardes et al. 2006; Plotz et al. 2002).

The complications described so far require major operations with at least a partial replacement of the prosthesis. Wear of the polyethylene bushing necessitates only minor surgical treatment (Mittermayer et al. 2001). Failure of the bushing is not as much a "complication" as a normal side effect of extensive usage, especially in young and active patients.

Wear of the polyethylene manifests in increasing instability of the joint. A repair should be performed early because the debris might induce aseptical loosening (Mittermayer et al. 2001, 2002).

The most common complication in proximal humerus replacement is the high dislocation rate (Table 4.1) due to resection of the rotator-cuff (Bos et al. 1987; Ross et al. 1987). It can be reduced by reattaching the remaining muscles to a MUTARS attachment tube (Asavamongkolkul et al. 1999; Kumar et al. 2003).

The dislocation rate in proximal femur replacement is reported in the literature with an incidence of up to 20% (Table 4.1; Bickels et al. 2000; Donati et al. 2001; Ilyas et al. 2002; Kabukcuoglu et al. 1999; Ward et al. 1995). In our department the use of a bipolar cup combined with the MUTARS attachment tube for reconstruction of the joint capsule and reattachment of the muscles (abductor muscles, iliopsoas muscle) reduced dislocation to 0% (Bickels et al. 2000; Gosheger et al. 2001; Morris et al. 1995).

Also in replacement of the proximal tibia, the attachment tube excelled as a reliable way to restore the extensor mechanism. Refixation of the patellar ligament to the tube—if necessary augmented with a gastrocnemius flap—leads to good functional results in active knee extension (Gosheger et al. 2006; Grimer et al. 1999; Fig. 4.3). A relevant weakening of the extensors, which occurs frequently if the tendon is directly fixed to the prosthesis, can be avoided (Bickels et al. 2001; Gosheger et al. 2006; Grimer et al. 1999).

4.5
Indications and Limits

Constant improvements of prostheses material and surgical techniques lead to a steadily increasing number of patients with limb-sparing procedures using modular tumor prostheses (Capanna et al. 1994; Fuchs et al. 1998; Sluga et al. 1999).

The typical indication for modular endoprostheses is a large osseous defect after resection of a malignant bone tumor of the meta-diaphyseal region of a long bone in the upper or lower extremity.

Involvement of major vessels by the tumor is still considered as a contraindication to limb salvage surgery (Lawrence 1988). But even in these cases patients can be saved from mutilating procedures. Limb salvage can nowadays be performed with modular endoprostheses and vascular reconstruction with good oncological and functional results. Thus the need for rotationplasty or amputation is decreasing (Leggon et al. 2001).

Another limitation for the usage of tumor prostheses is the infiltration of the extensor mechanism, especially in malignancies around the knee. If extraarticular resection becomes necessary the extensor muscles should be at least partially preserved. Otherwise defect

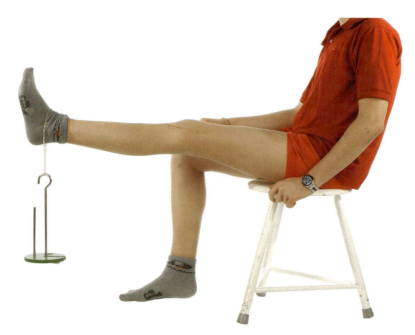

Fig. 4.3 Functional outcome after proximal tibia replacement and refixation of the patellar ligament to the attachment tube

coverage is hardly possible and limb function is unsatisfying. But even when large parts of the quadriceps femoris muscles have to be resected, the extensor mechanism can be augmented by a muscle flap of the biceps femoris and gastrocnemius reattached to a MUTARS attachment tube. If more stability is needed an additional orthosis with stance security can be prescribed.

Tumor prostheses reach their limits in cases of deep infections with poor soft tissue condition (e.g., extensive wound necrosis or skin induration due to irradiation). In patients with infections related to tumor prosthesis, limb salvage fails in approximately 30% of cases, depending on the soft tissue condition (Hardes et al. 2006). Even the new antibacterial silver coating is unable to countervail the poor soft tissue condition (Hardes et al. 2007) so that ablative surgery should be performed early to avoid repeated revision surgery (Hardes et al. 2006).

4.5.1
Tumor Prostheses in Children

Although reconstruction with modular endoprostheses has become the treatment of choice in adults, this cannot be transferred to bone tumors during childhood. Many surgeons still believe that the use of tumor prostheses is not a reasonable approach before the age of 11–13 (Cortes et al. 1974; Tunn et al. 2004). The combination of significant limb length discrepancies at maturity and the difficulties with participating in active rehabilitation programs for children compromised the good results achieved in adults. In very young patients limb ablation—including rotationplasty—is still a common procedure, because it is not usually accompanied by relevant surgical problems. As a one-step operation rotationplasty may be performed with good functional results (Hillmann et al. 1999;

Kotz et al. 1992; Kotz and Salzer 1982), but like amputation it is a mutilating procedure. Especially in children that are close to puberty its stigmatizing effect is not to be neglected. Nowadays this procedure should be reserved for selected cases. The reasonable alternative of osteoarticular allografts is accompanied by a very high complication rate and cannot prevent growth impairment (Mankin et al. 1996).

To date, endoprosthesis systems are still cautiously used in children due to complications caused by the limb length inequality and the frequent surgery necessary for elongation procedures. The invasive methods cause significant hospitalization time, time off from school, extensive scar formation, and increased risk of infection. In the worst cases this may finally lead to amputation (Capanna et al. 1994; Fuchs et al. 1998; Kawai et al. 1998; Renard et al. 1998; Ruggieri et al. 1993).

For almost 30 years modular expandable prostheses have been on the market. The basic technique for lengthening usually consists of a fixed stem with a screw extension mechanism, as in, for example, the Lewis expandable adjustable prosthesis (LEAP), introduced in 1983 (Kenan et al. 1991; Kenan and Lewis 1991; Lewis 1986) or later in the Howmedica Modular Reconstruction System (HMRS) with custom-made growth modules housed within the prosthesis (Kotz et al. 1990, 1991). The elongation is performed by insertion of a chuck key to turn the screw mechanism, thereby expanding the tubular portion of the prosthesis (Lewis et al. 1987). Other designs focus on modular systems in which a midsection is sequentially replaced by a longer one whenever elongation becomes necessary. But in both designs there is still the need for surgery with all the drawbacks mentioned above, including neurological compromise due to stretch injuries, vascular injury, and loss of motion (Babyn et al. 2001; Paley 1990; Renard et al. 2000). The maximal increase in length is limited to approximately 2 cm for each elongation procedure.

Perhaps the progress in modern growing prostheses such as the Phenix Growing Prosthesis (Phenix Medical, Paris, France) (Wilkins and Soubeiran 2001) or new generations of the HMRS (Krepler et al. 2003) will solve some of these problems. The mentioned prostheses usually consist of two hollow tubes containing a spring-loaded coil that is immobilized by a solid piece of plastic. When length adjustment is required the plastic is heated (for example by an external electromagnetic field), which melts it and releases the spring causing elongation until the plastic cools again. If possible minimal resurfacing using a press-fit prosthetic stem with a smooth surface can preserve the growth plate in the uninvolved side of the joint.

The new MUTARS Expand uses a similar approach. A motor housed in the prosthesis is connected to a subcutaneous receiver and can be activated and controlled by an external device, allowing exact length adjustment (up to 10 cm) without any surgery (Fig. 4.4). Both systems can be controlled in the outpatient clinic without hospitalization.

All these prostheses are designed to bear the corresponding loads over several years but they are only adjustable in length and do not grow concomitantly in strength and breadth. The devices might be at greater risk of breaking under the adult weight and finally would have to be replaced by a permanent implant.

After unsatisfying results at the beginning of the era of growing prostheses, the first experiences with the new systems are promising. But whether they will prove of value in practice can only be answered over time.

4.6
Functional Results

The functional results after reconstruction of bone defects in tumor surgery are promising and can be scored according to Enneking et al. (1993).

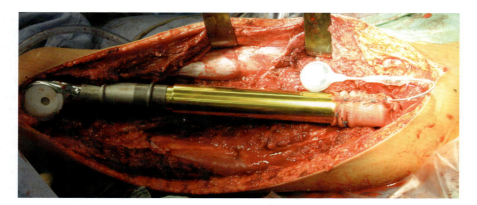

Fig. 4.4 MUTARS growing prosthesis in total femur replacement with attachment tube for capsular reconstruction of the hip joint. Note the small implant connected to an internal motor that is implanted subcutaneously and can be controlled by an external device

Herein subjective parameters (contentedness, pain, etc.) as well as functional parameters (range of motion, walking distance, use of walking aids, etc.) play a role. A score of 100% means unlimited function of the affected extremity. In the literature the average range shown is 60%–90% (Horowitz et al. 1993; Ilyas et al. 2002; Mittermayer et al. 2001; Plotz et al. 2002). We achieved the best results in patients with proximal tibia replacement (83%) followed by distal femur replacement (80%). Patients with proximal femur replacement achieved an average score of 70% (Gosheger et al. 2006). It has to be noted that, especially in elderly patients, they retain a Trendelenburg gait and most need a cane on the healthy side when performing longer walks, even if the gluteal muscles are reattached to the MUTARS attachment tube. Patients with replacement of the proximal humerus achieved an average of "only" 70%, which can be explained by the impaired range of motion of the shoulder joint. Due to resection of sizable parts of the rotator-cuff and deltoid muscle, which is unpreventable in removal of the tumor, patients can hardly elevate the arm more than 60° and abduct more than 30°. All patients are able to move their hand to their mouth (Gosheger et al. 2006). The new inverse shoulder prostheses might improve the functional outcome by restoring the function of the rotator-cuff, since it might be possible to preserve the axillary nerve and relevant parts of the deltoid muscle.

Summary

Limb salvage with tumor prostheses has become a routine procedure leading to excellent functional results. But especially in the case of young and active patients, who represent the "typical" bone-tumor patient, the material is pushed to its physical limits; mechanical complications seem to be almost unavoidable. Fortunately revision surgery of these complications is almost always successful.

The use of the MUTARS attachment tube can prevent dislocations after proximal femur replacement and lead to better functional results in reconstructions of the proximal tibia (Gosheger et al. 2006). The most severe complication besides local recurrence remains periprosthetic infection (Gosheger et al. 2006; Mittermayer et al. 2001). We hope that the use of the new antibacterial silver coating of MUTARS prostheses can significantly reduce the rate of infection without toxicological side effects (Gosheger et al. 2006; Gosheger et al. 2004; Hardes et al. 2007).

Due to constant improvements of prostheses material and surgical techniques, the indications and limits of limb salvage with modular tumor prostheses are continuously changing and to some extent might have to be reconsidered.

References

Asavamongkolkul A, Eckardt JJ, Eilber FR, Dorey FJ, Ward WG, Kelly CM, Wirganowicz PZ, Kabo JM (1999) Endoprosthetic reconstruction for malignant upper extremity tumors. Clin Orthop Relat Res 360:207–220

Babyn PS, Wihlborg CE, Tjong JK, Alman BA, Silberberg PJ (2001) Local complications after limb-salvage surgery for pediatric bone tumours: a pictorial essay. Can Assoc Radiol J 52:35–42

Bickels J, Meller I, Henshaw RM, Malawar MM (2000) Reconstruction of hip stability after proximal and total femur resections. Clin Orthop Relat Res 375:218–230

Bickels J, Wittig JC, Kollender Y, Neff RS, Kellar-Graney K, Meller I, Malawer MM (2001) Reconstruction of the extensor mechanism after proximal tibia endoprosthetic replacement. J Arthroplasty 16:856–862

Bos G, Sim F, Pritchard D, Shives T, Rock M, Askew L, Chao E (1987) Prosthetic replacement of the proximal humerus. Clin Orthop Relat Res 224:178–191

Capanna R, Morris HG, Campanacci D, Del Ben M, Campanacci M (1994) Modular uncemented prosthetic reconstruction after resection of tumours of the distal femur. J Bone Joint Surg Br 76:178–186

Cortes EP, Holland JF, Wang JJ, Sinks LF, Blom J, Senn H, Bank A, Glidewell O (1974) Amputation and adriamycin in primary osteosarcoma. N Engl J Med 291:998–1000

Donati D, Zavatta M, Gozzi E, Giacomini S, Campanacci D, Mercuri M (2001) Modular prosthetic replacement of the proximal femur after resection of a bone tumour a long-term follow-up. J Bone Joint Surg Br 83:1156–1160

Eckardt JJ, Eilber FR, Dorey FJ, Mirra JM (1985) The UCLA experience in limb salvage surgery for malignant tumors. Orthopedics 8:612–621

Enneking WF (1988) A system of staging musculoskeletal neoplasms. Instr Course Lect 37:3–10

Enneking WF, Dunham W, Gebhardt MC, Malawar M, Pritchard DJ (1993) A system for the functional evaluation of reconstructive procedures after surgical treatment of tumors of the musculoskeletal system. Clin Orthop Relat Res 286:241–246

Fuchs N, Bielack S, Epler D, Bieling P, Delling G, Korholz D, Graf N, Heise U, Jurgens H, Kotz R, Salzer-Kuntschik M, Weinel P, Werner M, Winkler K (1998) Long-term results of the co-operative German-Austrian-Swiss osteosarcoma study group's protocol COSS-86 of intensive multidrug chemotherapy and surgery for osteosarcoma of the limbs. Ann Oncol 9:893–899

Gosheger G, Hillmann A, Lindner N, Rodl R, Hoffmann C, Burger H, Winkelmann W (2001) Soft tissue reconstruction of megaprostheses using a trevira tube. Clin Orthop Relat Res 393:264–271

Gosheger G, Hardes J, Ahrens H, Streitburger A, Buerger H, Erren M, Gunsel A, Kemper FH, Winkelmann W, Von Eiff C (2004) Silver-coated megaendoprostheses in a rabbit model—an analysis of the infection rate and toxicological side effects. Biomaterials 25:5547–5556

Gosheger G, Gebert C, Ahrens H, Streitburger A, Winkelmann W, Hardes J (2006) Endoprosthetic reconstruction in 250 patients with sarcoma. Clin Orthop Relat Res 450:164–171

Grimer RJ, Carter SR, Tillman RM, Sneath RS, Walker PS, Unwin PS, Shewell PC (1999) Endoprosthetic replacement of the proximal tibia. J Bone Joint Surg Br 81:488–494

Grimer RJ, Belthur M, Chandrasekar C, Carter SR, Tillman RM (2002) Two-stage revision for infected endoprostheses used in tumor surgery. Clin Orthop Relat Res 395:193–203

Ham SJ, Schraffordt Koops H, Veth RP, van Horn JR, Molenaar WM, Hoekstra HJ (1998) Limb salvage surgery for primary bone sarcoma of the lower extremities: long-term consequences of endoprosthetic reconstructions. Ann Surg Oncol 5:423–436

Hardes J, Gebert C, Schwappach A, Ahrens H, Streitburger A, Winkelmann W, Gosheger G (2006) Characteristics and outcome of infections associated with tumor endoprostheses. Arch Orthop Trauma Surg 126:289–296

Hardes J, Ahrens H, Gebert C, Streitbuerger A, Buerger H, Erren M, Gunsel A, Wedemeyer C, Saxler G, Winkelmann W, Gosheger G (2007) Lack of toxicological side-effects in silver-coated megaprostheses in humans. Biomaterials 28:2869–2875

Hillmann A, Hoffmann C, Gosheger G, Krakau H, Winkelmann W (1999) Malignant tumor of the distal part of the femur or the proximal part of the tibia: endoprosthetic replacement or rotationplasty. Functional outcome and quality-of-life measurements. J Bone Joint Surg Am 81:462–468

Horowitz SM, Lane JM, Otis JC, Healey JH (1991) Prosthetic arthroplasty of the knee after resection of a sarcoma in the proximal end of the tibia. A report of sixteen cases. J Bone Joint Surg Am 73:286–293

Horowitz SM, Glasser DB, Lane JM, Healey JH (1993) Prosthetic and extremity survivorship after limb salvage for sarcoma. How long do the reconstructions last? Clin Orthop Relat Res 293:280–286

Ilyas I, Pant R, Kurar A, Moreau PG, Younge DA (2002) Modular megaprosthesis for proximal femoral tumors. Int Orthop 26:170–173

Jeys LM, Grimer RJ, Carter SR, Tillman RM (2003) Risk of amputation following limb salvage surgery with endoprosthetic replacement, in a consecutive series of 1261 patients. Int Orthop 27:160–163

Kabukcuoglu Y, Grimer RJ, Tillman RM, Carter SR (1999) Endoprosthetic replacement for primary malignant tumors of the proximal femur. Clin Orthop Relat Res 358:8–14

Kawai A, Backus SI, Otis JC, Healey JH (1998) Interrelationships of clinical outcome, length of resection, and energy cost of walking after prosthetic knee replacement following resection of a malignant tumor of the distal aspect of the femur. J Bone Joint Surg Am 80:822–831

Kenan S, Lewis MM (1991) Limb salvage in pediatric surgery. The use of the expandable prosthesis. Orthop Clin North Am 22:121–131

Kenan S, Bloom N, Lewis MM (1991) Limb-sparing surgery in skeletally immature patients with osteosarcoma. The use of an expandable prosthesis. Clin Orthop Relat Res 270:223–230

Kotz R, Salzer M (1982) Rotation-plasty for childhood osteosarcoma of the distal part of the femur. J Bone Joint Surg Am 64:959–969

Kotz R, Ritschl P, Kropej D, Capanna R (1990) Cementless modular prostheses. Basic concepts and evolution. Chir Organi Mov 75[Suppl 1]:177–178

Kotz R, Schiller C, Windhager R, Ritschl P (1991) Endoprostheses in children: first results. In: Langlais F, Tomeno B (eds) Limb salvage: major reconstructions in oncologic and nontumoral conditions. Springer Verlag, Berlin Heidelberg New York, pp 591–599

Kotz R, Ritschl P, Kropej D, Schiller C, Wurnig C, Salzer-Kuntschik M (1992) The limits of saving the extremity—amputation versus resection [in German]. Z Orthop Ihre Grenzgeb 130:299–305

Krepler P, Dominkus M, Toma CD, Kotz R (2003) Endoprosthesis management of the extremities of children after resection of primary malignant bone tumors [in German]. Orthopade 32:1013–1019

Kumar D, Grimer RJ, Abudu A, Carter SR, Tillman RM (2003) Endoprosthetic replacement of the proximal humerus. Long-term results. J Bone Joint Surg Br 85:717–722

Lawrence W Jr (1988) Concepts in limb-sparing treatment of adult soft tissue sarcomas. Semin Surg Oncol 4:73–77

Leggon RE, Huber TS, Scarborough MT (2001) Limb salvage surgery with vascular reconstruction. Clin Orthop Relat Res 387:207–216

Lewis MM (1986) The use of an expandable and adjustable prosthesis in the treatment of childhood malignant bone tumors of the extremity. Cancer 57:499–502

Lewis MM, Pafford J, Spires WJ (1987) The expandable prosthesis: tumor prosthesis in children. In: Coombs R, Friedlaender G (eds) Bone tumor management. Butterworths, London

Malawer MM, Chou B (1995) Prosthetic survival and clinical results with use of large-segment replacements in the treatment of high-grade bone sarcomas. J Bone Joint Surg Am 77:1154–1165

Mankin HJ, Gebhardt MC, Jennings LC, Springfield DS, Tomford WW (1996) Long-term results of allograft replacement in the management of bone tumors. Clin Orthop Relat Res 324:86–97

Mittermayer F, Krepler P, Dominkus M, Schwameis E, Sluga M, Heinzl H, Kotz R (2001) Long-term followup of uncemented tumor endoprostheses for the lower extremity. Clin Orthop Relat Res 167–177

Mittermayer F, Windhager R, Dominkus M, Krepler P, Schwameis E, Sluga M, Kotz R, Strasser G (2002) Revision of the Kotz type of tumour endoprosthesis for the lower limb. J Bone Joint Surg Br 84:401–406

Morris HG, Capanna R, Del Ben M, Campanacci D (1995) Prosthetic reconstruction of the proximal femur after resection for bone tumors. J Arthroplasty 10:293–299

Paley D (1990) Problems, obstacles, and complications of limb lengthening by the Ilizarov technique. Clin Orthop Relat Res 250:81–104

Picci P, Sangiorgi L, Rougraff BT, Neff JR, Casadei R, Campanacci M (1994) Relationship of chemotherapy-induced necrosis and surgical margins to local recurrence in osteosarcoma. J Clin Oncol 12:2699–2705

Plotz W, Rechl H, Burgkart R, Messmer C, Schelter R, Hipp E, Gradinger R (2002) Limb salvage with tumor endoprostheses for malignant tumors of the knee. Clin Orthop Relat Res 405:207–215

Renard AJ, Veth RP, Schreuder HW, Schraffordt Koops H, van Horn J, Keller A (1998) Revisions of endoprosthetic reconstructions after limb salvage in musculoskeletal oncology. Arch Orthop Trauma Surg 117:125–131

Renard AJ, Veth RP, Schreuder HW, van Loon CJ, Koops HS, van Horn JR (2000) Function and complications after ablative and limb-salvage therapy in lower extremity sarcoma of bone. J Surg Oncol 73:198–205

Roberts P, Chan D, Grimer RJ, Sneath RS, Scales JT (1991) Prosthetic replacement of the distal femur for primary bone tumours. J Bone Joint Surg Br 73:762–769

Ross AC, Wilson JN, Scales JT (1987) Endoprosthetic replacement of the proximal humerus. J Bone Joint Surg Br 69:656–661

Ruggieri P, De Cristofaro R, Picci P, Bacci G, Biagini R, Casadei R, Ferraro A, Ferruzzi A, Fabbri N, Cazzola A (1993) Complications and surgical indications in 144 cases of nonmetastatic osteosarcoma of the extremities treated with neoadjuvant chemotherapy. Clin Orthop Relat Res 295:226–238

Safran MR, Kody MH, Namba RS, Larson KR, Kabo JM, Dorey FJ, Eilber FR, Eckardt JJ (1994) 151 endoprosthetic reconstructions for patients with primary tumors involving bone. Contemp Orthop 29:15–25

Shin DS, Weber KL, Chao EY, An KN, Sim FH (1999) Reoperation for failed prosthetic replacement used for limb salvage. Clin Orthop Relat Res 358:53–63

Sluga M, Windhager R, Lang S, Heinzl H, Bielack S, Kotz R (1999) Local and systemic control after ablative and limb sparing surgery in patients with osteosarcoma. Clin Orthop Relat Res 358:120–127

Tunn PU, Schmidt-Peter P, Pomraenke D, Hohenberger P (2004) Osteosarcoma in children: long-term functional analysis. Clin Orthop Relat Res 421:212–217

Unwin PS, Cannon SR, Grimer RJ, Kemp HB, Sneath RS, Walker PS (1996) Aseptic loosening in cemented custom-made prosthetic replacements for bone tumours of the lower limb. J Bone Joint Surg Br 78:5–13

Ward WG, Dorey F, Eckardt JJ (1995) Total femoral endoprosthetic reconstruction. Clin Orthop Relat Res 316:195–206

Wilkins RM, Soubeiran A (2001) The Phenix expandable prosthesis: early American experience. Clin Orthop Relat Res 382:51–58

Wirganowicz PZ, Eckardt JJ, Dorey FJ, Eilber FR, Kabo JM (1999) Etiology and results of tumor endoprosthesis revision surgery in 64 patients. Clin Orthop Relat Res 358:64–74

Zeegen EN, Aponte-Tinao LA, Hornicek FJ, Gebhardt MC, Mankin HJ (2004) Survivorship analysis of 141 modular metallic endoprostheses at early followup. Clin Orthop Relat Res 420:239–250

Allograft Reconstruction in Malignant Bone Tumors: Indications and Limits

Kevin A. Raskin and Francis Hornicek

Abstract Advances in imaging studies and the growing effectiveness of chemotherapy have enabled musculoskeletal tumor surgeons to narrow their margins and employ limb-salvage surgery as the preferred method for managing bone sarcoma. The reconstructive options available to orthopedic oncologists range from allograft transplantation to endoprosthetic reconstruction to a combination of both. Bone allograft transplantation offers a biologic reconstruction that can restore bone stock and joint kinematics, while sparing the opposing articular surface. This chapter will discuss the limitations, complications, survival rates, and indications for using bone allografts.

5.1 Introduction

In 1881 MacEwen replaced two-thirds of a humeral shaft with an "inter-human osseous transplantation," undertaking the first intercalary allograft. Parrish furthered the field with his work in the 1940s and 1950s revitalizing the use of bone allograft transplantation to restore skeletal defects [13]. Procurement and storage of allografts [15] over the last 40 years has made handling bone allografts safer for the patients and has provided a wide range of allograft types for surgeon preference. Facility in managing bone allograft complications has also improved over recent years with better protocols for internal fixation and infection management. Enthusiasm for limb salvage has risen over the past 25 years from both the oncologic and functional perspectives. An equivalent survival and disease-free interval in patients treated with amputation versus wide resection and limb-salvage reconstruction has been demonstrated in past publications [14]. Functional outcomes after limb salvage continue to improve and rival those of well-functioning amputees. Both oncologic and functional gold standards are now met with limb-salvage surgery. The reconstructive options available in limb-salvage surgery range from bone allograft transplantation, to endoprosthesis, to a hybrid of both techniques [4, 5, 8, 9].

Bone allograft transplantation has been a mainstay in limb-salvage surgery after bone resection for both tumorous and nontumorous conditions. The advent of adjuvant chemotherapy, advanced

Kevin A. Raskin (✉)
Instructor, Orthopaedic Surgery
Harvard Medical School, Orthopaedic
Oncology Service,
Massachusetts General Hospital, 55 Fruit Street
Yawkey Outpatient Center Suite 3B
Boston, MA 02114, USA
E-mail: kraskina@partners.org

Table 5.1 Complications and revision rates in allograft transplantation

Complication	Average rate	Literature
Infection	12%	Lord et al. 1988 [8]
Fracture	16%	Berry et al. 1990 [1]
Nonunion	17%	Hornicek et al. 2001 [7]
Revision	25%–30%	Musculo et al. 2006 [11]

imaging modalities, and accurate staging techniques posits limb-salvage surgery as the preferred treatment for malignant neoplasms and benign conditions that leave large bone defects in the wake of their resections [14]. The reconstructive surgeon faces a multitude of options in fashioning a limb-salvage effort in treating these difficult problems. Bone allografts restore articular congruity, preserve bone stock, and provide musculotendinous attachment sites for host soft tissue structures, theoretically improving function [3, 8, 9, 12]. Osteoarticular allografts, intercalary, allograft arthrodesis, and allograft endoprosthetic composites are some of the applications authors have described in restoring large bone defects. Complications of allograft reconstruction have also been well described. Fracture, nonunion, and infection (Table 5.1) are common allograft complications that potentially threaten the procedure's success and longevity in patients [1, 6, 7].

5.1.1 Biology

Understanding the biology of allografts is important for their applications to skeletal defects. Allografts provide the potential for long-lasting reconstruction of large bony defects by providing a structural lattice for the ingrowth of the patient's own bone elements. The normal host bone slowly incorporates into the allograft by creeping substitution. Large segments of allografted bone do not completely fill with autogenous bone, potentially weakening the bone and leading to fracture over time. An inflammatory pannus-like tissue slowly replaces the articular cartilage and some patients may ultimately require joint resurfacing.

Allografts are available from tissue banks, and need to be matched to the size of the resected bone. Although bone is a relatively nonantigenic structure, matching for the class II major histocompatibility antigens results in better clinical outcomes. Freezing further decreases the likelihood of immune rejection, and the addition of glycerol or dimethylsulfoxide during freezing preserves the articular cartilage somewhat. Soft tissues are left attached to the allograft to increase function by providing a site of attachment for host soft tissues.

5.2 Indications and Types

When contemplating a limb-salvage surgery or skeletal reconstruction, allografts provide a versatile means with which to rebuild. Preoperative planning is essential. Accurate measurements of length, articular condylar width, and overall size of the graft are critically important when using allografts to restore anatomy.

5.2.1 Intercalary Allografts

For diaphyseal defects, intercalary allograft reconstruction (Fig. 5.1) is a straightforward modality that restores bone resected between articular surfaces and physes. After a diaphyseal defect is created, maintaining the length and rotation intraoperatively with a temporary plate

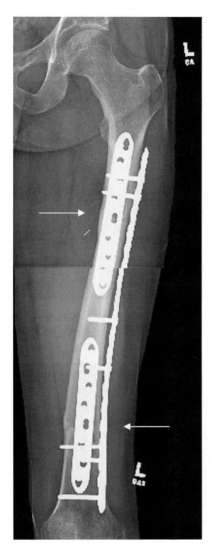

Fig. 5.1 a, b Intercalary allograft reconstruction for the femoral diaphysis. The *arrows* indicate the proximal and distal osteosynthesis sites

lary allografts can be with either plates and screws or intramedullary nails. The literature suggests a higher fracture rate with plates and screws and alternatively a lower union rate with intramedullary nails.

5.2.2
Osteoarticular Allografts

Around joints, osteoarticular allografts (Fig. 5.2) restore bone stock, allow for preservation of the opposite articular surface, and replace ligament and tendon attachment sites otherwise removed after surgery. Preparation for an osteoarticular allograft requires accurate measurement of the patient's articular surface. These measurements can be retrieved from the magnetic resonance imaging (MRI), computed tomography (CT), or plain film X-ray. When ordering the graft, one ought to stipulate the need for soft tissue attachments, requesting a graft with soft tissues intact. The proximal tibia is an example where soft tissue attachment is crucial. A proximal tibial allograft without its soft tissue attachments will not allow for reconstruction of the quadriceps extensor mechanism. An allograft harvested with its patellar ligament intact will provide a large soft tissue tether for extensor mechanism restoration. Further, good articular size matching is important to prevent incongruity at the articular surface and restore more normal joint kinematics. Fixation of osteoarticular allografts is typically performed with periarticular plates and screws. The host-donor osteosynthesis must be as flush as possible and fixation rigid to reduce nonunion rates and prevent periprosthetic fracture.

or external fixation sets up the reconstruction with the allograft. Bone banks can provide either an entire length of bone with the articular surfaces on either end or a preferred trimmed bone, without the articular surfaces, cut to the length required by the resection. Fixation for interca-

5.2.3
Allograft Arthrodesis

Using an allograft in conjunction with native bone to affect an arthrodesis is another tool in the armamentarium of the orthopedic oncologist. Large skeletal defects that span a joint, such as

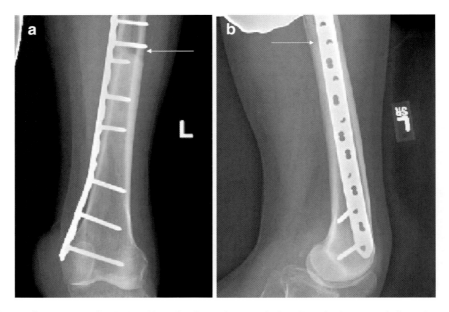

Fig. 5.2 a, b Anteroposterior (AP) and lateral radiograph osteoarticular allograft. The *arrows* indicate the proximal and distal osteosynthesis sites

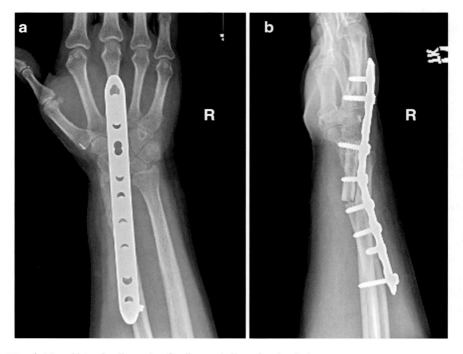

Fig. 5.3 a, b AP and lateral radiographs of radiocarpal allograft arthrodesis

an extraarticular resection, is a good indication for using an allograft to span the defect and fuse it to the neighboring bone. Other areas, such as the distal radiocarpal joint (Fig. 5.3), can be solidly reconstructed with an allograft arthrodesis, avoiding the complications of an osteoarticular allograft, and providing for excellent function without limiting supination or pronation of the forearm.

5.2.4
Allograft–Prosthetic Composites

Combining an allograft and an endoprosthesis is another novel way to utilize allografts. The proximal humerus (Fig. 5.4) and proximal femur are two areas where tendon attachments from an allograft play a critical role in joint kinematics; however, the skeletal defect might be reconstructed best with metal. By potting the endoprosthesis into the allograft, the surgeon gains the freedom of endoprosthetic modularity (size, length, rotation) and the inherent tendon attachments of the allograft (Fig. 5.5).

All in all, allografts are a reliable tool of limb-salvage surgery in patients with malignant bone tumors (Fig. 5.6).

5.3
Limits

Many authors have reported on specific allograft reconstructions, including proximal femur, proximal humerus, and intercalary [3, 6, 9, 10]. Additionally, the complications and survival data have been discussed, and most authors agree on certain givens when considering allografts. Infection has plagued allograft reconstruction from its outset. Lord et al. cited an 11.7% infection rate [8]. Surgical extent, soft tissue loss, and multiple operations left allografts precariously susceptible to infection in another series [6, 9], and the series reported from our institution reflects these conclusions. Allografts with adequate soft tissue coverage that was achieved early on, and efforts aimed at reducing the soft tissue cuff of normal tissue around tumors without compromising the oncologic goal, protected allografts from untoward infections. The most common pathogen in allograft infection is *Staphylococcus epidermidis*, a well-known skin pathogen [7]. Protecting an allograft with a cuff of vascular, viable tissue poised to fend off skin contaminants can therefore theoretically reduce allograft infections (Table 5.1).

Fracture and nonunion can individually and in tandem ruin an allograft reconstruction [1, 6]. The union of allografts relies on host bone cell proliferation, vascular supply, and repair potential to bridge the gap with the graft. Hornicek et al. examined the factors affecting nonunion in

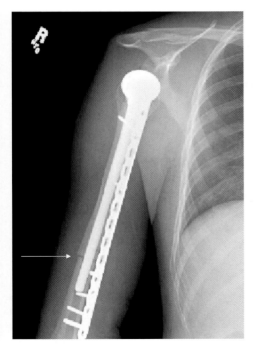

Fig. 5.4 Proximal humerus alloprosthetic composite. The *arrow* indicates the osteosynthesis site

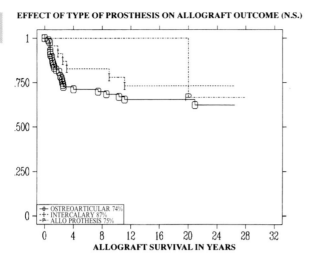

Fig. 5.5 Effect of type of prosthesis on allograft outcome (*N.S.*, not statistically significant)

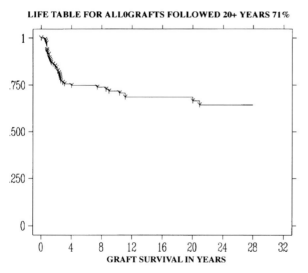

Fig. 5.6 Life table for allograft followed for more than 20 years, having 71% survival

allograft host junctions [7]. The authors report a nonunion rate of 17.2%, and implicate the type of allograft, initiation of chemotherapy, and infection as major contributors to nonunion and failure of the allograft. Intercalary allografts have been shown by this author (and elsewhere) to perform well and heal with predictable success [12]. Osteoarticular allografts perform less well; however, they do enjoy relative success in various reports [8]. Stiffness in the reconstructed joint with osteoarticular allografts may transmit untoward forces across the osteosynthesis site, creating excessive motion and higher rates of nonunion. Biologic healing of the osteosynthesis site relies on the extent of soft tissue resection, preservation of host periosteum, and compatibility between host and graft [2, 6].

Fracture in an allograft is also a devastating event. Osteosynthesis devices, plates, screws, and intramedullary rods have enjoyed greater and lesser success in healing graft–host junctions. Bicortical screw fixation has been held accountable for creating stress risers in allografts, leaving them susceptible to fracture. In addition, intramedullary nail fixation, albeit free from bicortical penetration of the allograft, lacks in stability what plates and screws offer. The advent of unicortical locking plates and screws may improve our rates of fracture by eliminating unnecessary stress risers in both. Furthermore, spanning the entire length of the allograft with internal fixation theoretically splints the graft, offering protection from bending and torsional forces causing fracture [16].

Summary

Allograft reconstruction offers patients a biologic reconstruction, which restores bone stock, joint mechanics, and soft tissue attachments. In young patients the need to restore bone stock and spare the opposing articular surface is important. Limb-salvage surgery implies complications and revision surgery in the young. As survival rates improve, our reconstructive efforts will begin to fail all patients as their lifespan approaches that of normal individuals. An allograft reconstruction restores limb bone stock such that the bone-depleting march of revision surgery is stalled and committing patients to endoprosthetic bone loss is slowed. Of course, complications inherent in allograft reconstruction can prove formidable. But with meticulous adherence to soft tissue coverage, rigid internal fixation, range-of-motion considerations, and appropriate patient selection, bone allograft transplantation will remain a viable and advantageous tool to the limb-salvage surgeon.

References

1. Berrey BH Jr, Lord CF, Gebhardt MC, Mankin HJ (1990) Fractures of allografts: frequency, treatment and end-results. J Bone Joint Surg Am 72:825–833
2. Capanna R, Donati D, Masetti C, Manfrin M, Panozzo A, Cadossi R, Campanacci M (1994) Effect of electromagnetic fields on patients undergoing massive bone graft following bone tumor resection: a double blind study. Clin Orthop Relat Res 306:213–221
3. Clohisy DR, Mankin HJ (1994) Osteoarticular allografts for reconstruction after resection of a musculoskeletal tumor in the proximal end of the tibia. J Bone Joint Surg Am 76:549–554
4. Eckardt JJ, Eilber FR, Rosen G, Mirra JM, Dorey FJ, Ward WG, Kabo JM (1991) Endoprosthetic reconstruction for Stage IIB osteosarcoma. Clin Orthop Relat Res 270:202–213
5. Eckardt JJ, Matthews JG, Eilber FR (1991) Endoprosthetic reconstruction of the proximal tibia. Orthop Clin North Am 22:149–159
6. Fox EJ, Hau MA, Gebhardt MC, Hornicek FJ, Tomford WW, Mankin HJ (2002) Long-term followup of proximal femoral allograft. Clin Orthop Relat Res 397:106–113
7. Hornicek FJ, Gebhardt MC, Tomford WW, Sorger JI, Zavata M, Menzner J, Mankin HJ (2001) Factors affecting nonunion of the allograft-host junction. Clin Orthop Relat Res 382:87–99
8. Lord CF, Gebhardt MC, Tomford WW, Mankin HJ (1988) Infection in bone allografts, incidence, nature, and treatment. J Bone Joint Surg Am 70:369–376
9. Mankin HJ, Doppelt SH, Sullivan HT, Tomford WW (1982) Osteoarticular and intercalary allograft transplantation in the management of malignant tumors of bone. Cancer 50:613–630
10. Mankin HJ, Gebhardt MC, Jennings LC, Springfield DS, Tomford WW (1996) Long-term results of allograft replacement in the management of bone tumors. Clin Orthop Relat Res 324:86–94
11. Musculo DL, Ayerz MA, Aponte-Tinao LA, Ranalletta M (2006) Use of distal femoral osteoarticular allografts in limb salvage surgery. Surgical technique. J Bone Joint Surg Am 88[Suppl 1]:305–321
12. Ortiz-Cruz EJ, Gebhardt MC, Jennings LC, et al (1997) The results of transplantation of

intercalary allografts after resection of tumors. A long-term follow-up study. J Bone Joint Surg 79A:97–106
13. Parrish FF (1973) Allograft replacement of all or part of the end of a long bone following excision of a tumor. J Bone Joint Surg Am 55:1–22
14. Simon MA, Aschliman MA, Thomas N, Mankin HJ (1986) Limb-salvage treatment versus amputation for osteosarcoma of the distal end of the femur. J Bone Joint Surg 68A:1331–1337
15. Kagan RJ (ed) (1999) Standards for tissue banking. American Association of Tissue Banking, McLean, VA
16. Thompson RC Jr, Pickvance EA, Garry D (1993) Fractures in large-segment allografts. J Bone Joint Surg Am 75:1663–1673

Expandable Endoprostheses in Malignant Bone Tumors in Children: Indications and Limitations

Rainer Baumgart and Ulrich Lenze

Abstract Expandable endoprostheses can be an option after resection of malignant bone tumors of the lower extremity in children and adolescents not only to bridge the resultant surgical defect but also to correct a residual limb length discrepancy. Small intramedullary diameter and short residual bone segments, as well as stress-shielding, are intrinsic technical limitations of fully implantable reconstructive devices. As a consequence, until recently, repeated operative interventions to reconstruct the limb and compensate for subsequent absence of growth within the affected limb were required to compensate for continued growth of the contralateral limb. Innovative expandable endoprosthetic devices are now available to help achieve equal limb length at maturity. One common device is a conventional endoprosthesis that is lengthened using a telescopic module, whereas the "bioexpandable" system lengthens the remaining bone using a lengthening nail as a modular part of the endoprosthesis. Both systems are equipped with motor drives that electromagnetic waves activate transcutaneously. One advantage of the "bioexpandable" endoprosthesis is that with sequential lengthening, the proportion of residual bone shaft to prosthesis length increases, thereby diminishing host bone-endoprosthetic lever arm forces.

6.1 Introduction

Of all malignant bone tumors, 80% occur in children and adolescents. About 60% of these are located around the knee joint, either at the distal femur or the proximal tibia, close to the most active growth plates (Schajowicz 1994; Wurster 2004). Due to modern, interdisciplinary therapy, 5-year survival rates of up to 60% have been achieved (Bielack et al. 2002; Grimmer et al. 2002; Sluga et al. 2002; Zalupski et al. 2004) with increasing tendency. With improved long-term survival, the functional impact of surgical treatment and subsequent reconstruction has to be even more carefully considered.

Rainer Baumgart (✉)
Zentrum für korrigierende und rekonstruktive Extremitätenchirurgie München (ZEM)
Limb Lengthening Center Munich/Germany
Nymphenburgerstr. 1
80335 Munich, Germany
E-mail: baumgart@zem.info

In adults, modular tumor endoprostheses are increasingly used for reconstructing the limb after surgical treatment of malignant bone tumors of the lower extremity. These modular endoprosthetics replace both the resected long bone shaft and the adjacent joint (Gosheger and Winkelmann 2000; Ilyas et al. 2002). Significant technical challenges present themselves when endoprosthetic reconstruction is considered in children after tumor surgery. These challenges include: the small dimensions of bone with respect to both overall length and intramedullary diameter; progressive subsequent limb length inequality due to continued growth of the contralateral limb; and stress-shielding within the residual bone segments as a biological response to the rigid intramedullary stem of the endoprosthetic device. Therefore, until recently, particularly in children, the cosmetically disturbing but functionally advantageous Van Ness–Borggreve rotationplasty has been preferred in many cases (Lindner et al. 1999). New concepts of fully implantable lengthening devices have now created new dimensions for reconstructive tumor surgery in children.

6.2 Principles of Expandable Tumor Endoprostheses

In technical terms the easiest way to perform limb lengthening is by acute distraction. Due to high complication rates associated with acute stretching of soft tissue, vessels, and nerves, the femur can typically be distracted only 2–3 cm, and the tibia only 1–2 cm at any one sitting. Lengthening of an endoprosthesis can be accomplished by replacing modular components; this necessitates large surgical approaches, however,

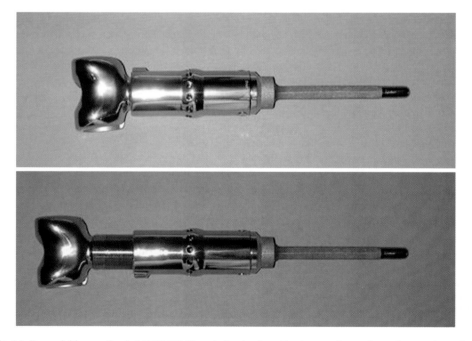

Fig. 6.1 Expandable prosthesis MUTARS Xpand classic. Lengthening can be performed up to 4cm via a small skin incision

and significant trauma to the surrounding soft tissues is unavoidable. As a consequence, the functional outcome is often unsatisfactory. A gradual mechanical lengthening mechanism, such as a double spindle mechanism MUTARS Xpand classic (Implantcast, Buxtehude; Fig. 6.1), which can be activated via small skin incisions, offers significant advantages over acute, open endoprosthetic lengthening. Using this device, the soft tissue trauma associated with lengthening is minimized and the patient is able to start with physiotherapy immediately after surgery. Another available device allows lengthening without open surgery. The ISEM (intercondylar stepless extendible module) as a part of the MHRS system (Stryker, Duisburg, Germany) is a modular device in which repeated hyperflexion of the knee joint leads to lengthening (Kotz et al. 2000). A drawback of this system is the need for general anesthesia to accomplish the required hyperflexion. The Repiphysis system (Wright, Arlington, USA) expands in small increments within a magnetic field and thus avoids soft tissue problems associated with substantial acute lengthening and open procedures (Gitelis et al. 2003). The most modern and recently available device combines a fully implantable motorized system for limb lengthening "Fitbone" (Wittenstein-intens, Igersheim) and a modular tumor endoprosthesis, MUTARS. These implants are available in two versions as described in more detail below.

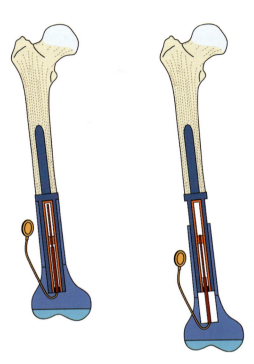

Fig. 6.2 Schematic view of the expandable prosthesis MUTARS Xpand. The fully implantable device is lengthened by an encapsulated motor drive

6.3
The Expandable Tumor Endoprosthesis MUTARS Xpand

The MUTARS Xpand (Fig. 6.2) combines the advantages of a modular endoprosthesis with a telescopic component and an encapsulated, powerful motor drive for lengthening purposes. The articular component of the endoprosthesis and the stem that fixes the prosthesis to the diaphysis are nearly the same as in conventional modular devices. However, between these two components a newly designed telescopic intermediate component is inserted, which can be incrementally expanded with a force of more than 1,500 N. This telescopic motor component consists of an encapsulated hermetic closed motor drive. Energy is transmitted by high-frequency signals from an external power unit to a reception antenna placed in the subcutaneous tissue, connected to the motor drive component of the endoprosthesis by a highly flexible cable. Thus, the whole system is fully implantable without any material connection to the outside. The motor component can be activated whenever a small leg length discrepancy is detected. The lengthening process can be done continuously or in small steps without any risk of injury to neurovascular structures or other soft tissues of the limb by excessive or acute distraction. The telescopic module with the motor drive remains in place until maturity, after which it should be replaced by a nonmotorized component.

6.4 The "Bioexpandable" Tumor Endoprosthesis MUTARS BioXpand

The latest and most innovative development of growing endoprostheses is the MUTARS BioXpand (Baumgart et al. 2005). While limb lengthening with the Xpand device seems to be much easier and safer compared to other endoprosthetic devices, all these devices share a problem of increasing leverage between the endoprosthesis and bone segments. This can result in potentially problematic loss of fixation between the prosthesis and the host bone, aggravated with each lengthening step. This problem can be understood by appreciating the ever-changing (and worsening) length-ratio of the prosthesis to the remaining bone with sequential lengthening of the device, and little or no comparable growth in the host bone segment. The concept of incremental lengthening of the "bioexpandable" endoprosthesis and its relationship to the host bone is quite different. Based on the method of callus distraction, bone growth is activated and the remaining bone lengthens, thus actually improving the endoprosthetic–host bone length ratio with time. The method of callus distraction was popularized by the work of Gavriil Ilizarov (1921–1992) who demonstrated that living tissue proliferates under continuous tension. After osteotomy, controlled distraction of the bone segments at a rate of about 1 mm/day will stimulate bone formation of high biological and mechanical quality within the distraction gap (Ilizarov 1992). The surrounding soft tissues limit bone segment lengthening, with a potential for joint stiffness or distraction injury to nerves and vessels. To stabilize and control distraction of the bone segments after osteotomy, Ilizarov and others traditionally used external fixators. These external fixation devices, with their continually transcutaneous contact with the bone and soft tissues by wires and/or half-pins, are associated with a high rate of local infection, discomfort, and pain. It is intolerable to entertain the use of external fixators in conjunction with an endoprosthesis, since bacterial contamination of an endoprosthetic device almost always necessitates its removal with catastrophic implications for limb reconstruction. The fully implantable motorized lengthening nail "Fitbone" (Fig. 6.3), commonly used for lengthening procedures of femora or tibiae to correct congenital or posttraumatic shortenings (Baumgart et al. 2006), offers new perspectives. Lengthening of more than 8 cm, axis correction, and bone transport can be performed without any external fixation. The new concept is to combine the Fitbone lengthening nail with a specially designed endoprosthesis. The energy supply of the system is the same as described above.

The modular design of the "bioexpandable" endoprosthesis MUTARS BioXpand consists of an articular component, a shaft substitute, and an anchoring component within the residual host bone segment. The articular component is similar to conventional tumor endoprostheses and is coupled to the corresponding articular surfaces. The shaft assembly is available in different lengths to bridge the bone defect resulting from tumor resection. An exchangeable shaft is used as the bone-anchoring component and is placed in the central cavity of the two prosthesis components (Fig. 6.4).

Immediately after tumor resection, a solid intramedullary nail is implanted as a preliminary fixation stem. The dimensions of this intramedullary nail are exactly the same as the fully implantable motorized lengthening nail (Fitbone). To prevent bony ingrowth, the shaft of the solid intramedullary nail has a polished surface. Two screws in a slotted hole prevent torsion of the

6 Expandable Endoprostheses in Malignant Bone Tumors in Children

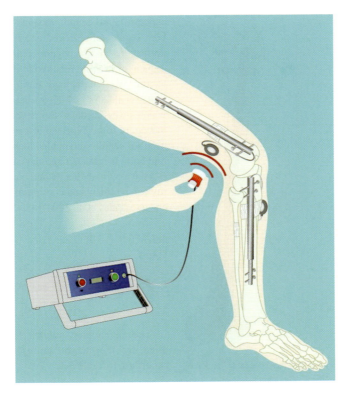

Fig. 6.3 Fully implantable motorized lengthening nails (Fitbone) in femur and tibia for limb lengthening. The receiver for transcutaneous energy transmission is placed in the subcutaneous tissue and is supplied by an induction transmitter placed on the overlying skin

implant. Once a leg length discrepancy of 3–4 cm resulting from normal contralateral limb growth is documented during postoperative follow-up, the solid intramedullary nail is exchanged for the active motorized lengthening nail and a cortical osteotomy performed. During distraction at a rate of 1 mm/day, the remaining bone is gradually lengthened using the principles of callus distraction, and new bone forms within the distraction gap. The energy that is necessary for the distraction process is supplied in the same way as described above by a small receiver placed subcutaneously. An antenna that transmits electromagnetic impulses is placed on the overlying skin three times a day for 90 s each, with no need for a direct connection between the distraction unit and the outside energy supply. Thus the skin is kept completely intact.

The lengthening procedure itself is painless. Physical therapy is necessary in order to reduce soft tissue tension and prevent decreased range of motion. Generally, with a distraction of about 4 cm, the new callus becomes adequate for full weight bearing after 4–6 months, on average. If necessary, the distraction procedure can be repeated as needed after several years if further leg length discrepancy develops. At maturity the expandable prosthesis has to be exchanged for a standard tumor endoprosthesis. The stem of this implant can then be definitively fixed within the newly formed, high-quality bone.

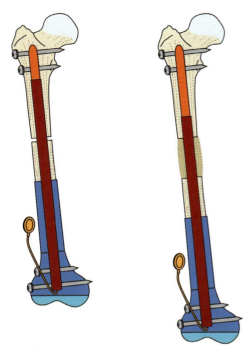

Fig. 6.4 Schematic view of the "bioexpandable" endoprosthesis MUTARS BioXpand. The length difference arising from physiological growth of the contralateral side is compensated by progressive, gradual callus distraction using the fully implantable motorized lengthening nail "Fitbone"

6.5 Indications

The surgical concept is part of the interdisciplinary treatment and is based on the nature of the bone tumor, the invasion of the surrounding soft tissue, and the longitudinal size and localization of the lesion as it is seen in the primary magnetic resonance imaging (MRI) studies before starting chemotherapy. Deciding if an expandable endoprosthesis is suitable or not, or which type is best indicated in individual cases, depends mainly on two questions: If the remaining bone was radiated for example in case of Ewing's Sarcoma, sufficient bone growth in that area may be delayed or completely suppressed using the "bioexpandable" endoprosthesis. Another question would be the expected limb length inequality resulting from both segmental resection and loss of subsequent normal growth. Calculations regarding loss of subsequent growth are required to make this determination. We recommend the multiplier method (Paley et al. 2000) which is easy to understand and which gives accurate estimation of limb length inequality to be expected at maturity without the need for serial radiographs. Starting with the current body height (H_c) and the current bone length (L_c) the total body height and bone length at maturity can be calculated considering the patient's sex and age (Paley et al. 2004).

6.5.1 Step 1

Calculation of the body height at maturity (H_m)

$$H_m = H_c \times M_H$$

The current body height (H_c) has to be multiplied by the height multiplier factor (M_H), according to Table 6.1.

6.5.2 Step 2

Calculation of the growth delay (ΔG) of the affected bone at maturity after tumor resection depends on the resected physis:

- Resection of the proximal femoral physis:

$$\Delta G = L_c (M_{LL} - 1) \times 0.29$$

- Resection of the distal femoral physis:

$$\Delta G = L_c (M_{LL} - 1) \times 0.71$$

- Resection of the proximal tibial physis:

$$\Delta G = L_c (M_{LL} - 1) \times 0.57$$

- Resection of the distal tibial physis:

$$\Delta G = L_c (M_{LL} - 1) \times 0.43$$

- Resection of distal femoral and proximal tibial physis:

$$\Delta G = L_c (M_{LL} - 1) \times 0.67$$

Table 6.1 Height multiplier M_H for boys and girls

a. Height multiplier M_H for boys

Age (yr+mo)	M_H	Age (yr+mo)	M_H	Age (yr+mo)	M_H
Birth	3.535	5+0	1.627	12+0	1.186
0+3	2.908	5+6	1.579	12+6	1.161
0+6	2.639	6+0	1.535	13+0	1.135
0+9	2.462	6+6	1.492	13+6	1.106
1+0	2.337	7+0	1.455	14+0	1.081
1+3	2.239	7+6	1.416	14+6	1.056
1+6	2.160	8+0	1.383	15+0	1.044
1+9	2.088	8+6	1.351	15+6	1.030
2+0	2.045	9+0	1.322	16+0	1.021
2+6	1.942	9+6	1.298	16+6	1.014
3+0	1.859	10+0	1.278	17+0	1.010
3+6	1.783	10+6	1.260	17+6	1.006
4+0	1.731	11+0	1.235	18+0	1.005
4+6	1.675	11+6	1.210	18+6	-

b. Height multiplier M_H for girls

Age (yr+mo)	M_H	Age (yr+mo)	M_H	Age (yr+mo)	M_H
Birth	3.290	5+0	1.514	12+0	1.082
0+3	2.759	5+6	1.467	12+6	1.059
0+6	2.505	6+0	1.421	13+0	1.040
0+9	2.341	6+6	1.381	13+6	1.027
1+0	2.216	7+0	1.341	14+0	1.019
1+3	2.120	7+6	1.309	14+6	1.013
1+6	2.038	8+0	1.279	15+0	1.008
1+9	1.965	8+6	1.254	15+6	1.009
2+0	1.917	9+0	1.229	16+0	1.004
2+6	1.815	9+6	1.207	16+6	1.004
3+0	1.735	10+0	1.183	17+0	1.002
3+6	1.677	10+6	1.160	17+6	-
4+0	1.622	11+0	1.135	18+0	-
4+6	1.570	11+6	1.108	18+6	-

From Paley et al. 2004

The current bone length, L_C, of the affected bone, in case of femoral and tibial resections of both bones, has to be multiplied by the lower limb multiplier factor (M_{LL}), listed in Table 6.2. The calculation is made considering the growth characteristics of the bone by factoring the growth contribution of the affected physis. The distal femoral physis contributes 71% to the total growth of the femur, whereas the proximal tibial physis contributes 57% to the total growth of the tibia (Anderson et al. 1963).

Using these calculations, the surgeon has to take into consideration other factors that might impact limb growth, particularly the inhibition of growth activity caused by chemotherapy.

6.6 Limitations

The primary biological limiting factor to using an endoprosthesis in children is the diameter of the host residual shaft diameter. Under long-term cyclical loading, even strong material will fail if the implant shaft diameter is less than 8 mm. Particularly in young children, the diameter of the bone may not allow sufficient reaming to accept an 8-mm implant without inducing unacceptable cortical weakening. Even more problematic is the remaining bone length after resection of the tumor. A conventional expandable prosthesis may not produce a favorable long-term result if the remaining shaft length is less than 8–10 cm. The metaphyseal and epiphyseal flare of long bones results in the tip of the anchorage stem being imbedded in soft intramedullary bone only, if inadequate shaft length is preserved. Furthermore, the amount of lengthening is limited by the prosthesis itself. If more length is needed, an exchange of the telescopic module is possible in most types. But in cases where substantial lengthening is anticipated, the surgeon must keep in mind that long-term results worsen with each lengthening step because the lever arm from the prosthesis to the remaining bone increases. That is why we recommend the "bioexpandable" prosthesis in cases in which substantial lengthening is anticipated and desirable.

The "bioexpandable" tumor prosthesis adds in addition to the above calculated fixation length another 3–5 cm for later bone transport. These are usually the limits in very small children with large tumor expansions. We recommend against using a "bioexpandable" prosthesis if the remaining bone length is less than 12 cm. Only in highly individualized cases where the residual bone length is below these dimensions may custom devices with a unique anchorage stem with screws be considered. Fortunately, this problem is overcome after the first successful lengthening step and subsequent stages are much easier to perform.

6.7 Clinical Cases

Consistent with ethical standards, the therapeutic concept and its experimental nature was discussed extensively with the patients and their families, obtaining full informed consent to the treatment, as well as the acquisition and publication of the following patients' data.

An 11-year-old boy with osteosarcoma of the right distal femur had an expected height at maturity of 162 cm. An epiphysiodesis of the contralateral side was not acceptable to the family. The distal femoral growth plate of the femur had to be resected with the tumor, with an anticipated limb length discrepancy at maturity calculated to be 3.8 cm. In this case a mechanical expandable endoprosthesis MUTARS Xpand classic was selected. Lengthening was performed in two stages of about 2 cm each. The first was done 3 years after resection of the tumor (Fig. 6.5) and the second 2 years after the

Table 6.2 Lower limb multiplier M_{LL} for boys and girls

Age (yr+mo)	M_{LL}	Age (yr+mo)	M_{LL}	Age (yr+mo)	M_{LL}
Lower limb multiplier (M_{LL}) for boys					
Birth	5.080	4+0	2.000	11+0	1.240
0+3	4.550	4+6	1.890	11+6	1.220
0+6	4.050	5+0	1.820	12+0	1.180
0+9	3.600	5+6	1.740	12+6	1.160
1+0	3.240	6+0	1.670	13+0	1.130
1+3	2.975	6+6	1.620	13+6	1.100
1+6	2.825	7+0	1.570	14+0	1.080
1+9	2.700	7+6	1.520	14+6	1.060
2+0	2.590	8+0	1.470	15+0	1.040
2+3	2.480	8+6	1.420	15+6	1.020
2+6	2.385	9+0	1.380	16+0	1.010
2+9	2.300	9+6	1.340	16+6	1.010
3+0	2.230	10+0	1.310	17+0	1.000
3+6	2.110	10+6	1.280	17+6	—
Lower limb multiplier (M_{LL}) for girls					
Birth	4.630	4+0	1.830	11+0	1.130
0+3	4.155	4+6	1.740	11+6	1.100
0+6	3.725	5+0	1.660	12+0	1.070
0+9	3.300	5+6	1.580	12+6	1.050
1+0	2.970	6+0	1.510	13+0	1.030
1+3	2.750	6+6	1.460	13+6	1.010
1+6	2.600	7+0	1.430	14+0	1.000
1+9	2.490	7+6	1.370	14+6	—
2+0	2.390	8+0	1.330	15+0	—
2+3	2.295	8+6	1.290	15+6	—
2+6	2.200	9+0	1.260	16+0	—
2+9	2.125	9+6	1.220	16+6	—
3+0	2.050	10+0	1.190	17+0	—
3+6	1.925	10+6	1.160	17+6	—

Paley (2002), p 701

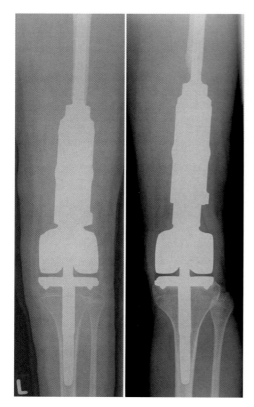

Fig. 6.5 Limb lengthening with the MUTARS Xpand classic; 2 cm of lengthening was performed via a small skin incision

first lengthening stage. At maturity, the patient's long standing radiographs show no limb length discrepancy (Fig. 6.6). Because this type of expandable prosthesis does not require exchange, the femoral anchoring stem has a rough surface to allow bony ingrowth into the stem increase stability. At maturity only the polished tibia shaft should be replaced by one with a rough surface.

A 9-year-old boy with osteosarcoma of the left distal femur had an expected height at maturity of about 170 cm and an expected limb length discrepancy of 8 cm. He had been treated 3 years previously in a different hospital by tumor resection and implantation of a tumor endoprosthetic prototype with a solid polished stem that had the option to be changed to a "bioexpandable" prosthesis. On presentation, he had a limb length discrepancy of 3.5 cm (Fig. 6.7), so a first-stage lengthening procedure was planned. The residual diaphyseal femur had a length of 20 cm and was osteotomized in a minimally invasive technique by a drill bit and a chisel, about 3 cm proximal to its distal end. The polished stem inside the modular joint replacing part was exchanged with a motorized lengthening nail "Fitbone" (Fig. 6.8), and distraction was performed at a rate of 1 mm/day (Fig. 6.9). Figure 6.10 shows good bone formation around the nail 4 months after the operation, and equal leg length. The anticipated development of a 4.5-cm leg length inequality with further growth will be treated in a similar fashion at maturity.

Both patients tolerated the procedure well without any intra- or postoperative complications.

6.8 Conclusion

In the pediatric population up to the present time, bone endoprosthetic implantation has played a minor role in reconstruction after resection of malignant bone tumors. This is due to the relatively small bone dimensions, difficult anchoring conditions, and, most importantly, the lack of growth after resection of the growth plate. Mechanically expandable endoprostheses only lengthen the prosthesis itself. In many cases with an expected limb length discrepancy of less than 4 cm, this type of prosthesis may be an option to compensate for both the defect and the limb length discrepancy itself. If expected bone growth is anticipated to result in a discrepancy of more than 4 cm, the "bioexpandable" endoprosthesis MUTARS BioXpand offers much better opportunities for long-term stability.

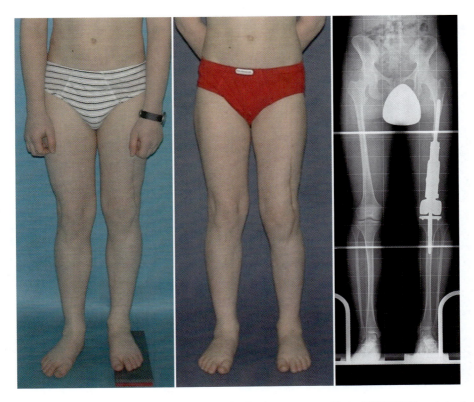

Fig. 6.6 Equal limb length at maturity after 4 cm lengthening in two stages with the MUTARS Xpand classic

Because the modular system works with the fully implantable, motorized distraction nail "Fitbone", there is no need for external fixation for lengthening and therewith a substantially reduced risk of infection. In contrast to all other growth endoprostheses, this new system can lengthen the remaining bone by gradual distraction. The technique of callus distraction with a fully implantable, programmable, motorized distraction nail (Fitbone) has been successfully employed worldwide in more than 700 cases, mainly for correction and lengthening of traumatic or congenital leg shortenings. The technique of forming bone of high quality may be also useful after en bloc resection of malignant bone tumors in children as well. The drawback of repeated surgical interventions [namely (1) implantation of the prosthesis, (2) exchange of the solid nail by the motorized lengthening nail, and (3) implantation of the final tumor endoprosthesis] is offset by the advantage of having new high-quality bone to stabilize the final endoprosthesis, which may improve long-term results dramatically. Because bone lengthening by the method of callus distraction is theoretically limitless, the procedure can be repeated as often as is needed to match the growth of the healthy contralateral leg. Furthermore, the gradual stretch

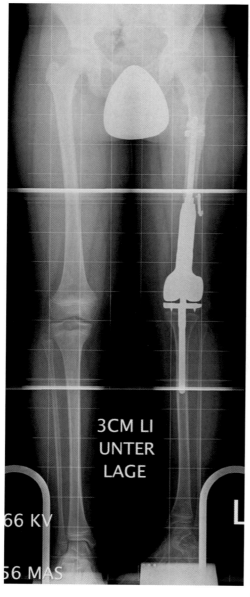
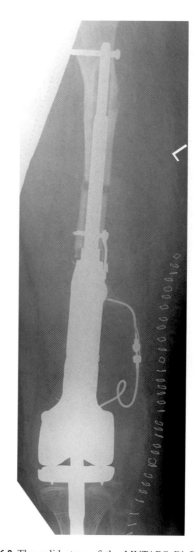

Fig. 6.7 Long standing radiograph 3 years after tumor resection. A limb length discrepancy of 3.5 cm was measured at the femur

Fig. 6.8 The solid stem of the MUTARS BioXpand was changed to a Fitbone nail and a diaphyseal osteotomy was performed using a minimally invasive technique. The receiver and cable can be seen in the subcutaneous tissue

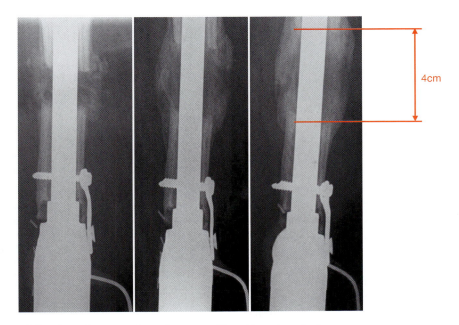

Fig. 6.9 Callus distraction was performed at a rate of 1 mm/day automatically

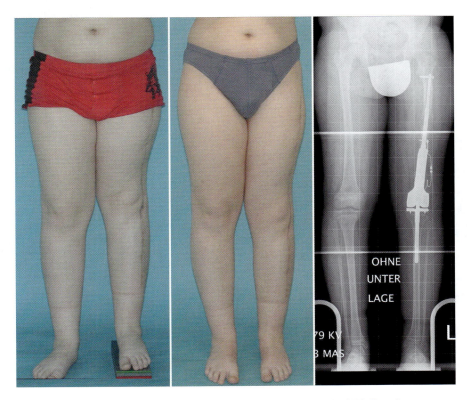

Fig. 6.10 Equal limb length after lengthening of the left femur with the MUTARS BioXpand

exerted on the soft tissue by this new technique is particularly gentle on the vessels and nerves, compared to conventional acute distraction procedures. This may also aid in postoperative mobilization and physical therapy.

Despite these advantages, there are still some obstacles to overcome. First, bone loss may occur at the site of prosthesis fixation due to impaired distribution of forces (stress-shielding). Children's bones are particularly sensitive to this phenomenon, which must be taken into consideration in the design of the prosthesis by improving the transition of force from the prosthesis to the surrounding bone.

Before starting the surgical treatment with an expandable prosthesis, all the above-mentioned thoughts and the geometrical calculations have to be taken into account. The use of ill-advised components in the primary reconstruction may prevent subsequent, more favorable reconstruction. The implantation of an expandable or a "bioexpandable" prosthesis is not much more extensive than a conventional endoprosthesis. Thus, children who do not require lengthening later are not burdened unnecessarily. In case of the "bioexpandable" prosthesis the surgeon has to recognize that considerable experience in limb lengthening and bone transport is required, particularly in these most challenging cases after tumor resection where vascularity is often compromised. This is why we recommend that treatment of such complex cases should be concentrated in highly specialized centers.

References

Anderson M, Green WT, Messner MB (1963) Growth and predictions of growth in the lower extremities. J Bone Joint Surg Am 45:1–14

Baumgart R, Hinterwimmer S, Krammer M, Muensterer O, Mutschler W (2005) The bioexpandable prosthesis: a new perspective after resection of malignant bone tumors in children. J Pediatr Hematol Oncol 27:452–455

Baumgart R, Thaller P, Hinterwimmer S, Krammer M, Hierl T, Mutschler W (2006) A fully implantable, programmable distraction nail (Fitbone)—new perspectives for corrective and reconstructive limb surgery. In: Leung KS, Taglang G (eds) The Principle of intramedullary locked nails. Springer, Berlin Heidelberg New York, pp 189–198

Bielack SS, Kempf-Bielack B, Delling G, Exner G, Flege S, Helmke K, Kotz R, Salzer-Kuntschik M, Werner M, Winkelmann W, Zoubek A, Jürgens H (2002) Prognostic factors in high-grade osteosarcoma of the extremities or trunk: an analysis of 1702 patients treated on neoadjuvant cooperative osteosarcoma study group protocols. J Clin Oncol 20:776–790

Gitelis S, Neel MD, Wilkins RM, Rao BN, Kelly CM, Yao TK (2003) The use of an expandable prosthesis for pediatric sarcomas. Chir Organi Mov 88:327–333

Gosheger G, Winkelmann W (2000) MUTARS: a modular tumor and revision system. Experiences at the Munster Tumor Center. Orthopade 29[Suppl] 1:54–55

Grimmer RJ, Taminiau AM, Cannon SR (2002) Surgical outcomes in osteosarcoma. J Bone Joint Surg Br 84:395–400

Ilizarov GA (1992) Transosseous osteosynthesis: theoretical and clinical aspects of the regeneration and growth of tissue. Springer, Berlin Heidelberg New York

Ilyas I, Pant R, Kurar A, Moreau P, Younge D (2002) Modular megaprosthesis for proximal femoral tumors. Int Orthop 26:170–173

Kotz R, Windhager R, Dominkus M, Robioneck B, Müller-Daniels H (2000) A self-extending paediatric leg implant. Nature 406:143–144

Lindner NJ, Ramm O, Hillmann A, Rodl R, Gosheger, Brinckschmidt C, Jürgens H, Winkelmann W (1999) Limb salvage and outcome of osteosarcoma. The University of Muenster experience. Clin Orthop 332:83–89

Paley D (2002) Principles of deformity correction. Springer, Berlin Heidelberg New York, p 701

Paley D, Bhave A, Herzenberg J (2000) Multiplier method for predicting limb length discrepancy. J Bone Joint Surg Am 82:1432–1446

Paley J, Talor J, Levin A, Bhave A, Paley D, Herzenberg J (2004) The multiplier method for prediction of adult height. J Pediatr Orthop 24:732–737

Schajowicz F (1994) Tumors and tumorlike lesions of bone. Springer, Berlin Heidelberg New York

Sluga M, Windhager R, Pfeiffer M, Ofner P, Lang S, Dominkus M, Nehrer S, Zoubek A, Kotz R (2002) Osteosarcoma and Ewing's sarcoma—the most frequent malignant bone tumors in children—therapy and outcome [in German]. Z Orthop Ihre Grenzgeb 140(6):652–655

Wurster K (2004) Knochentumoren und Weichteilsarkome. Empfehlung zur Diagnostik, Therapie und Nachsorge. Tumorzentrum, München

Zalupski MM, Rankin C, Ryan JR, Lucas DR, Muler J, Lanier KS, Budd GT, Biermann JS, Meyers FJ, Antman K (2004) Adjuvant therapy of osteosarcoma—a phase II trial: Southwest Oncology Group study 9139. Cancer 100:818–825

The Long-Term Risks of Infection and Amputation with Limb Salvage Surgery Using Endoprostheses

Lee Jeys and Robert Grimer

Abstract Endoprostheses are now an established technique to reconstruct defects following bone tumour resection. The long-term durability of the reconstruction is excellent, with limb salvage being maintained in the long term in 91% of patients at 20 years from surgery. The main reasons for secondary amputation were locally recurrent disease and deep periprosthetic infection. Infection remains one of the biggest threats to early failure of reconstructions with endoprostheses. Most series of reconstructions show a periprosthetic infection rate of approximately 10%. Infection most frequently occurs within 12 months from the last surgical procedure; however, the risk of infection is life-long. The commonest pathogenic organism is coagulase-negative Staphylococcus. The most effective treatment for deep infection is two-stage revision, with local treatments having little chance of curing deep infection. Research is on-going into surface treatments with silver and other materials to help to reduce the infection rates.

Lee Jeys (✉)
School House Farm
Purshull Green, Droitwich
Worcestershire WR90NL, UK
E-mail: lee.jeys@btclick.com

7.1 Introduction

Since the late 1960s, limb salvage surgery for primary bone tumours has evolved, with the use of endoprostheses (EPRs) becoming increasingly popular throughout the world. Since the routine use of neo-adjuvant chemotherapy in the 1980s, limb salvage surgery has become the standard treatment, with limb salvage rates above 90% in most major centres. As the long-term survival from primary bone tumours rose to 60%–70% at 10 years from diagnosis, the durability of reconstruction became increasingly important.

Endoprostheses have several advantages over biological reconstruction methods, being readily available in both custom-made and modular forms, initially reliable with low complication rates and allowing rapid return to full weight bearing with predicable function (normally 70% of normal). However, there have been concerns that the long-term risks of infection, locally recurrent disease, aseptic loosening and mechanical implant failure may lead to amputations due to the inability to revise the implant.

7.2 Long-Term Limb Salvage

The goal of any reconstruction for bone tumour surgery is to maintain a functional, painless limb in the long term. Jeys et al. [1] investigated the long-term risks of amputation in a consecutive series of 1,261 patients undergoing EPRs. They identified a subsequent amputation rate of 8.9% ($n=112/1,261$) with the 20-year limb salvage rate being 91%. The reasons for the amputations were: control of local recurrence ($n=71$; 63%), infection ($n=38$; 34%), mechanical failure of the prosthesis ($n=2$; 1.8%) and persistent pain ($n=1$; 0.8%). It was found that local recurrence was the single biggest risk factor affecting survival of the patient's limb. The 10-year survival of the limb fell to only 43% following local recurrence of the disease, and this was statistically significant ($p<=0.0001$) compared to the risk of amputation in patients without local recurrence. The risk of amputation following proven infection of an endoprosthetic replacement was 19%, compared to the risk for amputation with a local recurrence which was 36%.

For each endoprosthetic replacement site, local recurrence of tumour was the commonest cause of amputation, except for tibial endoprosthetic replacements, where infection played an equal role in causing amputation. The risk of amputation was lowest in the proximal femoral endoprosthetic replacements (5.5%) and highest in the tibial endoprosthetic replacements (15.1%). It was found that the patients with tibial endoprosthetic replacements had a statistically higher risk of amputation compared to patients with endoprosthetic replacements at other sites ($p=0.001$).

The time to amputation ranged from 2 days to 16½ years, with a mean of 31 months. The median time to amputation was 32 months for infection and 13 months for local recurrence. The risk of amputation decreased with time, although 10% of the amputations took place more than 5 years after insertion and late amputations occurred due to both infection and local recurrence (Fig. 7.1). Importantly there were no amputations for aseptic loosening, with both of the amputations for mechanical failure being for chronic implant instability. There were very few late amputations, with only 5% ($n = 5/112$) occurring after 10 years from implantation.

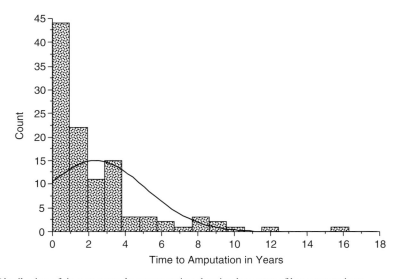

Fig. 7.1 Distribution of time to secondary amputation showing low rates of late amputations

The rate of amputation has reduced with time. Improved soft tissue cover for tibial EPRs, due to the routine use of gastrocnemius flaps, has led to significant reduction in infection rates and subsequent amputation. To date in our experience, the risk of amputation due to mechanical failure of the reconstruction with endoprostheses is negligible, with no amputations having to be performed due to aseptic loosening of implants. This suggests that reconstruction is a reliable long-term method of reconstruction.

Published results on amputation subsequent to limb salvage are quite scarce. Sim et al. [2] published a consecutive series of 50 endoprosthetic reconstructions around the knee performed between 1996 and 2005, with a mean follow-up of 2 years, with 3 subsequent amputations (6%). Sharma et al. [3] published a series of 77 distal femoral replacements performed between 1989 and 2004 with a mean follow up of 52 months. There were 5 (7%) subsequent amputations for control of local recurrence in 3 cases and infection in 2 cases. Ahlmann et al. [4] reported the outcome of endoprostheses of the lower limb in 211 patients performed between 1988 and 2003, with a mean follow-up of 14 months. There were 5 subsequent amputations (2.4%), 3 for control of infection and 2 for locally recurrent disease. Of 235 patients presenting with lower limb neoplasia, 24 (10%) underwent primary amputation. The literature is even more sparse when it comes to published limb salvage rates for new presentations of tumours, as units that have higher primary amputation rates theoretically should have less locally recurrent disease, and therefore lower secondary amputations.

Biological reconstructions are not immune to subsequent amputation. Futani et al. [5] compared endoprosthetic reconstruction to biological reconstruction for 40 skeletally immature patients with tumours of the distal femur. They found that 5 amputations were required, 1 for a skip metastasis and 4 secondarily to complications. The amputation was required in 1 of the 28 patients with an endoprosthesis (4%) compared to 3 of the 12 patients with a biological reconstruction (25%). Brigman et al. [6] reported the outcome of 116 patients under the age of 18 years who had undergone resection of a bone tumour about the knee and reconstruction with allograft. Amputation was required in 14 patients (12%), with a further 27% of patients having had a fracture and 34% having a non-union.

With modern surgical techniques and imaging, adjuvant therapy limb salvage is possible in the vast majority of patients presenting with a bone sarcoma. Endoprosthetic replacement has excellent long-term limb salvage results, despite increasing time-dependant complications. Infection and local recurrence remain the main threats to limb salvage.

7.3
Infection and Endoprostheses

Infection poses the largest iatrogenic risk to limb salvage, and controlling infection remains one the greatest challenges facing the limb salvage surgeon. Infection has always been the nemesis of orthopaedic implant surgery; however, infection rates in primary lower limb arthroplasty are currently low, typically reported to be 0.5%–2%, attributed to the use antibiotic loaded cement, antibiotic prophylaxis and clean air laminar flow theatres.

Infection of an implant is difficult to eradicate because of the adherent colonies of bacteria in a polysaccharide matrix, collectively called a biofilm [7]. This mode of growth has been implicated in a range of infections of medical devices, its importance in infection of orthopaedic implants being first noted by Gristina and Costerton [8]. Bacteria within biofilms are resistant to several hundred times the bactericidal concentrations of standard antibiotics [9]. The exact mechanism of resistance is not fully known, but hypotheses vary from protective effects of the enveloping polysaccharide to phenotypic variation of bacteria [10]. Infecting bacteria can remain dormant on the surface of an implant for a variable length of time. When conditions are right, clinical symptoms can be caused directly or indirectly by the local proliferation of bacteria shed by the biofilm. This may occur acutely, such as after fixation of a fracture, or several months or years after joint replacement when septic loosening occurs.

In a recent series of 1,254 patients receiving endoprostheses for musculoskeletal oncology, deep periprosthetic infection was identified in 136 (10.8%) patients [12]. The commonest pathogenic organisms were coagulase-negative Staphylococcus in 65 cultures (37%), *Staphylococcus aureus* in 35 cultures (20%), group D Streptococci in 16 cultures (9%) and *Escherichia coli* in 10 cultures (6%). These organisms are similar to ones found in published results for primary arthroplasty [13, 14]; multi-antibiotic resistant strains such as methicillin-resistant *Staphylococcus aureus* (MRSA) and vancomycin-resistant Staphylococcus epidermis (VRSE) were only isolated in 5 patients.

The risk of infection varied dramatically with the site of the endoprosthetic replacement with the highest risk in the tibia at 23% ($n = 57/247$), pelvis 22.9% ($n = 11/48$), distal femur 9.3% ($n = 48/519$) and proximal femur 6% ($n = 18/270$), and were lowest in the humerus at 1.1% ($n = 2/180$). Infection rates have decreased with time, with infection rates since 1995 being 2.7%.

Infection typically presented within 12 months from the last surgical procedure and at a mean of 2 years from insertion of the EPR. In keeping with research from Greidanus [11], the inflammatory markers of erythrocyte sedimentation rate (ESR) and C reactive protein (CRP) were often significantly raised at presentation (mean ESR = 74, mean CRP = 96 mg/l).

A number of host and surgical factors were identified as the presumed cause of infection; however, it was most commonly attributed to peri-operative bacteraemia attributed to indwelling central venous lines in 11% ($n = 15$) and revision surgery in 10.3% ($n = 14$). Preventable causes of deep infection, such as dental sepsis, ingrowing toenails and peri-operative throat infections, have previously accounted for 15.7% of infections. All patients prior to EPR surgery are now seen by a dentist and thoroughly examined for signs of infection pre-operatively and surgery is deferred until the patient's neutrophil count is above 1,200/mm^3.

Prophylaxis against infection is clearly important and the evidence on prophylaxis with antibiotic best practice is mixed. The standard prophylaxis in our unit for a primary EPR is a 1.5 g IV bolus of cefuroxime at induction followed by 3 post-operative doses of 750 mg cefuroxime in the 24 h following surgery. For revision surgery we favour a glycopeptide at induction, which continues for 5 days post-operatively until the results from samples taken at surgery are available. Antibiotic prophylaxis for patients with EPRs undergoing dental treatment is equally contentious. Guidelines from the British Orthopaedic Association for patients with total joint replacement is that no antibiotic prophylaxis is required; however, our advice to patients undergoing invasive procedures that risk bacteraemia is that they should have prophylaxis with amoxicillin (1 g IV or 3 g orally), which is the recommended regimen for patients with artificial heart valves.

Treatment for infection is arduous, time-consuming and expensive. The best treatment regime has been debated for primary arthroplasty, with both one-stage and two-stage revision having their advocates [16–19]. In our published series for EPRs [12], two-stage revision ($n = 58$), amputation ($n = 43$), surgical debridement ($n = 41$), one-stage revision ($n = 33$), coverage with a soft tissue flap ($n = 15$), antibiotic impregnated beads ($n = 11$), antibiotic impregnated cement ($n = 7$), excision arthroplasty ($n = 2$) and arthrodesis ($n = 1$) were all attempted. Local treatments, such as surgical debridement (2.4%; $n = 1/41$), arthroscopic washout (7.7%; $n = 1/13$), antibiotics alone

(6.8%; $n=8/117$) or impregnated beads/cement (11.1%; $n=2/18$) have little chance of curing deep infection. The limb salvage treatment with the best probability of curing deep infection was two-stage revision (70.7%, $n=41/58$), which was significantly more effective than one-stage revision (42.4%, Fig. 7.2). In our unit this entails removing the infected prosthesis with a thorough debridement of all the pseudocapsule (including the scar tissue behind the knee), inserting an antibiotic-impregnated cement spacer for a minimum of 7 weeks with parenteral antibiotics matched to the sensitivity of the isolated organism (Fig. 7.3). A new prosthesis can then be inserted if an aspirate taken from the peri-prosthetic cavity 4 weeks after the first stage revision (with no antibiotics for 1 week prior to aspiration) fails to grow any organism on extended cultures after 3 weeks. Multiple tissue samples are taken at the second stage of revision and the patient is kept on treatment antibiotics until the cultures are negative after 5 days incubation. If deep tissue samples are positive, intravenous antibiotics are continued for 6 weeks post-operatively.

Patients who have a deep infection have a significantly ($p<0.001$) higher risk of amputation (36.7%) compared with those without infection (6.2%); however, following the routine use of two-stage revision, the rate of amputation has reduced to approximately 25% for infections.

Several risk factors were identified that significantly increased the risk of deep infection and these were radiation therapy, subsequent patellar resurfacing, extendable prostheses, a tibial EPR site, a pelvic EPR site and subsequent operation to replace polythene bushings.

Recent published infection rates for tumour prostheses are similar to our results. Sharma et al. [3], published a series of 77 distal femoral EPRs with a mean follow-up of 52 months, with 6 deep infections (7.8%). Flint et al. [21] described a series of 44 uncemented proximal tibial EPRs with 7 deep infections (15.9%). Gosheger et al. [22] described one the largest series of 250 EPRs with a deep infection occurring in 30 patients (12%).

Infection is also a problem in biological reconstruction, in a series of 25 vascularized

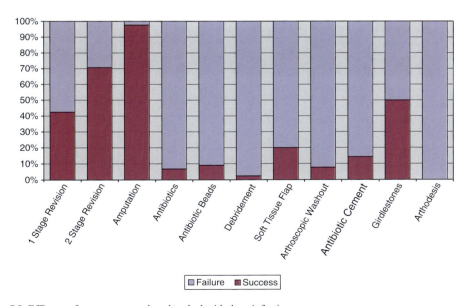

Fig. 7.2 Efficacy of treatments employed to deal with deep infection

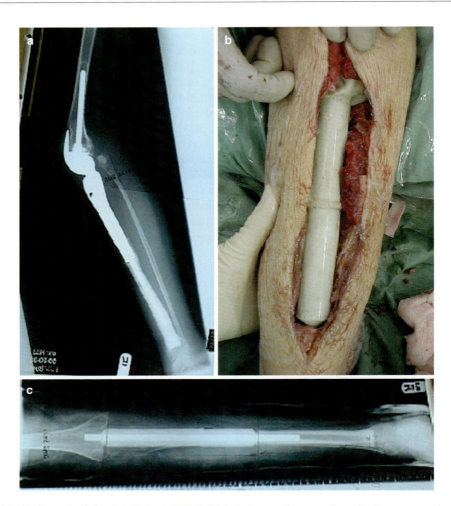

Fig. 7.3 a Radiograph of chronic infection in EPR. b Clinical photograph and c radiograph of cement space in situ

fibula strut grafts, Chen et al. [23], described 3 infections (12%). Muscolo et al. [24] described their experience of osteoarticular allografts of the distal femur; of the 62 patients available for review, 6 reconstructions failed due to infection (9.7%). Brigman et al. [6] showed a 16% infection rate in their series of 116 patients under the age of 18 years treated with allografts around the knee.

Some encouraging research from both animal [25, 26] and human studies [27] has shown that for patients with osteosarcoma, deep infection may have a survival benefit. In patients who had a deep early infection without metastases at presentation, the 10-year survival rate of 84.5% in the infected group compared to 62.2% in the non-infected group ($p=0.017$; Fig. 7.4). Deep infection had no effect on the development of

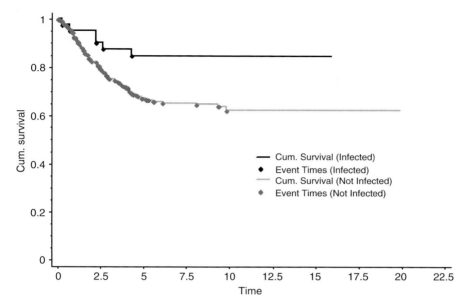

Fig. 7.4 Kaplan–Meier survival curves of survival rates for osteosarcoma for patients with and without deep infection using landmark analysis

locally recurrent disease ($p=0.56$) or distant metastases ($p=0.29$). There was a trend towards an increased time to metastases in the infected group but this was not significant ($p=0.09$, mean time for infected group=85 months, mean time for non-infected group=64 months). The postulated mechanisms for increased survival included stimulation of tumour necrosis factor (TNF)-α, cytotoxic cell-mediated tumour suppression and prevention of tumour neovascularization.

7.4 New Techniques to Combat Infection

With all types of reconstruction suffering similar significant levels of failure due to infection, the research efforts of several groups have identified ways that infection may be reduced, with the majority of emphasis being placed on prevention of infection rather than treatment.

7.4.1 Surface Treatments

Various chemicals are either bactericidal or bacteriostatic and considerable research is ongoing into how these could be incorporated into implants. The greatest interest is directed towards the coating of implants with silver. The anti-bacterial properties of silver have been known for thousands of years, dating back to ancient Greece. Silver, in its ionic form, binds to bacterial DNA, hindering bacterial replication and simultaneous deactivation of metabolic enzymes. Silver surface coatings have been used in a variety of medical devices from urinary catheters to cardiac valves. The sustained slow release of silver nanoparticles may prove to be important in the long-term effectiveness of this technology. Gosheger et al. [28, 29] have shown that silver coating of EPRs can reduce the infection rate in animal models and is non-toxic in humans. Other surface materials such as bioactive ceramics, antibiotic derivatives and surfactants to disrupt biofilms have all been investigated [30–33]. Antibiotics may be loaded into morcelized and allograft bone grafts in an attempt to reduce infection, and iontophoresis may be a novel technique to ensure high tissue levels of antibiotics in the perioperative period [34–36].

7.4.2
Antibiotic Prophylaxis

The bacteria implicated in peri-prosthetic infection has evolved from *Staphylococcus aureus* through coagulase-negative Staphylococcus to the emerging threat of multi-drug resistant organisms. Al-Maiyah et al. [37] showed that 9% of surgical gloves were contaminated during surgery, most frequently with coagulase-negative Staphylococcus, and that the majority of isolates were not sensitive to cefuroxime. This finding has been replicated when studying the organisms isolated at revision surgery for infection. Several authors have suggested that glycopeptides should be used in the routine prophylaxis of joint replacements, though the evidence for this is limited [38–41].

7.5
Conclusions

Limb salvage surgery with endoprostheses is established and has shown good long-term results, comparable with biological reconstructions. Amputation, on the other hand, poses a significant long-term risk, often due to locally recurrent disease or deep periprosthetic sepsis. Infection rates are widely reported to be approximately 10%, with treatment being arduous and time-consuming. In our experience, two-stage revision surgeries have the best chance of limb salvage with acceptable results. Technological advances, including surface coatings, may help to reduce the risk of infection.

References

1. Jeys LM, Grimer RJ, Carter SR, Tillman RM (2003) Risk of amputation following limb salvage surgery with Endoprosthetic replacement, in a consecutive series of 1261 patients. Int Orthop 27:160–163
2. Sim IW, Tse LF, Ek ET, Powell GJ, Choong PF (2007) Salvaging the limb salvage: management of complications following endoprosthetic reconstruction for tumours around the knee. Eur J Surg Oncol 2007 33:796–802
3. Sharma S, Turcotte RE, Isler MH, Wong C (2006) Cemented rotating hinge endoprosthesis for limb salvage of distal femur tumors. Clin Orthop Relat Res 450:28–32
4. Ahlmann ER, Menendez LR, Kermani C, Gotha H (2006) Survivorship and clinical outcome of modular endoprosthetic reconstruction for neoplastic disease of the lower limb. J Bone Joint Surg 88:790–795
5. Futani H, Minamizaki T, Nishimoto Y, Abe S, Yabe H, Ueda T (2006) Long-term follow-up after limb salvage in skeletally immature children with a primary malignant tumor of the distal end of the femur. J Bone Joint Surg Am 88:595–603
6. Brigman BE, Hornicek FJ, Gebhardt MC, Mankin HJ (2004) Allografts about the knee in young patients with high-grade sarcoma. Clin Orthop Relat Res 421:232–239
7. Pickering SAW (2003) Electromagnetic augmentation of antibiotic efficacy in infection of orthopaedic implants. J Bone Joint Surg Br 85:588–593
8. Gristina AG, Costerton JW (1984) Bacterial adherence and the glycocalyx and their role in musculoskeletal infection. Orthop Clin North Am 15:517–535
9. Nickel JC, Ruseska I, Wright JB, Costerton JW (1985) Tobramycin resistance of *Pseudomonas aeruginosa* cells growing as a biofilm on urinary catheter material. Antimicrob Agents Chemother 27:619–624
10. Gilbert P, Allison DG (1999) Biofilms and their resistance towards antimicrobial agents. In: Newman HN, Wilson M (eds) Dental plaque

revisited: oral biofilms in nature and disease. Bioline Publications, Cardiff, pp 125–143
11. Greidanus NV, Masri BA, Garbuz DS, Wilson SD, McAlinden MG, Xu M, Duncan CP (2007) Use of erythrocyte sedimentation rate and C-reactive protein level to diagnose infection before revision total knee arthroplasty. A prospective evaluation. J Bone Joint Surg Am 89:1409–1416
12. Jeys LM, Grimer RJ, Carter SR, Tillman RM (2005) Periprosthetic infection in patients treated for an orthopaedic oncological condition. J Bone Joint Surg Am 87:842–849
13. Fulkerson E, Valle CJ, Wise B, Walsh M, Preston C, Di Cesare PE (2006) Antibiotic susceptibility of bacteria infecting total joint arthroplasty sites. J Bone Joint Surg Am 88:1231–1237
14. Tsukayama DT, Estrada R, Gustilo RB (1996) Infection after total hip arthroplasty. A study of the treatment of one hundred and six infections. J Bone Joint Surg Am 1996 78:512–523
15. Reference deleted in proof
16. Raut VV, Siney PD, Wroblewski BM (1995) One-stage revision of total hip arthroplasty for deep infection. Long-term follow up. Clin Orthop Relat Res 321:202–207
17. Callaghan JJ, Katz RP, Johnston RC (1999) One-stage revision surgery of the infected hip. A minimum 10-year followup study. Clin Orthop Relat Res 369:139–143
18. Colyer RA, Capello WN (1994) Surgical treatment of the infected hip implant. Two-stage reimplantation with a one-month interval. Clin Orthop Relat Res 298:75–79
19. Younger AS, Duncan CP, Masri BA, McGraw RW (1997) The outcome of two-stage arthroplasty using a custom-made interval spacer to treat the infected hip. J Arthroplasty 12:615–623
20. Reference deleted in proof
21. Flint MN, Griffin AM, Bell RS, Ferguson PC, Wunder JS (2006) Aseptic loosening is uncommon with uncemented proximal tibia tumor prostheses. Clin Orthop Relat Res 450:52–59
22. Gosheger G, Gebert C, Ahrens H, Streitbuerger A, Winkelmann W, Hardes J (2006) Endoprosthetic reconstruction in 250 patients with sarcoma. Clin Orthop Relat Res 450:164–171
23. Chen CM, Disa JJ, Lee HY, Mehrara BJ, Hu QY, Nathan S, Boland P, Healey J, Cordeiro PG (2007) Reconstruction of extremity long bone defects after sarcoma resection with vascularized fibula flaps: a 10-year review. Plast Reconstr Surg 119:915–924
24. Muscolo DL, Ayerza MA, Aponte-Tinao LA, Ranalletta M (2006) Use of distal femoral osteoarticular allografts in limb salvage surgery. Surgical technique. J Bone Joint Surg Am 88[Suppl 12]:305–321
25. Lascelles BD, Dernell WS, Correa MT, Lafferty M, Devitt CM, Kuntz CA, Straw RC, Withrow SJ (2005) Improved survival associated with postoperative wound infection in dogs treated with limb-salvage surgery for osteosarcoma. Ann Surg Oncol 12:1073–1083
26. Thrall DE, Withrow SJ, Powers BE, Straw RC, Page RL, Heidner GL, Richardson DC, Bissonnette KW, Betts CW, DeYoung DJ (1990) Radiotherapy prior to cortical allograft limb sparing in dogs with osteosarcoma: a dose response assay. Int J Radiat Oncol Biol Phys 18:1351–1357
27. Jeys LM, Grimer RJ, Carter SR, Tillman RM, Abudu A (2007) Post operative infection and increased survival in osteosarcoma patients: are they associated? Ann Surg Oncol 14: 2887–2895
28. Gosheger G, Hardes J, Ahrens H, Streitburger A, Buerger H, Erren M, Gunsel A, Kemper FH, Winkelmann W, Von Eiff C (2004) Silver-coated megaendoprostheses in a rabbit model—an analysis of the infection rate and toxicological side effects. Biomaterials 25:5547–5556
29. Hardes J, Ahrens H, Gebert C, Streitbuerger A, Buerger H, Erren M, Gunsel A, Wedemeyer C, Saxler G, Winkelmann W, Gosheger G (2007) Lack of toxicological side-effects in silver-coated megaprostheses in humans. Biomaterials 28:2869–2875
30. Munukka E, Leppäranta O, Korkeamäki M, Vaahtio M, Peltola T, Zhang D, Hupa L, Ylänen H, Salonen JI, Viljanen MK, Eerola E (2007) Bactericidal effects of bioactive glasses on clinically important aerobic bacteria. J Mater Sci Mater Med [Epub ahead of print]
31. Lawson MC, Bowman CN, Anseth KS (2007) Vancomycin derivative photopolymerized to titanium kills S. epidermidis. Clin Orthop Relat Res 461:96–105
32. Price JS, Tencer AF, Arm DM, Bohach GA (1996) Controlled release of antibiotics from coated orthopedic implants. J Biomed Mater Res 30:281–286
33. Moussa FW, Gainor BJ, Anglen JO, Christensen G, Simpson WA (1996) Disinfecting agents for removing adherent bacteria from orthopaedic hardware. Clin Orthop Relat Res 329:255–262

34. Day RE, Megson S, Wood D (2005) Iontophoresis as a means of delivering antibiotics into allograft bone. J Bone Joint Surg Br 87:1568–1574
35. Michalak KA, Khoo PP, Yates PJ, Day RE, Wood DJ (2006) Iontophoresed segmental allografts in revision arthroplasty for infection. J Bone Joint Surg Br 88:1430–1437
36. Buttaro M, Comba F, Piccaluga F (2007) Vancomycin-supplemented cancellous bone allografts in hip revision surgery. Clin Orthop Relat Res 461:74–80
37. Al-Maiyah M, Hill D, Bajwa A, Slater S, Patil P, Port A, Gregg PJ (2005) Bacterial contaminants and antibiotic prophylaxis in total hip arthroplasty. J Bone Joint Surg Br 87:1256–1258
38. Periti P, Mini E, Mosconi G (1998) Antimicrobial prophylaxis in orthopaedic surgery: the role of teicoplanin. J Antimicrob Chemother 41: 329–340
39. Nehrer S, Thalhammer F, Schwameis E, Breyer S, Kotz R (1998) Teicoplanin in the prevention of infection in total hip replacement. Arch Orthop Trauma Surg 118:32–36
40. Periti P, Stringa G, Mini E (1999) Comparative multicenter trial of teicoplanin versus cefazolin for antimicrobial prophylaxis in prosthetic joint implant surgery. Italian Study Group for Antimicrobial Prophylaxis in Orthopedic Surgery. Eur J Clin Microbiol Infect Dis 18:113–119
41. de Lalla F (2001) Antibiotic prophylaxis in orthopedic prosthetic surgery. J Chemother 1:48–53

Reconstruction of the Pelvis After Resection of Malignant Bone Tumours in Children and Adolescents

Martin Dominkus, Eslam Darwish, and Philipp Funovics

Abstract The predominant tumour of the pelvic region in children and adolescents is Ewing's sarcoma followed by osteosarcoma. Both tumours are treated by chemotherapy and the best chance of survival is offered by wide tumour resection. Compared to surgical treatment on the extremities, the resection and reconstruction of pelvic sarcomas remains challenging. Surgery of pelvic sarcomas shows higher rates of local recurrence and complications and a lower functional outcome than other localisations. Especially in children and adolescents the reconstruction methods have to focus additionally on the growing skeleton. According to the different types of pelvic resections and therefore the need of different reconstruction methods, the following article is based on Enneking's surgical classification of pelvic resections. Type I resections are best reconstructed with autografts implanted between the supracetabular osteotomy and the sacrum. Patients show the best functional results after this reconstruction. Periacetabular resections (type II) in small children do best with iliofemoral arthrodesis or pseudarthrosis; in larger adolescents the use of the pedestal Schoellner cup showed superior results over the prior saddle prosthesis. Type III resections are not reconstructed. Complete internal hemipelvectomy represents the most difficult situation, in children as well as in adults. High complication rates after allograft and endoprosthetic reconstruction have recently favoured the renaissance of a flail hip reconstruction or the hip transpositionplasty.

8.1 Introduction

The pelvic area is a particular challenge for tumour orthopaedists, both in the diagnosis and in the therapy of primary malignant bone tumours. The most common tumour entities in children and adolescents are Ewing's sarcoma and osteosarcoma. These, as such, rare tumours are found in 9% [41] of the all Ewing's and osteosarcomas in the pelvic area. The diagnostic difficulty consists of the fact that these deep and

Martin Dominkus (✉)
Medical University of Vienna
University Clinic of Orthopaedics
Waehringer Guertel 18-20
1090 Vienna, Austria
E-mail: martin.dominkus@meduniwien.ac.at

centrally located tumours are only palpable when they are extremely large; furthermore, the clinical symptoms can be unspecific. Even in plain radiographs the tumours are diagnosed at a late stage, due to reduced image qualities by the inner organs. Thereby, from the surgical point of view, the frequent late diagnosis of a primary malignant tumour leads to exceptionally difficult conditions for an adequate tumour resection. This requires, as in the standard treatment of extremity tumours, a wide resection. Depending on the anatomical part of the pelvic bone involved by the tumour (ilium, ischium or pubis) and the age and physical demands of the patients, there are a number of different reconstruction options, all of which can be an oncological–surgical challenge due chiefly to the child's or adolescent's growing skeletal system. Therefore, in the following text, the necessary diagnostic measures and the possible reconstruction options for the individual resection sites will be discussed in detail.

8.2
Diagnosis

The predominant clinical symptom for tumours in the pelvic area is pain. As a rule this is diffuse and unspecific and can also simulate a radicular irritation as of a compression of the plexus parts or of the peripheral nerves. A palpable swelling—the second pathognomonic symptom of tumours—clinically appears very late, when the tumour's size is already very large. As applicable for tumours of the extremities, the first diagnostic tool is a plain X-ray. If the diagnosis from the X-ray is indistinct or if a definite lesion is not seen, then magnetic resonance (MR) tomography is indicated without delay. Furthermore, a bone scintigraphy is helpful to register very small lesions (e.g. osteoid osteoma). With these examinations a neoplastic occurrence can be confirmed or excluded with adequate certainty.

8.3
Biopsy

In the case of suspicion of a malignant bone tumour the next diagnostic step is the biopsy to secure the histological diagnosis. The biopsy, especially in the pelvic area, should only be carried out by an experienced tumour surgeon, as a tumour cell contamination in an adverse place can lead to inoperability and therewith usually lead to the death of the patient. In general, access to tumours of the os ilium have proved to be successful in the area of the iliac crest, whereby as a rule the biopsy can be performed subperiosteally on the medial wing side and covered by the iliac muscle. A biopsy of tumours of the os ischium is carried out preferably via a Ludloff approach and that of tumours of the os pubis can be carried out very well from the ventral side, medially of the femoral neurovascular bundle. Dependent on the histological diagnosis neoadjuvant chemotherapy according to standard protocols is carried out for osteosarcoma and Ewing's sarcoma. In childhood and adolescence, chondrosarcomas, which are not treated by chemotherapy, are very rare.

8.4
Preoperative Staging and Therapy

Later the patient receives a complete tumour staging, which usually comprises a lung/abdomen computed tomograph (CT), a whole body bone scintigraphy and a sonography of the inguinal and para-aortal lymph nodes. According to the localisation and extent of the tumour, further examinations may be necessary for the operative planning, such as an angiography or MR angiography, intravenous pyelography (IVP), cystoscopy or rectoscopy. Lately, in pre-operative management, the placing of a vena cava filter has been generally adopted to avoid thromboembolism, for which there is a clear increased risk in pelvic resections [19]. The classification of the pelvic resection types according to Enneking has proved efficient for the surgical resection treatment [12] (Fig. 8.1).

In the Vienna Bone Tumour Registry, which has been systematically registering all hospitalised patients treated for tumours of the skeletal system since 1966, there were 47 primary malignant bone tumours in children and adolescents under the age of 18 years (Table 8.1). Of these, 26 affected the os ilium (20 Ewing's sarcoma, 5 osteosarcoma, 1 chondrosarcoma), 11 the os pubis (10 Ewing's sarcoma, 1 osteosarcoma), 7 the os sacrum (3 Ewing's sarcoma, 4 osteosarcoma) and 3 the os ischium (2 Ewing's sarcoma, 1 osteosarcoma; see Table 8.2).

According to our data, Ewing's sarcoma is the numerically predominant type of tumour in the pelvic area in children and adolescents, and

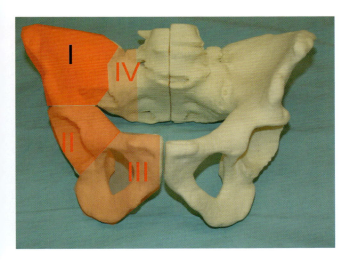

Fig. 8.1 Classification of pelvic resections according to Enneking. Type I refers to the supraacetabular ilium, type II to the periacetabular area, type III to the upper and lower pubic bone and type IV to the massa lateralis of the sacrum

Table 8.1 Distribution of primary malignant bone tumours of the pelvis below and over 18 years of age

Site	Total	≤18	>18
Ilium	127 (54.5%)	26	101
Ischium	11 (4.7%)	3	8
Pubis	39 (16.8%)	11	28
Sacrum	56 (24%)	7	49
Total	233 (100%)	47 (20.2%)	186 (79.8%)

Table 8.2 Distribution of the diagnosis according to the anatomic area

	Ilium ($n=26$)	Ischium ($n=3$)	Pubis ($n=11$)	Sacrum ($n=7$)
Ewing's sarcoma	20	2	10	3
Osteosarcoma	5	1	1	4
Chondrosarcoma	1			

osteosarcoma clearly occurs less frequently, in contrast to the extremities. The Ewing's tumours typically show a very large soft tissue tumour at diagnosis, which is usually reduced during the course of effective neoadjuvant chemotherapy, whereas, as a rule, one hardly notices any reduction in size in osteosarcoma during the neo-adjuvant chemotherapy. Therefore, the planning of the operation may change during chemotherapy, using regular MR controls of the tumour and its response to the chemotherapy.

Furthermore, the resection options and methods listed below should be set out according to Ennekings' classification.

8.5
Resection Type I: Os Ilium

8.5.1
Partial Resection of the Ilium Without Discontinuity of the Pelvic Ring

The most important feature in type I resections (Figs. 8.2 and 8.3) in respect to surgical reconstruction is the preservation or the interruptance of the pelvic continuity.

Small tumours in the region of the ala ossis ilii—which need a resection with a healthy, intra-osseous safety margin according to the MR tomography, without the continuity to the os sacrum being broken—can only be resected; in this case an osseous reconstruction is not necessary.

8.5.2
Complete Resection of the Os Ilium with Discontinuity of the Pelvic Ring

Tumours which affect the whole supraacetabular part of the os ilium (type I resection; Fig. 8.2) or those which approach the iliosacral joint or infringe into the massa lateralis of the sacrum (type I–IV resection; Fig. 8.4) require a complete supraacetabular resection of the iliac wing and as a rule are reconstructed biologically.

For this, autografts of the tibia (Figs. 8.5 and 8.6) or fibula are harvested, which are implanted supraacetabularly and in the iliosacral or sacral osteotomy area. As an alternative an iliosacral arthrodesis with allografts can be performed.

This reconstruction method achieves excellent functional results, with a minor rate of complications. As a rule the post-operative management is immobilisation in a pelvic cast

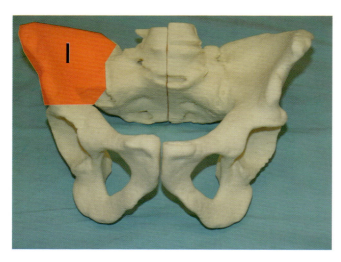

Fig. 8.2 Type I resection

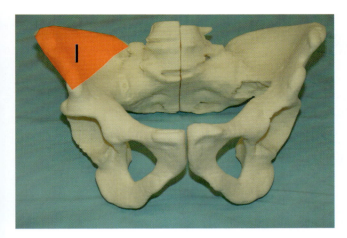

Fig. 8.3 Partial resection of the os ilium without discontinuity of the pelvic ring

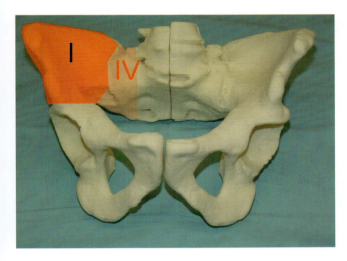

Fig. 8.4 Type I/IV resection

for at least 6 weeks with non-weight bearing mobilisation. After this the patient is mobilised with a removable pelvis–leg orthesis with a gradual release of movement in the hip joint for 3 months to half a year and a gradual increase in loading. Radiologically, thickening of the graft after bone consolidation is observed (Fig. 8.7). From this moment the patients are usually fully mobile without a walking aid and can, to a large extent, take part in sports activities. The length of the leg is well balanced or there can be a minimal shortening of 1–2 cm when the graft sinks in or the hip centre is raised. The functional result of a stable re-built pelvic ring depends on the degree of the resection of the gluteal muscles or the psoas muscle (Fig. 8.8).

8.6
Resection Type II: Acetabulum

For tumours in the region of the acetabulum (Fig. 8.9) or tumours of the proximal femur that show an extent of intra-articular involvement, a

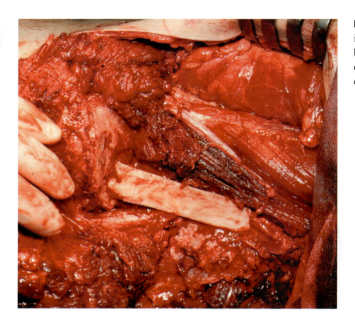

Fig. 8.5 Intra-operative view of interposition of a tibia autograft between the supraacetabular osteotomy and the sacral osteotomy

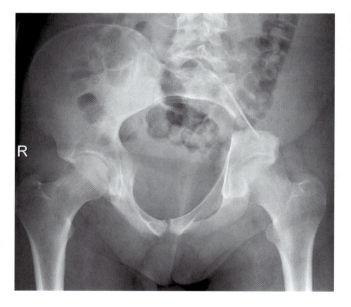

Fig. 8.6 Plain radiograph after a type I/IV resection of a Ewing's sarcoma in an 18-year-old boy with tibia autograft

resection of the acetabulum (type II) is necessary. These periacetabular resections require restoration of force transmission and weight bearing along the anatomic axis [11] and represent one of the most difficult situations in pelvic surgery. For reconstruction, either biological methods or endoprosthetic options are established.

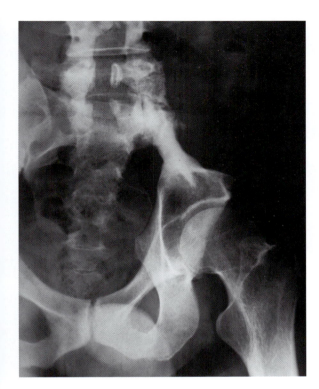

Fig. 8.7 X-ray 3 years post-operatively

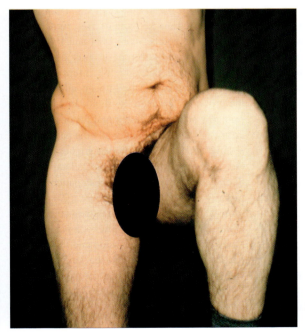

Fig. 8.8 Functional result after 3 years in the same patient

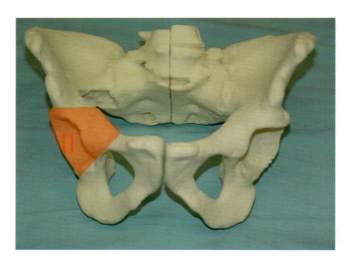

Fig. 8.9 Type II resection

8.6.1 Biological Reconstruction Methods

8.6.1.1 Iliofemoral Arthrodesis/Ischiofemoral Arthrodesis

Iliofemoral arthrodesis serves ideally for Enneking type II or Enneking type II and III resections, whereby the proximal osteotomy should be as near to the acetabulum as possible, in order to minimise the shortening of the leg and to achieve sufficient fusion. The fixation of the proximal femur or femoral head to the remaining ilium is made using plates; in addition, the trochanter major is fixed with the abductors. Furthermore, an iliac crest graft, which is also vascularly pedicled, can also be applied as an augmentation. Depending on the amount of pubis or ischium resection, additional arthrodesis and augmentation to the ischium or pubic bone can be performed (Fig. 8.10).

Using this method, the pelvic ring can be restored and patients achieve a partial limb function and a relief of pain [5]. In an attempt to preserve as much of the iliac bone as possible, to keep the leg shortening minimal, a high risk of local recurrence has been reported. Pseud-arthrosis may result as a failure after attempted fusion or as an option of a planned pseudarthrosis to preserve a partial motion of the hip joint (Figs. 8.11, 8.12, 8.13, 8.14 and 8.15) From the Mayo Clinic's experience on 60 patients treated from 1970 through 1985, 50% of the procedures resulted in a pseudarthrosis [32]. Fuchs et al. [14] reported on 32 patients who were treated with this method between 1981 and 1999. In 21 patients a solid arthrodesis was striven for, whereby for 5 patients the intention was a primary pseudarthrosis with an adaptation of the proximal femur to the ilium. In 14% of the primarily attempted iliofemoral fusions, a pseudarthrosis resulted. Functionally the patients with a solid fusion clearly showed higher values in the T score 76%, in Musculoskeletal Tumour Society (MSTS) score 71%, than patients with a primary pseudarthrosis (T score 52%; MSTS score 25%). In this group of patients there was a clinically noticeable mild low back pain, both in the patients with a solid fusion and those with a pseudarthrosis. The middle leg length discrepancy was 4.8 cm, which was compensated with a heightening of the shoe. The authors conclude that the iliofemoral arthrodesis is the reconstruction option of choice for young and active

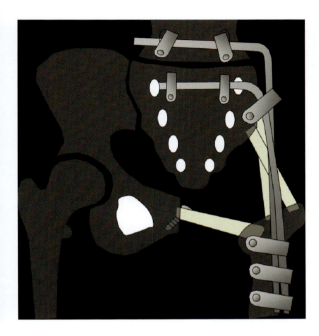

Fig. 8.10 Scheme of an iliofemoral and ischiofemoral arthrodesis with fibula-autografts and Isola Implants (AcroMed, Cleveland) instrumentation

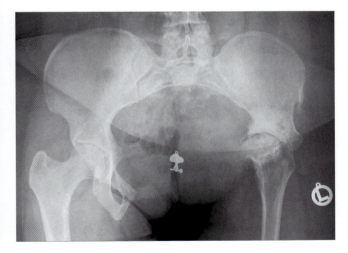

Fig. 8.11 Iliofemoral pseudarthrosis after a type II/III resection and osseous adaptation of a pseudoacetabulum in an 8-year-old girl after Ewing's sarcoma

patients with more activity requirements and the primary pseudarthrosis is ideal for patients who sit more.

Furthermore, iliofemoral arthrodesis' using microsurgical fibula flaps has been described [30, 37, 52, 55]. The advantage of this technically more demanding procedure is earlier bone healing and reliable results in the restoration of the pelvic ring. Only a mild limb length shortening of 2 cm, with satisfactory functional results and without operative complications, is reported in a small series [55].

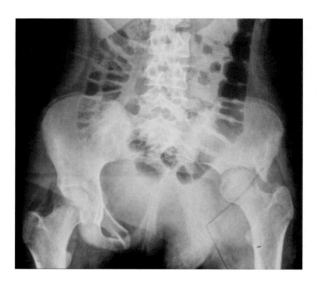

Fig. 8.12 Evolution of the remodelled acetabulum over time

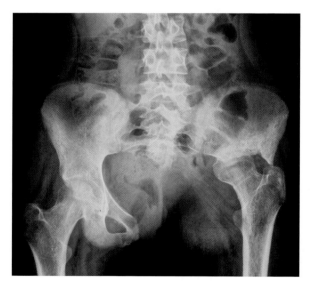

Fig. 8.13 Evolution of the remodelled acetabulum over time

An analysis comparing the costs of three different reconstruction methods—external hemipelvectomy with its need of an orthotic device, internal hemipelvectomy with endoprosthetic reconstruction and iliofemoral arthrodesis—clearly demonstrated the advantage of the latter method [4].

8.6.1.2
Implantation of an Acetabulum Allograft

For the biological reconstruction of a type II acetabular defect, autoclaved or irradiated bone as an autograft, or the use of an allograft, is specified (Figs. 12, 13 and 14) [2, 10, 17, 25, 28,

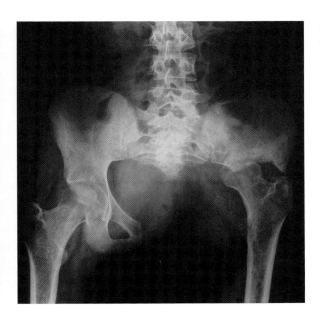

Fig. 8.14 Evolution of the remodelled acetabulum over time

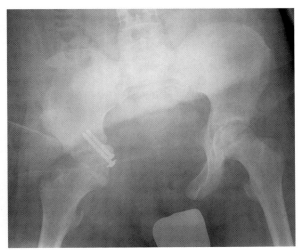

Fig. 8.15 Reconstruction after an intra-acetabular osteotomy with a pelvic crest in a 12-year-old boy after Ewing's sarcoma of the right pubic bone

33, 39, 42]. The advantage of using an allograft is the possibility of individual bone preparation and the full restoration of movement, in order to avoid an arthrodesis or a flail hip situation. However, a high rate of infection and mechanical failures have been reported [17, 33, 41]. In a study between 1985 and 2003 of 24 patients, Delloye et al. reported a 46% complication rate, all of whom needed an operation (11 patients); 9 patients had to be re-operated due to complications of the reconstruction [8]. Regarding functional results, an MSTS score of 73% was given whereby results were clearly better in patients under the age of 20 years. One has to point out that there were 25% neurological complications in periacetabular resections. The high infection rates given in the literature could be reduced by impregnating the allografts with rifampicin [9]. Non-union rates appeared, especially when the fit of the allograft was inadequate and large inter-fragmentary cracks formed. More than half of these patients were mobile without crutches. Children and adolescent patients showed a significantly better MSTS score (82%) when compared to adult patients (65%).

8.6.2 Endoprosthetic Reconstruction Methods

Many different techniques of endoprosthetic reconstruction of the pelvis after tumour resection have been reported [1, 15, 24, 26, 29, 31, 35, 40, 41, 44, 47–49]. The most important implants will be discussed in detail in the following chapter.

8.6.2.1 Saddle Prosthesis

The use of saddle prostheses after a peri-acetabular resection goes back to the original indication for reconstruction of patients with a large bone defect after a hip endoprosthesis or infections [31]. Since the end of the 1980s, experience has been gathered worldwide in the use of saddle prostheses after peri-acetabular tumour resection [1, 26, 35]. A lot of design-related complications such as loosening, loss of motion, dislocation and fractures have been addressed by modifications of the implant. The advantage is the modular construction of the prosthesis combined with a conventional hip shaft and the possibility to adjust any possible leg length difference. Aboulafia et al. [1] reported on 17 patients between 1988 and 1991 who were reconstructed with a saddle prosthesis after peri-acetabular tumours. Regarding the functional results, 12 out of 17 were assessed as excellent or good, 5 were fair or poor. The complications described were wound healing disorders and infections, but mostly prosthesis dislocation (53% of the complications). In the long term, one notices that there is often a cranial migration (Fig. 8.16) of the saddle or a snapping of the ilium. The basic requirement for good functional results is to create an adequate notch in the ilium and to achieve sufficient tension between the pelvis and the femur with an interposition of the correct implant length, in order to achieve well-balanced muscle tension via iliopsoas and

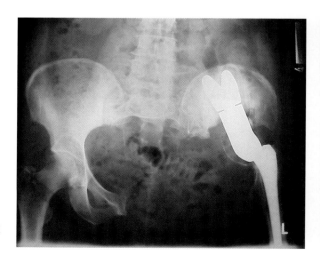

Fig. 8.16 Saddle prosthesis after a type II/III resection with a severe cranial migration

abductor. The absence of the iliac bone, as well as the condition after resection of the psoas and the abductor muscles is described as a contraindication [1].

8.6.2.2 Modular Pelvic Prosthesis

The high rates of infection and complications after allograft reconstructions and the desire for better functional results led to the development and widespread use of endoprosthetic reconstruction methods in the middle of the 1990s [20, 41, 49]. A 3D CT pelvis model of the patient was made pre-operatively to construct a modular custom-made pelvic endoprosthesis on which the exact resection margins of the tumour were marked and simulated (Fig. 8.17).

On the basis of this pre-operative planning, the custom-made pelvic prostheses were produced (Fig. 8.18) and these aimed at a restoration of the pelvic ring as well as the anatomical hip rotation. Intra-operatively, the resection simulated on the model was copied as exactly as possible in order to obtain an optimal fit for the prosthesis (Figs. 8.19 and 8.20). However, after good functional results at the beginning, the use of these mega-implants showed a high rate of prosthesis loosening, broken screws and migration of the prosthesis. The large cavity left after reconstructing the pelvic ring probably led to the high rate of post-operative haematoma and infection. Therefore, at the beginning of the third millennium the use of these custom-made mega-pelvic prostheses was widely abandoned [41].

However, the subtle pre-operative planning, which was necessary for the production of these pelvic prostheses, has led to a clear reduction in the rate of local relapse and a higher rate of adequately resected tumours [15].

8.6.2.3 Schoellner Pedestal Cup

More recently new socket designs have found acceptance. Initially the need for a revision [40] of severe acetabular defects after failed conventional hip arthroplasties encouraged the development of the pedestal socket (Schoellner cup, Zimmer, Warsaw, USA) which has more recently proved to be especially useful in the reconstruction of acetabular defects after tumour resection [44]. This relatively small implant requires only

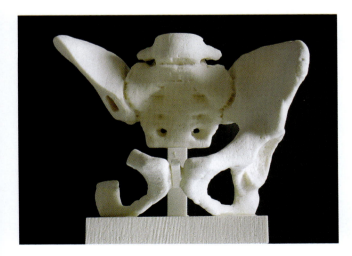

Fig. 8.17 Preoperative 3D CT model with the simulated tumour resection

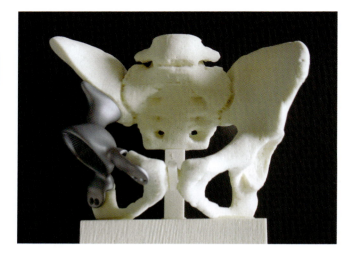

Fig. 8.18 Custom-made pelvis prosthesis with its exact fit

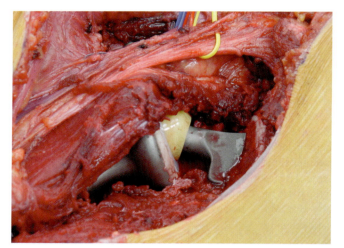

Fig. 8.19 Intra-operative situs after implantation

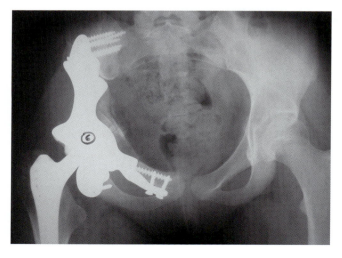

Fig. 8.20 Post-operative X-ray, 4 years after implantation. The pelvic prosthesis is covered by a periprosthetic ossification

a cranial part of the remaining os ilium and is implanted into it according to the load transferring lines of the iliosacral joint. Moreover, different lengths of sockets enable an extensive reconstruction of the hip rotation centre. Closing the pelvic ring by means of the prosthesis is not necessary due to the axial load transfer to the socket. Due to the small size of the implant as compared to the custom-made pelvic prostheses, good soft tissue coverage and a reduction of the wounds' dead space is easily possible, which has led to a clear reduction in the infection and complications rate [44]. The functional results correspond to those of conventional hip arthroplasties, depending, however, on the extent of the resection of the gluteal and psoas muscles. Due to the fact that this is a standard, commercially available implant, pre-operative time is no longer necessary for planning and implant production, as was the case for custom-made prostheses. These features have made the implant this author's reconstruction of choice in patients where a part of the iliac bone could be preserved (Figs. 8.21, 8.22, 8.23 and 8.24).

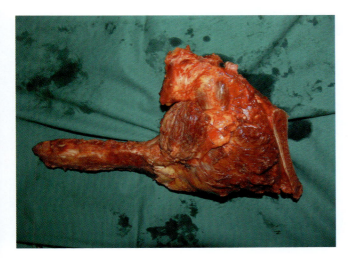

Fig. 8.21 Resected specimen after proximal femur resection with closed hip joint and acetabulum

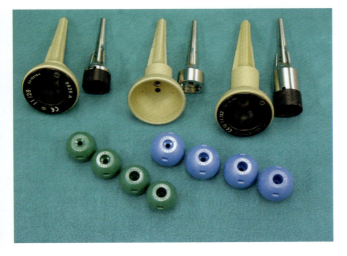

Fig. 8.22 Trial prosthesis of the "Schoellner" pedestal cup. Three different lengths of the socket are available for adjustment of the hip centre

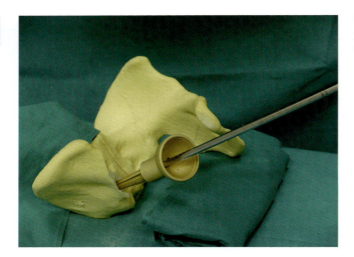

Fig. 8.23 Simulation of the prosthesis' insertion into the remaining ilium

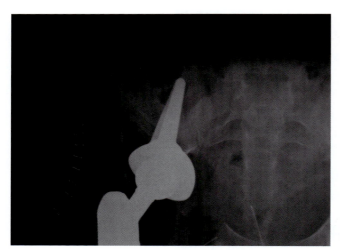

Fig. 8.24 Postoperative X-ray after implantation

8.6.2.4 Composite Allograft/Allograft Reconstruction

After tumour resection of the periacetabular region, a further option is the use of a pelvic allograft [2, 16] or an autograft, recycled by heating [3, 27], freezing [46, 53, 54] or irradiation [6, 42] in combination with a conventional hip prosthesis [23]. The most obvious advantage of an autograft is its perfect fit and easy accessibility. For both methods the most common complications are infection, fracture, loosening and local recurrence. The infection rate varies widely between 15% and 50% [2, 20, 25] and mainly depends on the extent of soft tissue resection, the remaining dead space after reconstruction and the need of adjuvant therapy such as chemotherapy or radiation therapy. Poor bone quality resulting from the recycling process of the autografts has been suggested to be responsible for graft fracture or loosening [23].

8.7
Resection Type I–II +/– IV

Acetabular/supra-acetabular tumours, which also affect large parts of the os ilium (resection type I–II +/–IV; Fig. 8.25) are the most common and difficult situations in large pelvic tumours. Depending on whether a cranial part of the os ilium can be preserved, there are a number of different reconstruction methods (Fig. 8.26 and 8.27).

8.7.1
Allograft

The use of allografts of the pelvic bone is a well-known method of reconstruction of every type of pelvic resection. Good functional results in the early follow-up are reported. However, high complication rates such as non-union, infection and fracture have not yet been solved. Significantly better results have been reported in patients below 20 years of age compared to older patients [8].

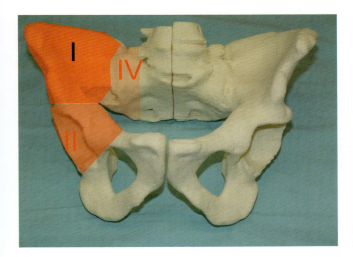

Fig. 8.25 Type I–II +/– IV resection

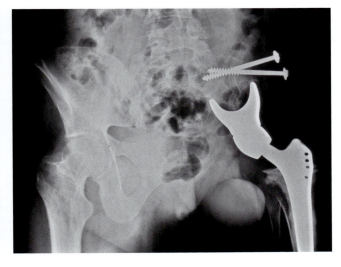

Fig. 8.26 A rare reconstruction after total femur resection and type I, II, III resection of the pelvis with rotationplasty and saddle prosthesis

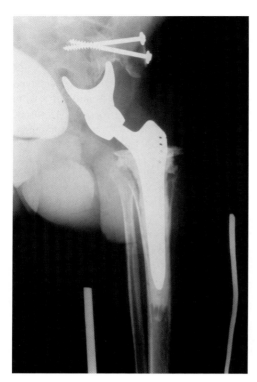

Fig. 8.27 A rare reconstruction after total femur resection and type I, II, III resection of the pelvis with rotationplasty and saddle prosthesis

8.7.2
Autograft

The resected specimen after tumour resection may serve as an autograft when the tumour is definitely denaturated. This can be achieved by autoclavation, pasteurisation, freezing or extracorporal irradiation. After complete removal of the soft tissues and the bony tumour bulk, the graft can be replanted. This procedure has some advantages compared to allografts. First, as autografts are directly resected, the shape of the graft is identical to the resection, so there is an optimal fit. Second, there are no foreign infectious or immunogenic agents which may influence the ingrowth of the graft [13, 42, 45].

Furthermore, there is no need of a bone bank [15, 18, 29].

However, a recent series of 15 patients reported a complication rate of 13/15 patients, mostly related to mechanical failures of hip arthroplasties, but also infection (3/15) and a high rate of local recurrences (7/15). The functional scores were fair.

8.7.3
Flail Hip

In the early days of limb salvage surgery an alternative to hindquarter amputation was the preserving of the leg after internal hemipelvectomy without reconstruction [38]. The indication was the possibility of preserving the nerve and muscle function of the leg after wide resection of the pelvic tumour. The remaining femur was left in place without reconstruction. This flail hip situation resulted in a leg length shortening of up to 10 cm, but the patients had a remaining leg function when the leg length was corrected by shoes. The functional results correlated with the amount of the ilium resection [43]. Lower complication rates and favourable wound healing compared to technically more demanding reconstruction methods have led to a renaissance of this reconstruction method. By introduction of textile implants the remaining head or even a part of a remaining acetabulum could be fixed to the sacral osteotomy with very good functional results [50]. This technique is called hip transpositionplasty.

8.7.4
Hip Transpositionplasty

In this variant the femur head is adjusted and fixed to the proximal, sacral osteotomy region with soft tissue or textile implants. As a rule this causes a considerable shortening of the leg. With an adequate orthopaedic shoe, these patients indicate a satisfactory, functional result and also show a lower complication rate. Methods of subsequent osteodistraction treatment for lengthening of the femur have been described [36].

The incidence of complications and the number of revisions were reported to be the lowest compared to endoprosthetic reconstruction or allograft reconstruction (Figs. 8.28, 8.29 and 8.30) [20, 21].

8.8 Resection Type III

Tumours of the upper or lower pubic bone, which do not involve the acetabulum, require a resection of the upper or lower pubic bone (Fig. 8.31). In these cases there is no need for a bone reconstruction.

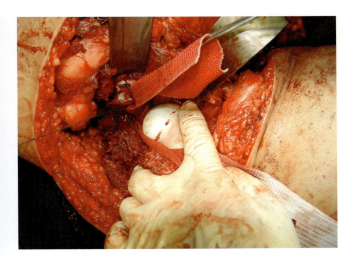

Fig. 8.28 Transposition of the femoral head to the sacral osteotomy. A polyester band (LARS, Dijon, France) is fixed by transosseous sutures to the sacrum

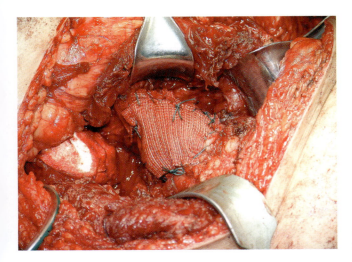

Fig. 8.29 Fixation of the femoral head by closing the LARS band

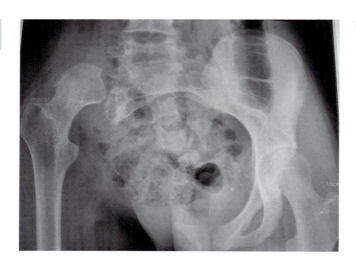

Fig. 8.30 Post-operative X-ray

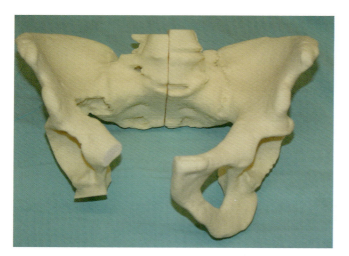

Fig. 8.31 Type III resection

8.9
Resection Type II, III

Tumours of the upper and lower pubic bone, which additionally affect the acetabulum, require an intra-acetabular or supra-acetabular resection (type II–III; Fig. 8.32). The reconstruction is in keeping with the sole type II resection.

8.10
Resection Type I–III/IV

Tumours which affect the total hemipelvis (type I–III/IV; Fig. 8.33) require a complete resection of the hemipelvis.

This can be carried out as an internal or external hemipelvectomy. An external hemipelvectomy is

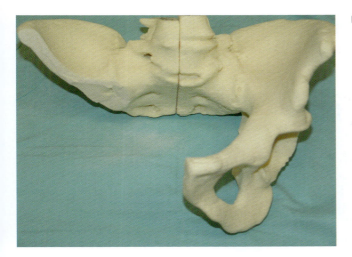

Fig. 8.32 Type II/III resection

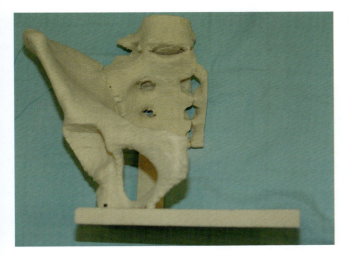

Fig. 8.33 Type I–III/IV resection

indicated when an oncologically adequate resection would result in a major resection of the nervus femoralis and nervus ischiadicus or a resection of the sacral nerve roots is necessary, which would lead to an unusable leg. Furthermore, the indication for an external hemipelvectomy has to result as a non-reconstructable vascular resection of the iliac vessels.

If an internal hemipelvectomy is oncologically and technically possible, then reconstruction methods covered in the following sections apply.

8.10.1
Flail Hip: No Reconstruction

8.10.1.1
Hip Transpositionplasty

8.10.1.1.1
Custom-Made Pelvic Prostheses

In some patients, spontaneous periprosthetic ossification were seen (Fig. 8.20), in others additional bone grafting was performed during

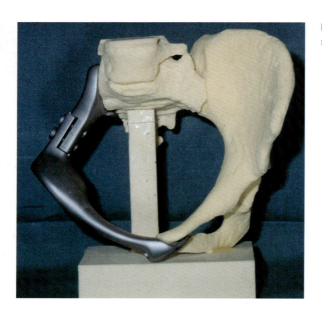

Fig. 8.34 Custom-made prosthesis for the right hemipelvis

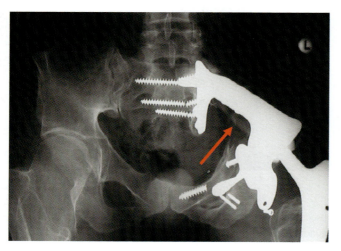

Fig. 8.35 Six-year follow-up after resection of the left hemipelvis. Lateral migration of the custom-made prosthesis with fracture of all screws and dislocation of the prosthesis occurred after 3 years postoperatively. Bone grafting with allografts was performed, which led to a stable periprosthetic ossification and stabilised the prosthesis (*arrow*)

surgical revision without changing the prosthesis's position. In these patients, loosening did not occur or the dislocation process stopped due to the stabilising effect of the ossification (Figs. 8.34 and 8.35).

8.10.2
Hemipelvis Allograft

Allografts offer the advantage of biological restoration of the pelvis and enable easier muscle reattachment (Figs. 8.36, 8.37, 8.38 and 8.39).

8 Reconstruction of the Pelvis After Resection of Malignant Bone Tumours in Children and Adolescents

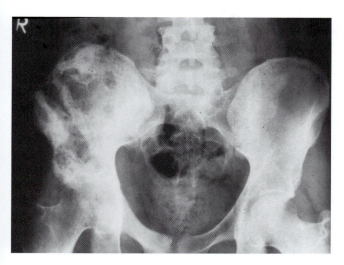

Fig. 8.36 Ewing's sarcoma of the entire hemipelvis

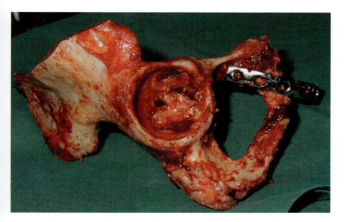

Fig. 8.37 Allograft of the hemipelvis

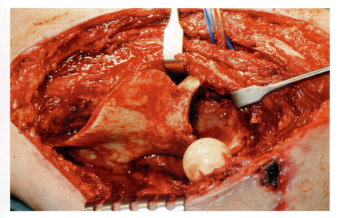

Fig. 8.38 Intra-operative situs of the implanted allograft

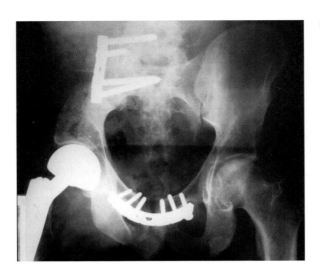

Fig. 8.39 Postoperative X-ray

8.11 Future Aspects

Oncological follow-up has shown that patients with primary malignant tumours of the pelvic area clearly have a worse prognosis than a comparable statistical population with tumours of the extremities. This is due to the fact that these tumours very often are discovered at a late stage, having spread extensively, and also that the local recurrence rate in pelvic resections clearly exceeds those of extremity resections. Especially the 3D planning and performance of an adequate tumour resection is a formidable task for the orthopaedic surgeon. The use of pre-operative planning on a 3D CT pelvis model has already proved efficient with a significant reduction of inadequate margins [15], and further development of computer-assisted navigation techniques based on CT and MR images will hopefully improve the rate of adequate resections in the pelvic region [7, 22, 34, 51].

Summary

Modern technical and surgical developments also favour limb salvage procedures as the preferred treatment of pelvic sarcomas in children and adolescents. However, surgery in the pelvic area represents an especially difficult task for the oncological orthopaedist seeking to achieve adequate margins. Many different techniques of reconstruction have been described according to the pelvic resection types and some differences can be seen in complication rates and the patients' functional outcome. The choice of the reconstruction method has to take into consideration the patients' age, amount of bone and soft tissue resection, the attempted functional outcome and the possible complication rate of the method.

Summing up the presented options, the younger the child, the more that biological reconstructions attempting solid pelvico-femoral fusions are indicated. In older patients, endoprosthetic reconstruction of the hip joint, preferably by the use of the pedestal cup (Schoellner cup), offers an excellent functional outcome with a very low complication rate. The method of choice after complete internal hemipelvectomy seems to be the hip transpositionplasty because of its predictable low complication rate and acceptable functional outcome.

References

1. Aboulafia AJ, Buch R, Mathews J, Li W, Malawer MM (1995) Reconstruction using the saddle prosthesis following excision of primary and metastatic periacetabular tumors. Clin Orthop Relat Res 314:203–213
2. Bell RS, Davis AM, Wunder JS, Buconjic T, McGoveran B, Gross AE (1997) Allograft reconstruction of the acetabulum after resection of stage-IIB sarcoma. Intermediate-term results. J Bone Joint Surg Am 79:1663–1674
3. Bohm P, Springfeld R, Springer H (1998) Re-implantation of autoclaved bone segments in musculoskeletal tumor surgery. Clinical experience in 9 patients followed for 1.1–8.4 years and review of the literature. Arch Orthop Trauma Surg 118:57–65
4. Bruns J, Luessenhop S, Behrens P (1998) Cost analysis of three different surgical procedures for treatment of a pelvic tumour. Langenbecks Arch Surg 383:359–363
5. Capanna R, Guernelli N, Ruggieri P (1987) Periacetabular pelvic resections. In: Enneking WF (ed) Limb salvage in musculoskeletal oncology. Churchill Livingstone, New York, pp 141–146
6. Chen TH, Chen WM, Huang CK (2005) Reconstruction after intercalary resection of malignant bone tumours: comparison between segmental allograft and extracorporeally-irradiated autograft. J Bone Joint Surg Br 87:704–709
7. Krettek C, Geerling J, Bastian L, Citak M, Rücker F, Kendoff D, Hüfner T (2004) Computer aided tumor resection in the pelvis. Injury 35[Suppl 1]:79–83
8. Delloye C, Banse X, Brichard B, Docquier PL, Cornu O (2007) Pelvic reconstruction with a structural pelvic allograft after resection of a malignant bone tumor. J Bone Joint Surg Am 89:579–587
9. Delloye C (2000) Bone banking in orthopaedic surgery. In: Gallinaro P, Lemaire R (eds) Surgical techniques in orthopaedics and traumatology. Elsevier, Paris, pp 55–61
10. Delloye C, de Nayer P, Allington N, Munting E, Coutelier L, Vincent A (1988) Massive bone allografts in large skeletal defects after tumor surgery: a clinical and microradiographic evaluation. Arch Orthop Trauma Surg 107:31–41
11. Enneking WF, Dunham WK (1978) Resection and reconstruction for primary neoplasms involving the innominate bone. J Bone Joint Surg Am 60:731–746
12. Enneking WF, Spanier SS, Goodman MA (1980) A system for the surgical staging of musculoskeletal sarcoma. Clin Orthop Relat Res 153:106–120
13. Friedlaender GE (1991) Bone allografts: the biological consequences of immunological events. J Bone Joint Surg Am 73:1119–1122
14. Fuchs B, O'Connor MI, Kaufman KR, Padgett DJ, Sim FH (2002) Iliofemoral arthrodesis and pseudarthrosis: a long-term functional outcome evaluation. Clin Orthop Relat Res 397:29–35
15. Gradinger R, Rechl H, Hipp E (1991) Pelvic osteosarcoma. Resection, reconstruction, local control, and survival statistics. Clin Orthop Relat Res 270:149–158
16. Guest CB, Bell RS, Davis A, Langer F, Ling H, Gross AE, Czitrom A (1990) Allograft-implant composite reconstruction following periacetabular sarcoma resection. J Arthroplasty 5 Suppl:25–34
17. Harrington KD (1992) The use of hemipelvic allografts or autoclaved grafts for reconstruction after wide resections of malignant tumors of the pelvis. J Bone Joint Surg Am 74:331–341
18. Harrington KD, Johnston JO, Kaufer HN, Luck JV Jr, Moore TM (1986) Limb salvage and prosthetic joint reconstruction for low-grade and selected high-grade sarcomas of bone after wide resection and replacement by autoclaved [corrected] autogenetic grafts. Clin Orthop Relat Res 211:180–214 Erratum in: Clin Orthop 216:312
19. Helmberger T (2007) Vena cava filter [in German]. Radiologe 47:439–442
20. Hillmann A, Hoffmann C, Gosheger G, Rödl R, Winkelmann W, Ozaki T (2003) Tumors of the

pelvis: complications after reconstruction. Arch Orthop Trauma Surg 123:340–344
21. Hoffmann C, Gosheger G, Gebert C, Jürgens H, Winkelmann W (2006) Functional results and quality of life after treatment of pelvic sarcomas involving the acetabulum. J Bone Joint Surg Am 88:575–582
22. Hüfner T, Kfuri M Jr, Galanski M, Bastian L, Loss M, Pohlemann T, Krettek C (2004) New indications for computer-assisted surgery: tumor resection in the pelvis. Clin Orthop Relat Res 426:219–225
23. Jeon DG, Kim MS, Cho WH, Song WS, Lee SY (2007) Reconstruction with pasteurized autograft-total hip prosthesis composite for periacetabular tumors. J Surg Oncol 96:493–502
24. Johnson JT (1978) Reconstruction of the pelvic ring following tumor resection. J Bone Joint Surg Am 60:747–751
25. Langlais F, Lambotte JC, Thomazeau H (2001) Long-term results of hemipelvis reconstruction with allografts. Clin Orthop Relat Res 388:178–186
26. van der Lei B, Hoekstra HJ, Veth RP, Ham SJ, Oldhoff J, Schraffordt Koops H (1992) The use of the saddle prosthesis for reconstruction of the hip joint after tumor resection of the pelvis. J Surg Oncol 50:216–219
27. Manabe J, Ahmed AR, Kawaguchi N, Matsumoto S, Kuroda H (2004) Pasteurized autologous bone graft in surgery for bone and soft tissue sarcoma. Clin Orthop Relat Res 419:258–266
28. Mankin HJ, Doppelt S, Tomford W (1983) Clinical experience with allograft implantation. The first ten years. Clin Orthop Relat Res 174:69–86
29. Mnaymneh W, Malinin T, Mnaymneh LG, Robinson D (1990) Pelvic allograft. A case report with a follow-up evaluation of 5.5 years. Clin Orthop Relat Res 255:128–132
30. Nagoya S, Usui M, Wada T, Yamashita T, Ishii S (2000) Reconstruction and limb salvage using a free vascularised fibular graft for periacetabular malignant bone tumours. J Bone Joint Surg Br 82:1121–1124
31. Nieder E, Elson RA, Engelbrecht E, Kasselt MR, Keller A, Steinbrink K (1990) The saddle prosthesis for salvage of the destroyed acetabulum. J Bone Joint Surg Br 72:1014–1022
32. O'Connor MI, Sim FH (1989) Salvage of the limb in the treatment of malignant pelvic tumors. J Bone Joint Surg Am 71:481–494
33. Ozaki T, Hillmann A, Bettin D, Wuisman P, Winkelmann W (1996) High complication rates with pelvic allografts. Experience of 22 sarcoma resections. Acta Orthop Scand 67:333–338
34. Reijnders K, Coppes MH, van Hulzen AL, Gravendeel JP, van Ginkel RJ, Hoekstra HJ (2007) Image guided surgery: new technology for surgery of soft tissue and bone sarcomas. Eur J Surg Oncol 33:390–398
35. Renard AJ, Veth RP, Schreuder HW, Pruszczynski M, Keller A, van Hoesel Q, Bokkerink JP (2000) The saddle prosthesis in pelvic primary and secondary musculoskeletal tumors: functional results at several postoperative intervals. Arch Orthop Trauma Surg 120:188–194
36. Rödl R, Gosheger G, Leidinger B, Lindner N, Winkelmann W, Ozaki T (2003) Correction of leg-length discrepancy after hip transposition. Clin Orthop Relat Res 416:271–277
37. Sakuraba M, Kimata Y, Iida H, Beppu Y, Chuman H, Kawai A (2005) Pelvic ring reconstruction with the double-barreled vascularized fibular free flap. Plast Reconstr Surg 116:1340–1345
38. Salzer M (1965) Hemipelvectomy (amputation interileo-abdominalis, hindquarter amputation). Wien Klin Wochenschr 77:330–331
39. Satcher Jr RL, O'Donnell RJ, Johnston JO (2003) Reconstruction of the pelvis after resection of tumors about the acetabulum. Clin Orthop Relat Res 409:209–217
40. Schoellner C, Schoellner D (2000) Pedestal cup operation in acetabular defects after hip cup loosening. A progress report. Z Orthop Ihre Grenzgeb 138:215–221
41. Schwameis E, Dominkus M, Krepler P, Dorotka R, Lang S, Windhager R, Kotz R (2002) Reconstruction of the pelvis after tumor resection in children and adolescents. Clin Orthop Relat Res 402:220–235
42. Von Sys G, Uyttendaele D, Poffyn B, Verdonk R, Verstraete L (2002) Extracorporeally irradiated autografts in pelvic reconstruction after malignant tumour resection. Int Orthop 26:174–178
43. Takami M, Ieguchi M, Takamatsu K, Kitano T, Aono M, Ishida T, Yamano Y (1997) Functional evaluation of flail hip joint after periacetabular resection of the pelvis. Osaka City Med J 43:173–183
44. Toma C, Kubista B, Funovics P, Abdolvahab F, Dominkus M, Kotz R (2005) Pedestal cups for acetabular and pelvic defects following tumor resection. A new approach to an old problem. Abstract book, 13th ISOLS Korea, p 148

45. Tomford WW, Thongphasuk J, Mankin HJ, Ferraro MJ (1990) Frozen musculoskeletal allografts. A study of the clinical incidence and causes of infection associated with their use. J Bone Joint Surg Am 72:1137–1143
46. Tsuchiya H, Wan SL, Sakayama K, Yamamoto N, Nishida H, Tomita K (2005) Reconstruction using an autograft containing tumour treated by liquid nitrogen. J Bone Joint Surg Br 87:218–225
47. Uchida A, Myoui A, Araki N, Yoshikawa H, Ueda T, Aoki Y (1996) Prosthetic reconstruction for periacetabular malignant tumors. Clin Orthop Relat Res 326:238–245
48. Walker RH (1993) Pelvic reconstruction/total hip arthroplasty for metastatic acetabular insufficiency. Clin Orthop Relat Res 294:170–175
49. Windhager R, Welkerling H, Kastner N, Krepler P (2003) Surgical therapy of pelvis and spine in primary malignant bone tumors. Orthopade 32:971–982
50. Winkelmann W (1988) A new surgical method in malignant tumors of the ilium. Z Orthop Ihre Grenzgeb 126:671–674
51. Wong KC, Kumta SM, Chiu KH, Cheung KW, Leung KS, Unwin P, Wong MC (2007) Computer assisted pelvic tumor resection and reconstruction with a custom-made prosthesis using an innovative adaptation and its validation. Comput Aided Surg 12:225–232
52. Yajima H, Tamai S (1994) Twin-barrelled vascularized fibular grafting to the pelvis and lower extremity. Clin Orthop Relat Res 303:178–184
53. Yamamoto N, Tsuchiya H, Tomita K (2003) Effects of liquid nitrogen treatment on the proliferation of osteosarcoma and the biomechanical properties of normal bone. J Orthop Sci 8:374–380
54. Yokobayashi Y, Shingaki S, Nakajima T (1988) Reimplantation of frozen-thawed autogenous mandible after resection of an ameloblastoma. J Oral Maxillofac Surg 46:490–493
55. Yu G, Zhang F, Zhou J, Chang S, Cheng L, Jia Y, Li H, Lineaweaver WC (2007) Microsurgical fibular flap for pelvic ring reconstruction after periacetabular tumor resection. J Reconstr Microsurg 23:137–142

Methods of Biological Reconstruction for Bone Sarcoma: Indications and Limits

9

Pierre Kunz and Ludger Bernd

Abstract Therapy of bone sarcoma has dramatically changed over the past few decades. Several successful interdisciplinary treatment strategies have led to an increase of the survival rates from 20% to 60%–80%. Consequently new demands on the operative treatment of bone and soft tissue sarcoma have arisen. Nowadays limb salvage can be achieved in 80%–90% using tumour megaprostheses or biological reconstruction procedures. In this article we outline the indications and limitations of biological reconstruction procedures after bone tumour resection. We therefore introduce the different biological approaches such as free autologous bone grafting, reimplantation of extracorporeal devitalized autografts or distraction osteogenesis and summarize the currently available data on the individual procedures. Our analyses demonstrate a wide applicability of biological procedures in tumour situations. Although accompanied by considerable complications in the early postoperative phase, biological reconstructions clearly demonstrate the potential of having excellent long-term durability and functionality.

9.1 Introduction

Bone sarcomas represent approximately 10% of all malignancies in growing patients and 1% of malignancies in adults. Therapy of these rare sarcomas has changed considerably; within the past few decades several successful interdisciplinary treatment strategies have been established [15, 70]. The introduction and improvement of adjuvant chemo- and radiotherapy in bone and soft tissue sarcoma has led to an increase of the survival rates from 20% to 60%–80% [4, 74, 95].

Consequently, additional demands are being placed on the operative treatment of bone and soft tissue sarcoma: Whereas formerly the most important therapeutic consideration was the amputation height of the affected extremity, standards for surgical procedures of bone sarcomas are considerably higher today. Without affecting the (still necessary) radicality of tumour resection for oncological reasons, a long-lasting stability and durability as well as a maximum degree of

Pierre Kunz (✉)
Stiftung Orthopädische Universitätsklinik Heidelberg
Schlierbacher Landstrasse 200a
69118 Heidelberg, Germany
E-mail: Pierre.Kunz@ok.uni-heidelberg.de

functionality, analgesia and emotional acceptance is expected by the reconstruction procedures.

Thanks to improvements in local and systemic tumour control through chemotherapy, a more precise radiological description of the tumour situation, and a better understanding of tumour biology and staging, as well as an improvement of microsurgical techniques, the new demands can often be accommodated. Thus a variety of limb salvage surgical procedures have been advanced and implemented in different oncological centres throughout the world in the last 30 years. These procedures nowadays enable the experienced surgeon to avoid amputation in 80%–90% and to select a reconstruction procedure adapted to the long-term functional demands of the mostly young patients [5, 7, 78].

The most common procedures to bridge bony defects after tumour resection are megaprostheses, massive allografts, endoprosthesis/allograft-composites or biological reconstructions. The latter are characterized by the integration of autografts and/or the initiation of de novo bone formation for defect reconstruction. There is no common consent about the definition of the terminus, especially regarding a possible affiliation of allografts [114]. Due to the integration and partial substitution of an allograft by the host and the biological nature of the implant, the implantation of an allograft could also be considered to be a biological reconstruction. However, they will not be discussed individually in this chapter.

This article will dwell on common biological reconstruction procedures of bony defects after bone tumour resection and discuss their indications and limits.

Within the scope of orthopaedic oncology, we differentiate the following biological reconstruction procedures:

- Transplantation of vital bone—vascularized or non-vascularized autografts
- Implantation of avital bone—extracorporeal devitalized autograft (or allograft)
- De novo bone synthesis by distraction osteogenesis

Cancellous bone grafting—which is, strictly speaking, a biological reconstruction—is widely used in orthopaedic oncology and has proved its value in various indications. Nevertheless, due to its inability to be used for cortical bone reconstructions, it will not be discussed in this context.

Although the above-mentioned procedures have their distinct indications, there is an overlap in many tumour situations. In order to select the right method, a stringent consideration of various aspects is indispensable. Besides the localization of the reconstruction—intercalary/articular, joint replacement/preservation, upper/lower extremity—and the size of the defect, the expected soft tissue damage, age of the patient (growth reserve), functional demands on the patient and prognosis always have to be considered; weighing these factors is essential to achieve a tumour situation-adapted compromise regarding the stability, durability and functionality of the reconstruction.

9.2 Biological Reconstruction Procedures and Outcome

9.2.1 Transplantation of Vital Autografts

Several autologous bones are used nowadays to reconstruct bone defects. Fibula grafts [7, 31, 47], clavicula grafts [37, 106, 115], iliac crest grafts [47, 69, 118], scapula grafts [1] and rib grafts [99, 102] can be transplanted either as a pedicled bone graft (exempli gratia fibula pro tibia, clavicula pro humero) or a free bone graft (exempli gratia fibula pro humero). Although these procedures have retained their special indications, the fibula—due to its anatomical structure regarding length, straightness and cortical strength—is the preferable vital bone graft [1, 14, 22]. It represents one of the most common biological reconstruction procedures in orthopaedic oncology following bone tumour resection and can be performed as a pedicled bone graft, a free vascularized bone graft and a non-vascularized bone graft.

The first pedicled fibula graft, used to reconstruct a bony defect after tibial pseudarthrosis, was described by Hahn in 1884 [44]. While the transfer of a free non-vascularized fibula has been performed since 1911 [112] for defect reconstructions, it took another 70 years, with the improvements within the field of microsurgical techniques, to enable the transfer of a free vascularized fibula graft with an arterial and venous vessel anastomosis at the recipient site [101].

Along with a number of other reconstruction procedures, this technique has now been established at most orthopaedic oncological centres and is used in a variety of indications including bone reconstruction after pseudarthrosis, infection, trauma and tumour resection. Among the available reconstruction procedures for bone defects, the transplantation of a vascularized bone graft, preserving its endosteal and periosteal blood supply, has one unique advantage: if you treat it right, it has the potential to behave like a normal vital bone [32, 41, 42].

A vascularized graft is therefore not only able to incorporate by the laws of fracture healing [32], it is also capable of remodelling and can react to changes of mechanical loading by hypertrophy [1, 22, 27, 97] and has an unharmed resistance to infection [32]. It is therefore also suitable for use in pre-damaged recipient sites. In growing patients, the plasticity reserve after simultaneous transfer of the epiphysis even supports longitudinal growth as well as adaptation to the articular shape of the recipient site after transplantation [13, 59, 60].

There are also, however, serious drawbacks. Since harvesting and transplanting a vascularized fibula is a surgical procedure of high demands, a second operating team is often needed and the operation time is prolonged by hours. In order to gain the above-mentioned advantages, all sections of the graft require a maintaining perfusion at the recipient site.

Taking into consideration that the blood supply of the fibula is complex and individualized [77, 82], an exact anatomical knowledge of the nutrient vessels of different segments of the fibula is an essential prerequisite for a successful graft transfer. Postoperative thrombosis of the vessel anastomoses of the graft is a common side-effect and requires—if recognized—a re-intervention [51, 52, 76]. Due to a lack of primary stability, free autologous bone grafts require additional fixation devices and a longer postoperative immobilization than other reconstruction techniques such as megaprostheses. The harvest of the fibula is usually performed by a lateral approach [7, 113] or a posterior approach initially described by Taylor et al. [101]. The above-mentioned attributes make the fibula an ideal bone graft for intercalary defects of up to 30 cm. Vascularized and non-vascularized fibular grafts are therefore widely used to reconstruct intercalary defects of the humerus [7, 38, 39, 110], radius, ulna [7, 60, 77], tibia or the femur [7, 47, 120]. It is also used for resection arthrodesis of the knee and shoulder [2, 87, 110], in which it constantly presents good functional outcomes, as well as for reconstructions of the pelvis [66, 92]. Articular defects—although the main domain of megaprostheses—can be partly reconstructed by fibular grafts [7, 38, 60, 77, 110].

Depending on the mechanical forces at the defect site, a fibular graft often has to be supported by additional bone grafts in order to obtain sufficient initial mechanical strength [50, 80]. A solely fibular graft is therefore primarily used to reconstruct defects of the radius, ulna and the humerus (see Figs. 9.1 and 9.2). In the lower extremity, the fibular graft is often combined with either an allograft as described by Capanna and colleagues [18], an extracorporeal devitalized autograft (see Fig. 9.3), a second vital autologous bone graft, or it is used in a double barrel technique (see Fig. 9.4) [65, 80, 120, 123]. Fixation of the graft is usually conducted by spanning plates, blade plates, cortical screws, K-wires or intramedullary nails.

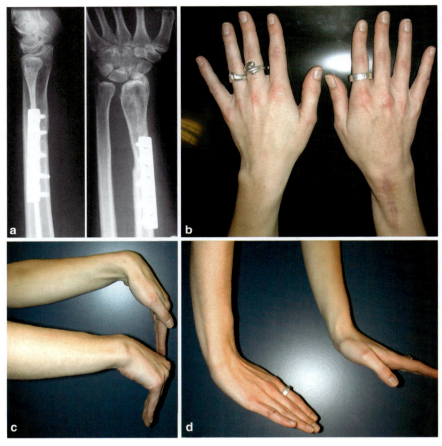

Fig. 9.1 Articular reconstruction of the distal radius by transplantation of a vascularized fibular graft including the fibular head (**a**), showing excellent functional outcome (**b, c, d**)

9.2.1.1
Outcome of Vital Bone Grafts

Evaluation of the outcome of vital bone grafts include critical parameters such as:

- Graft union—rates and time to union
- Graft adaptation—hypertrophy
- Functional outcome
- Complication rate (fracture, non-union, infection rate, failure rate)

In vital autograft, these aspects depend on factors such as the localization of the reconstruction, cause of the defect (tumour resection/infection/pseudarthrosis), fixation device, length of the graft, adjuvant therapy, whether a vascularized or a non-vascularized graft is used, persisting perfusion of a vascularized graft, local and systemic tumour staging and the condition of the recipient bed.

The following results include our own data of 31 free vascularized fibular grafts after tumour resection.

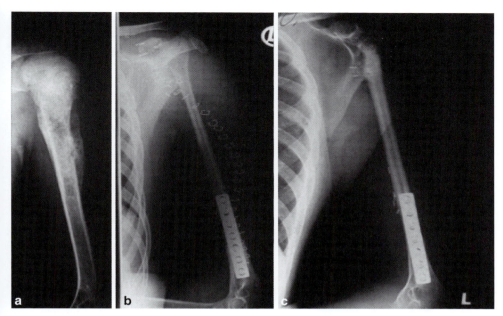

Fig. 9.2 Bone sarcoma of the proximal humerus including the shoulder joint (**a**); osteoarticular reconstruction with a vascularized fibula graft and external fixation (**b**); and solid union and hypertrophy of the graft combined with atrophy of the fibular head (**c**)

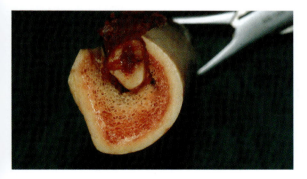

Fig. 9.3 Extracorporeal irradiated autograft combined with a vascularized fibular graft

9.2.1.1.1
Union of Vital Bone Grafts

The overall primary union rate after a reconstruction procedure using a free bone graft—vascularized or non-vascularized—ranges from 61% to 100%. Most of the published series reach final union rates of 90%–100% after suitable re-intervention within 2–12 months [2, 7, 31, 32, 35, 38, 39, 47, 55, 60, 66, 76, 77, 80, 82, 87, 110, 111, 119, 120, 123].

Union rates of free bone grafts are significantly higher in case of a reconstruction of defects after tumour resection compared to a reconstruction of a defect caused by infection [47, 76, 117].

123]. In non-vascularized fibular grafts, Enneking et al. and Yadav et al. showed a union in approx. 60% of their patients after 10–12 months [35, 119], while Krieg and Hefti achieved an 89% union rate within 24 weeks [66].

Upper limb reconstructions have a significant [47] higher union rate (primary/finally 74%–91%/93%–100%) [7, 31, 38, 47, 60, 77, 82, 87, 110, 123] than lower limb reconstructions (69%–86%/78%–100%) [2, 7, 22, 31, 47, 111, 120, 123]. Time to union seems to be achieved faster in the upper extremity [60, 82, 123].

Extramedullary fixation of the graft tends to achieve higher union rates compared to intramedullary fixation [47].

Although not significant in other publications, additional cancellous bone grafting at the graft/host junction has been shown to significantly increase union rate in de Boers collective [27, 47, 124]. No differences regarding union rate were reported for different lengths of fibular grafts.

9.2.1.1.2 Adaptation of Vital Bone Grafts: Hypertrophy in Free Vascularized Bone Graft

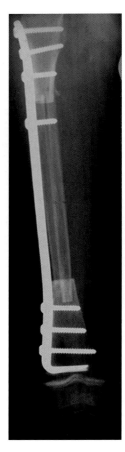

Fig. 9.4 Combined vascularized and non-vascularized fibual graft with external fixation for intercalary femoral reconstruction

Not considering a postoperative perfusion control, the overall final union rates of vascularized bone grafts after tumour resection ranges from 71% to 100% [2, 7, 32, 38, 39, 47, 55, 60, 77, 87, 110, 111, 113, 116, 123] and from 60% to 89% for non-vascularized fibular grafts [35, 66, 119]. Vascularized grafts with a positive postoperative perfusion control show a significant higher union rate compared to those with a negative perfusion control [47]. Time to union averages from 2–12 months in vascularized grafts [2, 31, 38, 39, 55, 60, 76, 80, 82, 87, 110, 111, 120,

Hypertrophy as a sign of adaptation of the graft is commonly evaluated after de Boer et al. or Weiland et al. [27, 113]. Both methods are based on radiological evaluation of the diameter of the recipient's and the grafted bone. De Boers hypertrophy index of the host and graft bone diameter allows for a 20% interval due to false radiological projection.

Graft hypertrophy is reported in up to 86% of the cases. The hypertrophy rate is significantly higher in the lower extremity due to the higher mechanical load [22, 27, 31, 55, 68]. A significant difference has also been described for different methods of fixation; the best hypertrophy results were achieved without fixation (combined with the highest fracture rates), and the poorest by using intramedullary fixation [27].

9.2.1.1.3
Functional Outcome of Vital Bone Grafts

Functional outcome is mostly evaluated by the revised Musculoskeletal Tumour Society (MSTS) score, the former Enneking score, or the Mankin score [33, 34, 72]. The revised MSTS score assigns numerical values from 0 to 5 for six categories, including pain, function and emotional acceptance in upper and lower extremities. Results are expressed in numerical scores and percentage rating. The four Mankin categories are excellent, good or fair results and failure.

In general, functional outcome of biological reconstructions using a free bone graft show good to excellent long-term results after union and re-convalescence. Publications using the revised MSTS score report average scores from 68%–97% for the upper extremity, and 76%–87% for the lower extremity. Other publications report 14%–61% of the patients achieving excellent results, 34%–86% good results, 4%–25% fair results and 0%–8% a poor results/failure [7, 22, 39, 55, 66, 82, 87, 110, 111, 123]. Average time to full weight bearing of the corresponding lower limb is 5–18 months after operation [40, 91, 124].

9.2.1.1.4
Complications and Failures Using Vital Bone Grafts

The most common complications at the recipient site include fracture of the graft, non-union/delayed union and infection. Overall complication rates of vital bone grafts (fibula, clavicula, scapula etc.) range from 0% to 52% [2, 7, 47, 55, 60, 66, 76, 82, 111, 120].

Looking at transplanted fibulae, fracture rates of the currently published series range from 0% to 58% [7, 22, 35, 38, 47, 55, 111]. Fracture rates after transplantation to the upper extremity are 12%–50% [7, 22, 87, 110, 120], transplantation to the lower extremity fracture in 0%–22% of cases [2, 7, 56, 94]. However fracture rates as high as 60%–100% are seen in the lower extremity, if the fibular graft is used solely without any supportive allograft (Capanna), autograft or in a double barrel technique [22, 111]. Using an intramedullary fixation device, the fracture rate is significantly lower than using an extramedullary fixation device [27].

No differences regarding fracture rates were observed between vascularized and non-vascularized fibular grafts, but the moment of fracture seems to be primarily within the first year in vascularized grafts and after 2 years in non-vascularized grafts [27, 35]. Longer grafts fracture more often than shorter grafts [35, 76]. Non-union occurs in 3%–19% and delayed union in up to 40%, depending on the recipient site [35, 39, 47, 55, 76].

Donor site complications are reported in 0%–25% of the patients after harvesting a free fibular graft. Complications include transient peroneal nerve palsy, contraction of the long flexor of great toe, compartment syndrome of the lower limb, knee instability and valgus deformity of the ankle joint. The majority of complications regarding recipient and donor site are successfully treated without negative effects on the long-term outcome of the reconstruction. Failure rates, resulting in late amputation or a change of the reconstruction procedure are described in 3%–13% [7, 47, 55].

9.2.2
Implantation of Avital Bone: Extracorporeal Devitalized Autografts

The basic idea behind implanting avital bone is to re-implant the resected bone after extracorporeal devitalization of the tumour. It can therefore be best compared to the implantation of a massive allograft.

Different methods of devitalization using irradiation, autoclaving, pasteurization or liquid nitrogen (LN) have been described [11, 62, 88,

105]. These devitalization treatments significantly influence the mechanical properties of the bone graft [23, 46, 48, 89, 109]. Among the common devitalization procedures, irradiation seems to be superior over heat devitalization regarding the integrity of the collagenous matrix and the preservation of intrinsic osteoinductive proteins. Nevertheless, irradiation has also been shown to negatively influence mechanical strength regarding maximum load and wear to fracture of the bone in high doses [23, 109]. To our knowledge, one series has been presented using LN, offering theoretical advantages regarding biomechanical properties over heat devitalization procedures [105, 121].

Extracorporeal devitalized autografts have distinct advantages over other reconstruction procedures. Just like massive allografts, they offer initial mechanical strength as well as a frame structure for a slow creeping substitution. Devitalized autografts and massive allografts are used for intercalary or osteoarticular defects, being especially suitable to reconstruct anatomically difficult tumour sites such as the pelvis [24, 54, 88] and to preserve joint surfaces as well as stabilizing ligaments and tendons in joint reconstructions [3, 105]. In contrast to an allograft, however, a devitalized autograft is bioinert, non-allergenic and guarantees a perfect fit with a maximal contact area at the interface between host and graft (see Fig. 9.5). There is no need for a complex, expensive bone bank and it can therefore be performed at most institutions. Using a devitalized autograft, the risk of contamination by an allograft, which can occur at any of the times of harvesting, processing and storing, is considerably lower. The risks for transmission of infections as well as for an immunological response, harming the integration of the graft, are absent [3, 20, 105]. Last but not least, cultural objections to allografts can be avoided.

Nevertheless, especially if compared to vital autografts, the disadvantages of these procedures are obvious: The re-implant can only function as a frame structure without the capability to respond to changing biomechanical demands or immunological challenges. Integration of the graft is exclusively driven by the recipient bed, which is often weakened by chemotherapy, radiation and a lack of soft tissue coverage due to tumour resection. As a logical consequence, the most common complications using avital bone grafts are infection and non-union, as well as fractures caused by wear. Another disadvantage is the unavailability of the en bloc tumour for pathological analyses in cases of neoadjuvant and adapted postoperative chemotherapy protocols.

In order to compensate for some of these disadvantages, devitalized autografts and allografts are frequently combined with vascularized bone grafts (see Figs. 9.3 and 9.6) or endoprosthetic devices [21].

First described in 1970 by Spira and Lubin [96], intraoperative extracorporeal irradiated and re-implanted (IEIR) autologous bone grafts are a commonly used type of devitalized graft. Compared to vital bone grafts, however, they are considerably less frequently used; fewer publications focus on this issue, showing controversial results [3, 11, 21, 24, 54, 65, 100, 105, 107]. The following current results focus on IEIR and LN devitalized autografts. Except for pelvic reconstructions, cases of autograft/endoprosthetic composites were excluded. IEIR has been used at our institution since 1996 [88, 89].

9.2.2.1
Outcome of Extracorporeal Devitalized Autografts

The outcome of extracorporeal devitalized autografts depends on the size of the replant, location of the reconstruction site, fixation device, recipient bed, combination with other reconstructive procedures and tumour staging.

Similar to vital bone grafts, critical parameters for the evaluation of the outcome include:

- Graft union—rates and time to union
- Functional outcome

9 Methods of Biological Reconstruction for Bone Sarcoma: Indications and Limits 121

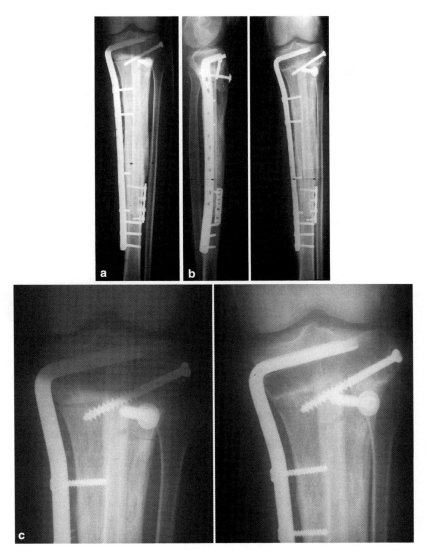

Fig. 9.5 Reconstruction of a defect of the proximal tibia after tumour resection using an intraoperative extracorporeal irradiated and re-implanted (IEIR) autograft combined with a vascularized fibular graft, demonstrating the perfect fit of the graft with maximal contact area (**a**); solid union of the junction after 8 months (**b**); proximal junction 1 week after operation (*left*) and 8 months after operation (*right*) (**c**)

- Complication rate (fracture, non-union, infection rate, failure rate)

Hypertrophy as a sign of graft adaptation cannot be observed in avital bone grafts; in cases of a combined use of a devitalized graft with a vascularized vital graft, hypertrophic adaptation is seen in 62% of the vital grafts [65].

Table 9.1 shows a summary of the currently available data of IEIR and LN-devitalized autografts.

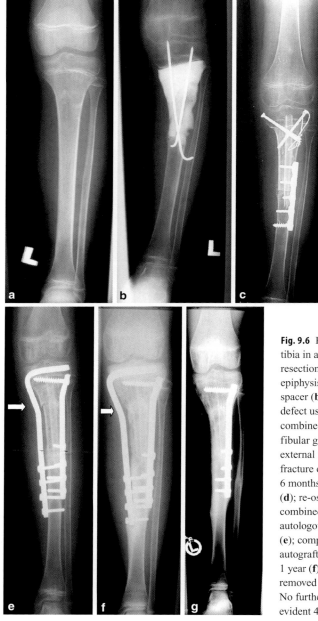

Fig. 9.6 Ewing sarcoma of proximal tibia in an 11-year-old patient (**a**); resection under preservation of epiphysis and implantation of a spacer (**b**); reconstruction of the defect using IEIR autograft combined with a vascularized fibular graft with insufficient external fixation (**c**), resulting in fracture of the IEIR autograft 6 months after implantation (*arrow*) (**d**); re-osteosynthesis using a combined double plate and autologous cancellous bone grafting (**e**); complete healing of the IEIR autograft fracture occurred within 1 year (**f**) and the blade plate was removed after another year (**g**). No further complications are evident 4 years later

9.2.2.1.1
Union in Extracorporeal Devitalized Autografts

Overall union rates in IEIR or LN-devitalized autografts range from 54% to 100% [3, 9, 20, 24, 54, 65, 88, 100, 105] with an average time to union of 6–10 months [3, 54, 65, 105] (see Table 9.1).

Union rate is significantly higher if the devitalized graft is combined with a vascularized fibular graft [65]. Controversial data are shown regarding intercalary and osteoarticular grafts. While Araki et al. [3] presented a primary union rate of 64% of the junctions in intercalary defects (*n*=14) and a 100% union rate in osteoarticular grafts (*n*=11), Krieg et al. [65] found a primary/final union rate of 84%/100% in their intercalary femur group (*n*=16).

There is a tendency towards higher union rates using extramedullary fixation devices.

9.2.2.1.2
Functional Outcome in Extracorporeal Devitalized Autografts

Functional outcomes were mostly evaluated using the revised MSTS score, which ranged from 68% to 92% [3, 9, 20, 24, 65, 88]. Authors using the former Enneking evaluation score report excellent results in 71%, good results in 11%, fair results in 11% and poor results in 7% (see Table 9.1). The functional outcome in this heterogeneous group seems to be strongly dependent on the localization of the reconstruction. Similar to other reconstruction techniques, higher functional scores are seen in the upper extremity [3] (see Table 9.2).

9.2.2.1.3
Complications of Extracorporeal Devitalized Autografts

Common complications in extracorporeal devitalized autografts include infection, non-union/ delayed union, fracture and epiphyseal slip in younger patients [3, 9, 20, 24, 88, 105]. In patient populations including pelvic reconstruction, complication rates are reported in up to 87% of the cases, resulting in failure of the reconstruction procedure in up to 46% [88, 100]. Excluding publications focussing on the most fragile pelvic reconstructions, complication rates are much lower, in the moderate range (25%–60%), and average around 48% [3, 9, 20, 65, 105] (see Table 9.2).

The average infection rate is around 11%, while persisting non-union appeared in up to 23% in the presented series, averaging at 8% [3, 88, 105]. Fracture rates are reported in up to 20% of the cases, averaging at 7% [3, 9, 11, 20, 24, 65, 88, 100, 105] (see Table 9.2). Consolidation is usually achieved by plating, cancellous bone grafting and immobilization. Failure of extremity reconstructions is reported in 7% of the patients [20, 21, 24, 105] (see Table 9.2).

9.2.3
De Novo Bone Formation: Distraction Osteogenesis

Among the conducted biological reconstructions, distraction osteogenesis seems to be the "most biological" reconstruction. In distraction osteogenesis, the defect is reconstructed by de novo bone formation at the defect site [25, 45, 58]. It is therefore possible to achieve a defect-specific regeneration suiting the exact demands of the defect site regarding strength and diameter of the bone. Nevertheless, although this technique for bony defects is widely used in the treatment of leg lengthening, pseudarthrosis and osteomyelitis [57, 58], it is not very common in tumour situations yet. To our knowledge, only about 110 cases in total have been published to date, and they are limited to defects of the lower extremity [30, 36, 67, 75, 81, 83, 90, 103, 104, 108].

Table 9.1 Currently published series of IEIR and liquid nitrogen-devitalized autografts

	Böhm et al. [9]	Araki et al. [3]	Chen et al. [20]	Sys et al. [100]	Krieg et al. [65]	Tsuchiya et al. [105]	Sabo et al. [88]	Davidson et al. [24]	Hong et al. [54]	Uyttendaele et al. [107]
n	6[c]	20	15	15	16	28	13	18 (23)[e]	13 (16)[d]	17
Mean age (in years)	25	36	32.3	38	17	31.1	21.3	28.3	16.5	19.6
Mean follow-up (in months)	66	45	76.2	54.3	49.7	28.1	32	40.8	24.3	44.8
Functional outcome	92%	73%	86.9%	54%[f]	85%	20–3–3–2	68%	77.5%	4–6–1–0	0–10–2–0
Union	10/10[a]	23/29[a]	29/30[a]	14/15[b]	32/32[a]	26/28[b]	19/19[a]	18/20[a]	7/13[b]	16/17[b]
Complications severe	2/6	12/20	5/15	13/15	7/16	7/28	11/13	9/18	6/13	8/17
Pseudarthrosis	–	6/29	–	–	–	2/28[b]	–	2/20[a]	3/13[b]	1/17[b]
Infection rate	0/8	4[a]/20	0/15	4[a]/15	0/16	3/28	4/13	2/18	0/13	2/17
Fracture rate	1/6	1/20	3/15	0/15	1/16	2/28	2/13	1/18	0/13	1/17
Failure	1/6	2/20	1/15	2/15	0/16	3/28	6/13	2/18	1/13	4/17
+Vascularized graft	–	–	–	–	13	–	3	2	–	–
DOD	0/6	3/20	3/15	7/15	0/15	6/28	4/13	5/23	0/13	4/17

[a]Graft/host junctions
[b]Patients
[c]Two patients excluded due to knee arthrodesis
[d]Three patients excluded due to short follow-up
[e]Out of originally 50 patients in this series, 10 were excluded due to autograft/endoprosthetic composite, the femoral cases are presented in Krieg et al. [65], five of the remaining patients died of disease and functional results were not provided [1–10]
[f]EMSOS score

9 Methods of Biological Reconstruction for Bone Sarcoma: Indications and Limits

Table 9.2 Results of IEIR and nitrogen devitalized autografts sorted by tumour site (cases where detailed information about tumour location is presented within the publication)

	Overall	Humerus total	Humerus intercalary	Humerus osteoartic.	Femur total	Femur intercalary	Femur osteoartic.	Tibia total	Tibia intercalary	Tibia oste-oarict.	Pelvis
n	161	13	3	7	67	39	12	20	15	5	44 (49–5)[a]
Mean age (years)	27.4	21.4	24	24.4	23.5	26.1	22.5	23	21.7	27	31.9
Mean follow-up (months)	43.8	43.2	73.7	42	41.6	45	30.8	43.1	45.74	35.4	36.3
Functional outcome	75.5% (108)	88.3% (6)	93.3%	83.3% (3)	79.7% (38)	81.6% (33)	67.4% (5)	88.5% (11)	92.6% (9)	70% (2)	~60%
	24-19-6-0	2–3–0–1		2–0–1–0	11–5–1–0	5–0–0–0	5–1–0–0	4–0–0–0	1–0–0–0	3–0–0–0	
Union (%)	91%	88.4%	83.3%	100%	91.3%	96%	91.6%	94.98%	93.3%	100%	88.6%
Complication sev. (%)	48.2%	38.4%	66.6%	28.5%	47.70%	44%	66.6%	35%	40%	20%	64%
Pseudarthrosis (%)	8.4%	11.5%	16.6%	-	7%	4%	8.3%	5%	6.6%	-	11.4%
Infection (%)	10.6%	15.3%	-	28.5%	1.5%	2.5%	-	6.7%	2.2%	20%	22.7%
Fracture (%)	7.2%	7.7%	33.3%	0%	12%	10%	33.3%	1.7%	2.2%	-	2.3%
Failure (%)	12.7%	-	-	-	8.9%	2.7%	16.7%	3.3%	4.4%	-	25%

[a]Five patients who died of the disease (DOD) were excluded since functional outcome was not available [1–10]

Three procedures are differentiated for tumour defect reconstruction:

1. Segment transport after an osteotomy proximal and/or distal to the defect (mono- or bifocal lengthening)
2. Shortening-distraction without additional osteotomy
3. Segment transport or shortening-distraction along an intramedullary nail

Distraction is usually started 7–14 days after the osteotomy or the shortening, with a rate of 1 mm/day [57]. After distraction over the length of the defect has been completed, maturation of the newly formed bone requires approximately twice the time of distraction.

Distraction osteogenesis can theoretically be applied to defects of any length and diameter. Although its indication is limited to the reconstruction of intercalary defects and cannot be used to reconstruct articular sites such as allografts, autografts and megaprostheses, it can be used to preserve a joint after epiphyseal tumour resection as close as 0.5 cm to the joint surface [103].

The downsides of this procedure are first and foremost the long duration for bone formation as well as the need of a bi- or unilateral external fixation system for about 30 days/cm of bone formation. Depending on the defect length, this results in reduced mobilization of the patient for several months. Achieving full weight bearing sometimes takes years. Therefore compliance and a very close doctor–patient relationship are of particular importance. In addition, complication rates are high, including delayed ossification and maturation, pseudarthrosis at the docking site, pin infection, skin invagination, bone resorption, pes equinus and rotational and axis deviations [63, 83, 103, 104]. Another disadvantage of distraction osteogenesis is an often-required second operation for cancellous bone grafting to avoid pseudarthrosis at the docking site [63, 103].

9.2.3.1
Outcome of Distraction Osteogenesis

The following results include 80 out of, to our knowledge, 109 published cases of distraction osteogenesis after tumour resection [36, 63, 83, 103, 104, 108]. 29 patients of Case reports, series of two and publications not providing data on the individual patients were excluded.

Critical parameters for the evaluation of the outcome include:

- External fixation index and distraction index
- Functional outcome
- Complications and failure

9.2.3.1.1
External Fixation Index and Distraction Index

The external fixation index (EFI) is defined by the duration of external fixation per centimetre of bridged bone defect. The distraction index (DI) describes the duration of distraction per centimetre.

The mean EFI of the published series ranges from 8.1 days/cm to 95 days/cm, resulting in an arithmetic mean of 27.7 days/cm in all 80 cases. The high variation between the series is caused by the use of an additional intramedullary nail in some of the series, resulting in considerably shorter external fixation time [108]. Considering that defect lengths of up to 27 cm were treated, external fixation time can exceed 2 years.

Since bone lengthening is commonly conducted at 1 mm/day, DI varies from 8.6 days/cm to 14.1 days/cm [36, 63, 83, 103, 104, 108] (see Table 9.3). Existing differences in the distraction index are due to partly conducted bifocal, double-elongation distraction. In these cases, two segments of bone—one proximal and one distal—are transported at the same time in order to shorten the procedure in large bone defects.

Table 9.3 Current publications using distraction osteogenesis after tumour resection

	Mean age (years)	Mean follow-up (months)	EFI (days/cm)	DI (days/cm)	Complications	Functional outcome	Failure	DOD
Tsuchiya et al. [104] n=19	29	37	33.8	17.5	9/19	12–5–2–0	0/19	3/19
Kapukaya et al. [63] n=9	17	22	33.3	13.4	3/9	4–3–2–0	0/9	1/9
Erler et al. [36] n=9	19.3	59	31.5	11.2	6/9	4–3–1–1	1/9	0/9
Tsuchiya et al. [103] n=11	21.5	54	33	14.1	7/11	97.4%	1/11	1/11
Ozaki et al. [83] n=5	23	48	95	?	5/5	0–0–3–2	2/5	1/5
Vidyadhara et al. [108] n=27	35.5	65	8.1	8.6	6/27	12–9–6–0	0/27	0/27
Total n=80	27.4	50	27.7	12.6	36/80	42–20–15–3	4/80	6/80

9.2.3.1.2
Functional Outcome

Functional outcome was surveyed by the revised MSTS score and the former Enneking score, respectively [33, 34]. Out of 80 patients, 42 showed excellent results, 20 achieved good results, 15 fair and three poor results (see Table 9.3).

9.2.3.1.3
Complications and Failure

The most common complications using this method are pseudarthrosis at docking site, pin infection, skin invagination, bone resorption, pes equinus and rotational or axis deviations [63, 83, 103, 104]. Major complications occur in 22.2%–100% [83, 108] of the patients with a total average of 45%, excluding the common pin infections. Failure of the procedure is described in only 5% of the cases (see Table 9.3).

9.3
Discussion

In 80%–90% of all malignant bone tumours today, limb preservation can be achieved using vital or avital autografts, distraction osteogenesis, megaprostheses, composite procedures or rotationplasty. The introduction of tumour megaprostheses for articular reconstruction offered previously unsurpassed early postoperative results regarding functionality and stability in bone tumour patients. Combined with the short operation time, low rates of early complications and a considerably easier procedure for reconstruction, megaprostheses have without doubt strong indications within orthopaedic oncology and currently constitute the most common reconstruction procedure following bone tumour resection. More than 30 years after their introduction, however, the downsides of megaprostheses are becoming increasingly obvious. In patients with a long survival, they often seem to be less than a worthwhile investment in the future. Overall 10-year survival rates of megaprostheses are reported as low as 67%, and as low as 50% after knee reconstruction [8, 16, 64, 71]. Complications and failure rates of the procedure rise with time, total risk for aseptic loosening and late infection, necessitating a removal of the prosthesis, increases over its lifetime.

Biological reconstructions, on the other hand, represent the opposite virtues. Once integrated, they are meant to last. Offering considerably high complication rates and major restrictions in the early postoperative phase, biological reconstructions are highly demanding for the patient and the surgeon, and yet they offer decreasing complication rates over time, showing very few complications following the initial 3 years after operation [7, 72, 108]. Their primary strength is therefore longevity.

A multitude of factors have to be considered before indicating either one of the available reconstruction procedures after tumour resection. Besides the oncological prognosis, the surgeon has to consider the special pitfalls, complications and critical factors influencing the outcome of the chosen reconstruction procedure. This might be taken for granted, but in case of biological reconstructions after tumour resection, this standard is hard to achieve: Not only are biological reconstructions highly demanding regarding the surgical procedure and postoperative management, but the limited numbers of published series and the strong heterogeneity of the presented study populations regrettably allow for suggestions rather than precise conclusions. Thus, various outcome-relevant aspects in biological reconstructions are not finally clarified.

Considering the currently published data and our own 25-year experience in this field, we would like to emphasize and discuss important aspects of the individual biological reconstruction procedures.

Important common aspects of biological reconstruction procedures are the general condition and the age of the patient as well as the recipient bed. This becomes apparent by pointing out the common principle of biological reconstructions: they utilize the patient's own ability to integrate, adapt, regenerate and substitute bone structures. These processes are strongly driven by the recipient bed. There is consent that a good blood circulation as well as good soft tissue coverage is important for solid integration and consecutively for a good outcome. Age is important, since younger patients possess higher regenerative capabilities. Controversially discussed, however, is the impact of adjuvant therapy on this process. Various studies have dealt with the influence of chemotherapy on the integrative and regenerative capabilities of bone. While Subasi et al. [98] found no reduction in osteogenesis in a rabbit model after application of chemotherapy, most authors of clinical studies show trends towards a negative impact of chemotherapy [61, 63, 85]; nevertheless, due to the small study populations, no significant differences concerning integration of the bone could be shown in patients with or without chemotherapy. It seems logical that an adjuvant therapy, based on the reduction of cell growth and activity, would not support a regeneration process. Nevertheless, other reconstruction procedures are faced with the same problem and, secondly, adjuvant therapy is the most crucial factor affecting improved survival rate in bone sarcoma; we will therefore have to accept this potential handicap.

Besides those general aspects, each reconstruction procedure shows individual factors influencing integration processes such as union, fracture or pseudarthrosis.

9.3.1
Vital Bone Grafts: Vascularization

The theoretical advantages of vital bone grafts regarding healing properties and infection resistance have been pointed out earlier. Notably, the potency of vascularized bone grafts seems to be exceptional. Comparing the published results for vascularized and non-vascularized fibular grafts, overall results of vascularized fibular grafts regarding integration parameters such as union rate, time to union, pseudarthrosis and hypertrophy are without doubt superior over non-vascularized grafts. But the differences are not as impressive as we would expect. Union rates in different study populations with a vascularized fibular graft have been reported to tend towards 100% and average time to union has been reported as short as 8 weeks [47]. These results come close to the theoretical expectations of normal bone healing. Compared to the best union rates of 89% within 24 weeks in non-vascularized fibular grafts, shown by Krieg and Hefti [66], the potential of vascularized grafts can clearly be seen. At the same time, though, several series of vascularized fibular grafts present average union rates of 70%–90% with a time to union of up to 12 months [2, 39, 87]. These results seem to be less than superior to the Krieg and Hefti [66] non-vascularized grafts. One simple explanation for the diversity of this data could be the suggestion that many of the vascularized grafts loose their initial perfusion postoperatively due to thrombosis of the vessel anastomoses, resulting in a regenerative potential comparable to a non-vascularized transplant. In an exceptional series of 160 vascularized grafts, Han et al. [47] presented a failure of 25% of the anastomoses in 91 patients, where a perfusion control using technetium 99m bone scans within the first postoperative week was performed. They were able to show a significant difference in primary union rate (71% compared to 41%) as well as the overall union rates (91% compared to 64%) in patients with a positive postoperative perfusion control compared to those with a negative postoperative perfusion control. Unfortunately, only a few other authors have performed perfusion controls at all, and hardly any of them in their total series [79, 117, 122]. Additionally, the reliability of bone scans for postoperative perfusion controls is not finally answered.

Publications focussing on this issue present controversial results. While Bos [12] suggests a control within the first week will give reliable results, Shaffer et al. [93] conclude that a a representative result can be ascertained only within the first days. However, other authors presented 37.5% false-positive results in a dog model using this method within the first week [17]. The actual failure rate of the anastomoses of vascularized bone transfer, therefore, has to be considered even higher than the reported 25%.

Anyhow, functionality of the anastomoses is not the only issue regarding the vascularization. Just as important is the question whether the correct vessel has been harvested. The difficulty of preparing the donor site results from the complexity and variability of the blood supply of the fibula [73, 77, 82, 84, 86]. In most patients the diaphyseal part is primarily supplied by the peroneal artery with their aa. nutriciae, the proximal part of the diaphyseal section additionally by the anterior tibial artery, and the fibula head primarily by the inferior lateral genicular artery [43, 51, 101]. This becomes important in case of long fibular transfers or in epiphyseal transfers, especially if closure of the epiphyseal plate is not completed. Most authors use the anterior tibial artery or the peroneal artery in fibular grafts, regardless of a possible fibula head transfer. The high numbers of transplants developing either fibular head atrophy (in up to 62%) or a temporary atrophy of sections of the fibula could be explained by an insufficient segmental blood supply [7, 66]. Ono et al. [82] suggest that in the latter case of epiphyseal/fibular head transfer two vessels should be harvested; the inferior lateral genicular artery to preserve the vitality of the epiphysis and the head in order to enable longitudinal growth, plus either the peroneal artery or the anterior tibial artery for meta-/diaphyseal sections.

We agree on the importance of the vessel anatomy and recommend putting effort into the selection of the according vessels, including a preoperative angiography. Harvesting the proper vessels depending on the utilized section of the fibula, as well as maintaining the anastomoses, in our opinion represents the key to the advantages of vascularized bone grafts. Experience is of great importance in this matter.

9.3.2 Biomechanical Aspects in Free Bone Grafts: Union, Hypertrophy, Fracture

As described above, integration processes of bone grafts are influenced by the general condition of the patient, the recipient bed and possibly by adjuvant therapy. Besides those factors though, union of the graft/host interface, hypertrophy and fracture of the graft are all strongly constrained by the biomechanical load on the graft.

In summary, increased loading of mechanical force on the fibular graft results in a strong stimulus for union and hypertrophy, with the risk of fracture in case of repetitive load exceeding the strength of the bone; reduced loading of mechanical force results in decreased fracture rates, associated with increased rates of delayed- and non-union, and a reduced hypertrophic adaptation.

The mechanical load bearing of the bone graft itself depends on the transplantation site (upper/lower extremity) and can be controlled by different types of fixation devices (intramedullary/extramedullary) and supporting bone grafts (Capanna's method/double barrel technique).

Rigid intramedullary fixation as well as additional autografts or allografts reduce the mechanical load on the fibula, resulting in significantly lower fracture rates, lower hypertrophy indices as well as higher non-union rates [27, 31, 55]. Extramedullary fixation provides lesser load absorption as well as high forces at the screw holes in plates; combined with solely transplanted fibular grafts, the highest hypertrophy indices, union rates and fracture rates are observed [1, 7, 22, 27, 31, 47, 111, 120, 123]. Although the natural biomechanical forces in the upper extremity are smaller than those in the lower extremity, significantly higher union rates, but also a higher fracture rate, have been presented in the upper extremity [7, 38, 47]. This putative contradiction can be explained by the operation techniques: In the upper extremity, most authors use the fibular graft solely with an extramedullary fixation device [7, 31, 47, 60, 77]. In the lower extremity though, the fibula is commonly supported by either a combination with an additional autograft or allograft, or the use of a double barrel technique; rigid intramedullary fixation is accomplished when feasible [50, 80, 123]. The additional graft and the rigid fixation by an intramedullary nail absorb a considerable amount of the biomechanical load, leaving limited load to the fibular graft itself. The stimulus for graft adaptation is therefore reduced, resulting in lower union rates and fracture rates of approximately 10% [55, 120, 123]. We had no fractures in our own patients in the lower extremities using Capanna's method [50]. Solely fibular grafts, however, reach fracture rates of 12%–50% even in the upper extremity [7, 22, 87, 110, 120]. Looking at solely transplanted bone grafts in the lower extremity, fracture rates in some series exceed 60%–100%, outlining the importance of the use of supporting graft or a double barrel technique in the lower extremity [22, 55, 111]. Deviating from these results, Amr et al. [2] presented only two fractures in their series of 23 patients with resection arthrodesis of the knee using a sole fibular graft with extramedullary fixation. These data can be explained by the fact that postoperative weight bearing was strictly adapted to the results of the radiological controls in order to prevent biomechanical overload of the graft.

Whether it is beneficial to use additional cancellous bone grafts in order to improve union and integration is still controversial, showing significant differences in some series and none in others [26, 116, 124]. We have favoured the use of cancellous bone grafting in our patients.

The presented results comprise many variables in small patient populations in the currently published series. In our opinion, they are not suitable to identify certain procedures as being superior to others, but rather to sensitize the surgeon to the importance of a thoughtfully adapted postoperative management regimen.

9.3.3
Complications and Functional Outcome in Vital Grafts

Most complications of vital bone grafting can be cured with moderate effort. Therefore, despite considerable fracture and primary non-union rates, functional outcome is hardly influenced by the occurring complications.

The higher functional scores in the upper extremity are concomitant with other biological reconstruction procedures. Tumour staging and associated resection procedure seems to be more important for the functional outcome than the type of reconstruction [72].

9.3.4
Extracorporeal Devitalized Grafts

A general initial concern regarding a possible higher rate of local or systemic tumour recurrence caused by insufficient devitalization could not be confirmed by the currently existing data. Uyttendaele and colleagues even suggest a positive immune stimulus caused by the release of intracellular tumour proteins after reimplantation [107]. Different devitalization methods using heat, radiation or cryo-application have been reported [11, 62, 88, 105]. These procedures variably influence the properties of the graft. Compared to heat devitalization, biomechanical strength and osteoinductivity of the graft seem to be better preserved using extracorporeal irradiation applying a dose of 50–300 Gy [10, 23, 109]. These results can be explained by the increased denaturing of matrix proteins and osteoinductive proteins caused by heat application. The impact on biomechanical properties performing a devitalization using fluid nitrogen is not yet clarified.

Considering the similarity of extracorporeal devitalized autografts and allografts regarding their indication spectrum, theoretical advantages and integration properties, these results about bone integrity demonstrate that the potential disease transfer in allografts also hides a biomechanical problem; in order to achieve sufficient reduction of bacterial and viral load in allografts, different conditioning steps are carried out for allografts in tissue banks, involving heat treatment or high doses of irradiation. As described above, heat results in a denaturation of matrix and osteoinductive proteins; after high-dose irradiation (kGy), Currey et al. have shown a dose-dependent decrease of impact energy absorption and bending capacity as well as a brittle behaviour of bone grafts [23].

Integration of avital bone grafts proceeds by creeping substitution originating in the recipient bed. Although union is achieved in a high percentage of patients after reasonable time, partial substitution of the whole graft takes years, and a transformation into physiological bone remains incomplete. Due to the slow integration and its initial biomechanical properties, fractures primarily occur after the first 1–2 years by wear of the graft rather than by initial overload (in contrast to vital graft, where fractures usually occur within the first year [27, 72]).

The avitality of devitalized autografts and allografts causes a relatively high infection rate of approximately 11% in devitalized autografts, and 15%–71% in allografts [19, 28, 29, 72]. Reaching up to 50%, infection rates are especially high at poor vascularized recipient sites such as the pelvis, often resulting in failure of the graft [24, 88]. In extremity reconstructions, IEIR grafts show low infection rates of about 5%.

Since integration processes of IEIR autografts as well as allografts can be significantly improved if combined with a vital bone graft (e.g. Capanna), this procedure is recommended if applicable [24, 65, 88].

Comparing allografts and IEIR autografts, a significantly higher rate of non-union can be found in allografts, ranging from 15% to 71% [19, 20, 28, 29, 72]. This is probably caused by two factors. First, autografts offer a perfect fit and therefore a maximal area of graft–host interface, thereby supporting integration. Second, allografts are suspected to cause a light immunological rejection of the graft, resulting in delayed integration [3, 105].

The biggest problem in identifying further entrapments of irradiated and LN-treated autografts is the fact that, to the best of our knowledge, only 166 cases in total have been published, primarily represented in small, heterogeneous series. We have summarized the currently available publications (see Table 9.1) and sorted the available data by tumour site (see Table 9.2).

Most cases of IEIR autografts at extremity sites show good to excellent functional results (depending on soft tissue coverage). Especially intercalary reconstructions achieve MSTS scores around 90%. In the upper extremity, a better functional outcome can be seen with higher union rates. As expected, intercalary reconstructions achieve significantly better functional results than osteoarticular reconstructions. The reported osteoarticular grafts of the extremities have achieved an MSTS score of 72.7% in 10 patients; patients evaluated using former evaluation scores report 9 excellent results, 3 good results and 1 poor result. This functional outcome is similar to allograft reconstructions [72].

Compared to early results after endoprosthetic reconstruction of the knee joint, functional scores are inferior, but the failure rate of endoprosthetic reconstructions rises with time; the failure rate of IEIR autografts or allografts strongly declines after 3 years, and the reconstruction is then expected to last.

Despite high complication rates, the failure rate of the presented devitalized autografts is only 12.7% in total and only about 4% after extremity reconstruction with a median follow-up of 44 months; the most fragile period of time in biological reconstructions has therefore often already passed.

The worst results are seen in pelvic reconstructions, presenting failure rates of approximately 25%, often caused by infection due to the poor recipient site. However, the available alternative procedures for pelvic reconstructions are also unreliable; pelvic megaprostheses glare with even higher complication and failure rates, while pelvic allografts with a good-fit are difficult to obtain [53]. One benefit of pelvic reconstructions, however, seems to be the excellent long-term functional results in patients without failure of the reconstruction.

Another advantage of using devitalized autografts is the ability to reconstruct even small joints such as the ankle joint or complex bone formations such as the carpus [3]; in these locations, suitable allografts are very rare and megaprosthetic devices are not available.

A general evaluation comparing allografts and extracorporeal devitalized autografts is very difficult. Chen et al. demonstrated a significantly higher complication rate his in his allograft group, directly comparing IEIR autografts and allografts [20]. Considering the presented data for IEIR and a review of allograft results, we share the impression that replanted IEIR autografts in general trend to better results; however, the differences are not major and results seem strongly dependent on the experience of the performing team.

9.3.5 Distraction Osteogenesis

Distraction osteogenesis is yet not very common in the reconstruction of bone defects after tumour resection. The absence of sufficient literature and evaluation criteria limits the power of the presented results more than in vital and avital bone grafting.

Although all biological reconstructions are associated with a relatively long immobilization period, this issue is clearly the crucial downside of distraction osteogenesis. On the other hand, distraction osteogenesis represents the ethnic idea of a biological reconstruction, inducing de novo bone synthesis originated by the patient. Once the newly formed bone has matured, it provides physical biomechanical strength, immune-reactive abilities and normal regenerative potential. Performing this reconstruction procedure, the patient's organism undertakes the highest demands of integration and adaptation. The condition of the patient as well as the soft tissue at the defect area are therefore of essential importance [83]. Conducting distraction without shortening, osteogenesis is conducted away from the defect area, supplying intact soft tissue and an unharmed periosteal tube at the bone construction site.

Besides immobilization, prolonged external fixation time seems to be an important aspect in distraction osteogenesis. A reduction results in decreased complication rates [30, 103, 104]. Two procedures are described to achieve this goal. (1) Distraction along an intramedullary nail allows finishing external fixation after the distraction period, stabilizing the maturation process by the nail [30, 104]. (2) Using bifocal elongation, distraction time can almost be halved [108].

The backside poses an increased risk for late infection in cases of intramedullary nailing and creates a more complex procedure in the guiding of two bone segments using bifocal distraction.

A promising new procedure is the implantation of a fully implantable, motorized intramedullary nail with the ability of distraction without any external fixation [6].

The presented overall results regarding functional outcome in distraction osteogenesis seem to be superior over other reconstruction procedures; however, due to the exclusive application in intercalary defects of the extremities, these results need to be put into perspective. Total complication and failure rates are similar to other biological reconstruction procedures (see Table 9.3).

9.3.6
Indications and Limitations

In our opinion, based on the existing data no legitimate, stringent indication or limitation can be pronounced preferring either one of the biological reconstruction procedures. Due to the plurality of influencing parameters in oncological patients, the decision for a reconstruction procedure stays individual. Current results rather allow a surgeon to properly assess some of the influencing factors.

The most important factors are probably tumour staging and tumour location [72]. Since biological reconstruction procedures present their disadvantages, including delayed mobilization of the patient and high complication rates, within the first years after an operation, on the one hand, and feature excellent and lasting long-term results, on the other hand, they are an excellent investment in the future. In patients with a good prognosis, especially in children, these are exactly the attributes we strive for; in a patient with a poor future perspective due to an advanced tumour stage, however, these attributes are unlikely to prove beneficial.

The functional outcome of a reconstruction procedure is mostly dependent on the tumour location, associated with the mechanical requirements and the soft tissue condition of the defect site. The type of reconstruction procedure seems to define the outcome subsequently [72]. In intercalary defects, all of the presented biological procedures have shown good to excellent long-term results; in patients with favourable prognosis, a biological approach is to our understanding therefore the first choice. In patients with a poor or unclear prognosis, intercalary prostheses may be used as a spacer and may be replaced by a biological reconstruction later on [123].

In articular defect reconstruction it is catchier; they generally present worse functional outcomes and biological approaches are limited. In the upper extremity, the most common tumour sites are the proximal humerus and the distal radius. If the shoulder joint is affected in a proximal humerus lesion, biological reconstructions and megaprostheses can be used for articular reconstruction, depending on the tumour extension [110]; if the rotator cuff can be salvaged, better function of the shoulder joint can be achieved using a megaprostheses. If substantial parts of the rotator cuff have to be resected, however, the primary goal is shoulder stability to achieve good function in the elbow and hand. We would therefore prefer a biological reconstruction (primarily vascularized fibula graft) due to the low failure rates of biological reconstruction at that site and the risk of aseptic loosening and infection over time in megaprostheses.

Excellent results have been reported for distal radius reconstructions performing an epiphyseal transfer in children or fibular head transfer in adults (see Fig. 9.1). Prostheses do not represent an equivalent alternative at this site [60, 77].

In the lower extremity, most common tumour locations are the proximal femur, the distal femur and the proximal tibia. In joint-involving defects, megaprostheses are the mostly used reconstructions if the motor of the joint can be salvaged. In hip reconstructions they offer reliable and good survival rates and excellent functional outcome. In these cases we also prefer the implantation of a megaprosthesis [49].

Reconstructions of the knee joint after tumour resection, on the other hand, represent challenging procedures with an insecure outcome. At this defect site there are currently no satisfying solutions. Megaprostheses offer good early functional outcome but present failure rates of up to 50% after 10 years [8]. In these cases, osteoarticular allografts and replanted autografts are a true alternative. Although early function is clearly inferior compared to a reconstruction with a megaprosthesis, they offer low failure rates and reasonably functional long-term results of the joint [72, 105]. At the same time, megaprostheses remain a strategic withdrawal in case of failure of a biological reconstruction approach, whereas reverse is not practicable.

Considering the above-mentioned possible indications, biological reconstructions can be used at most bone tumour sites. However, biological reconstructions are considerably more demanding regarding surgical skills as well as postoperative management than the implantation of megaprostheses. In case of an inadequate biological reconstruction procedure, the favourable attributes of a long-lasting outcome are likely to prove elusive.

Presenting similar failure and complication rates, as well as functional outcome, no biological reconstruction procedure can be considered superior over another. If a defect site can be reconstructed by different biological approaches, best results are most likely achieved by the procedure the surgeon is most experienced in.

9.4 Conclusion

Among the presented procedures, biological reconstructions represent the most elegant form of defect reconstruction after bone tumour resection and can be applied at numerous defect sites. Although being highly demanding, they offer unique possibilities, being the only ones—assuming proper indications—that offer the prerequisites for a *restitutio ad integrum*.

Further studies will help to improve our understanding of critical outcome influencing aspects in biological reconstruction approaches. Due to the unmatched long-term-results of these procedures, the reported high complication rates in the beginning and the prolonged immobilization should be seen—in our opinion, especially in young patients with good oncological prognosis—as a good investment for the future.

References

1. Amin SN, Ebeid WA (2000) Shoulder reconstruction after tumor resection by pedicled scapular crest graft. Clin Orthop Relat Res 397:133–142
2. Amr SM, El-Mofty AO, Amin SN, Morsy AM, El-Malt OM, Abdel-Aal HA (2000) Reconstruction after resection of tumors around the knee: role of the free vascularized fibular graft. Microsurgery 20:233–251
3. Araki N, Myoui A, Kuratsu S, Hashimoto N, Inoue T, Kudawara I, Ueda T, Yoshikawa H, Masaki N, Uchida A (1999) Intraoperative extracorporeal autogenous irradiated bone grafts in tumor surgery. Clin Orthop Relat Res 368:196–206
4. Bacci G, Briccoli A, Rocca M, Ferrari S, Donati D, Longhi A, Bertoni F, Bacchini P, Giacomini S, Forni C, Manfrini M, Galletti S (2003) Neoadjuvant chemotherapy for osteosarcoma of the extremities with metastases at presentation: recent experience at the Rizzoli Institute in 57 patients treated with cisplatin, doxorubicin, and a high dose of methotrexate and ifosfamide. Ann Oncol 14:1126–1134
5. Bacci G, Ferrari S, Lari S, Mercuri M, Donati D, Longhi A, Forni C, Bertoni F, Versari M, Pignotti E (2002) Osteosarcoma of the limb. Amputation or limb salvage in patients treated by neoadjuvant chemotherapy. J Bone Joint Surg Br 84:88–92
6. Baumgart R, Hinterwimmer S, Krammer M, Muensterer O, Mutschler W (2005) The bioexpandable prosthesis: a new perspective after resection of malignant bone tumors in children. J Pediatr Hematol Oncol 27:452–455
7. Bernd L, Sabo D, Zahlten-Hinguranage A, Niemeyer P, Daecke W, Simank HG (2003) Experiences with vascular pedicled fibula in reconstruction of osseous defects in primary malignant bone tumors [in German]. Orthopade 32:983–993
8. Biau D, Faure F, Katsahian S, Jeanrot C, Tomeno B, Anract P (2006) Survival of total knee replacement with a megaprosthesis after bone tumor resection. J Bone Joint Surg Am 88:1285–1293
9. Böhm P, Fritz J, Thiede S, Budach W (2003) Reimplantation of extracorporeal irradiated bone segments in musculoskeletal tumor surgery: clinical experience in eight patients and review of the literature. Langenbecks Arch Surg 387:355–365
10. Bohm P, Scherer MA (1997) Incorporation of devitalised autografts in dogs. Int Orthop 21:283–290
11. Bohm P, Springfeld R, Springer H (1998) Re-implantation of autoclaved bone segments in musculoskeletal tumor surgery. Clinical experience in 9 patients followed for 1.1–8.4 years and review of the literature. Arch Orthop Trauma Surg 118:57–65
12. Bos KE (1979) Bone scintigraphy of experimental composite bone grafts revascularized by microvascular anastomoses. Plast Reconstr Surg 64:353–360
13. Bowen CV, O'Brien BM, Gumley GJ (1988) Experimental microvascular growth plate transfers. Part 2. Investigation of feasibility. J Bone Joint Surg Br 70:311–314
14. Brown KL (1991) Limb reconstruction with vascularized fibular grafts after bone tumor resection. Clin Orthop Relat Res 64–73
15. Campanacci M, Bacci G, Pagani P, Giunti A (1980) Multiple-drug chemotherapy for the primary treatment of osteosarcoma of the extremities. J Bone Joint Surg Br 62-B:93–101
16. Cannon SR (1997) Massive prostheses for malignant bone tumours of the limbs. J Bone Joint Surg Br 79:497–506
17. Canosa R, Gonzalez del Pino J (1994) Effect of methotrexate in the biology of free vascularized bone grafts. A comparative experimental study in the dog. Clin Orthop Relat Res 291–301
18. Capanna R, Bufalini C, Campanacci C (1993) A new technique for the reconstruction of large metadiaphyseal bone defects. Orthop Traumatol 2:159
19. Cara JA, Lacleriga A, Canadell J (1994) Intercalary bone allografts. 23 tumor cases followed for 3 years. Acta Orthop Scand 65:42–46
20. Chen TH, Chen WM, Huang CK (2005) Reconstruction after intercalary resection of malignant bone tumours: comparison between segmental allograft and extracorporeally-irradiated autograft. J Bone Joint Surg Br 87:704–709
21. Chen WM, Chen TH, Huang CK, Chiang CC, Lo WH (2002) Treatment of malignant bone

22. Chew WY, Low CK, Tan SK (1995) Long-term results of free vascularized fibular graft. A clinical and radiographic evaluation. Clin Orthop Relat Res 258–261
23. Currey JD, Foreman J, Laketic I, Mitchell J, Pegg DE, Reilly GC (1997) Effects of ionizing radiation on the mechanical properties of human bone. J Orthop Res 15:111–117
24. Davidson AW, Hong A, McCarthy SW, Stalley PD (2005) En-bloc resection, extracorporeal irradiation, and re-implantation in limb salvage for bony malignancies. J Bone Joint Surg Br 87:851–857
25. De Bastiani G, Aldegheri R, Renzi-Brivio L, Trivella G (1987) Limb lengthening by callus distraction (callotasis). J Pediatr Orthop 7:129–134
26. de Boer HH (1988) The history of bone grafts. Clin Orthop Relat Res 292–298
27. de Boer HH, Wood MB (1989) Bone changes in the vascularised fibular graft. J Bone Joint Surg Br 71:374–378
28. Donati D, Capanna R, Campanacci D, Del Ben M, Ercolani C, Masetti C, Taminiau A, Exner GU, Dubousset JF, Paitout D, et al (1993) The use of massive bone allografts for intercalary reconstruction and arthrodeses after tumor resection. A multicentric European study. Chir Organi Mov 78:81–94
29. Donati D, Di Liddo M, Zavatta M, Manfrini M, Bacci G, Picci P, Capanna R, Mercuri M (2000) Massive bone allograft reconstruction in high-grade osteosarcoma. Clin Orthop Relat Res 186–194
30. Dormans JP, Ofluoglu O, Erol B, Moroz L, Davidson RS (2005) Case report: reconstruction of an intercalary defect with bone transport after resection of Ewing's sarcoma. Clin Orthop Relat Res 258–264
31. Eisenschenk A, Lautenbach M, Rohlmann A (1998) Free vascularized bone transplantation in the extremities [in German]. Orthopade 27:491–500
32. Eisenschenk A, Lehnert M, Weber U (1994) Die freie, gefäßgestielte Fibulatransplantation zur Überbrückung von Knochendefekten. Operative Orthopäd Traumatol 6:117–118
33. Enneking WF (1987) A system for functional evaluation of the surgical management of musculoskeletal tumors. In: Enneking WF (ed) Limb salvage in musculoskeletal oncology. Churchill Livingstone, New York, p 5–16
34. Enneking WF, Dunham W, Gebhardt MC, Malawar M, Pritchard DJ (1993) A system for the functional evaluation of reconstructive procedures after surgical treatment of tumors of the musculoskeletal system. Clin Orthop Relat Res 241–246
35. Enneking WF, Eady JL, Burchardt H (1980) Autogenous cortical bone grafts in the reconstruction of segmental skeletal defects. J Bone Joint Surg Am 62:1039–1058
36. Erler K, Yildiz C, Baykal B, Atesalp AS, Ozdemir MT, Basbozkurt M (2005) Reconstruction of defects following bone tumor resections by distraction osteogenesis. Arch Orthop Trauma Surg 125:177–183
37. Fritz W, Ullmann T (1996) Initial experiences with Winkelmann "clavicula pro humero" operation in malignant bone tumors of the proximal humerus in childhood [in German]. Langenbecks Arch Chir Suppl Kongressbd 113:1102–1107
38. Gao YH, Ketch LL, Eladoumikdachi F, Netscher DT (2001) Upper limb salvage with microvascular bone transfer for major long-bone segmental tumor resections. Ann Plast Surg 47:240–246
39. Gebert C, Hillmann A, Schwappach A, Hoffmann C, Hardes J, Kleinheinz J, Gosheger G (2006) Free vascularized fibular grafting for reconstruction after tumor resection in the upper extremity. J Surg Oncol 94:114–127
40. Gidumal R, Wood MB, Sim FH, Shives TC (1987) Vascularized bone transfer for limb salvage and reconstruction after resection of aggressive bone lesions. J Reconstr Microsurg 3:183–188
41. Goldberg VM, Shaffer JW, Field G, Davy DT (1987) Biology of vascularized bone grafts. Orthop Clin North Am 18:197–205
42. Goldberg VM, Stevenson S (1987) Natural history of autografts and allografts. Clin Orthop Relat Res 7–16
43. Guo F (1981) Observations of the blood supply to the fibula. Arch Orthop Trauma Surg 98:147–151
44. Hahn E (1884) Eine Methode, Pseudarthrosen mit großem Defekt zur Ausheilung zu bringen. Zentralblatt Chir 21:337–341
45. Hamanishi C, Yoshii T, Totani Y, Tanaka S (1994) Lengthened callus activated by axial shortening. Histological and cytomorphometrical analysis. Clin Orthop Relat Res 250–254

46. Hamer AJ, Strachan JR, Black MM, Ibbotson CJ, Stockley I, Elson RA (1996) Properties of cortical allograft bone using a new method of bone strength measurement A comparison of fresh Biochemical (1996) fresh-frozen and irradiated bone. J Bone Joint Surg Br 78:363–368
47. Han CS, Wood MB, Bishop AT, Cooney WP 3rd (1992) Vascularized bone transfer. J Bone Joint Surg Am 74:1441–1449
48. Harrington KD, Johnston JO, Kaufer HN, Luck JV Jr, Moore TM (1986) Limb salvage and prosthetic joint reconstruction for low-grade and selected high-grade sarcomas of bone after wide resection and replacement by autoclaved [corrected] autogeneic grafts. Clin Orthop Relat Res 180–214
49. Heisel C, Kinkel S, Bernd L, Ewerbeck V (2006) Megaprostheses for the treatment of malignant bone tumours of the lower limbs. Int Orthop 30:452–457
50. Hennen J, Sabo D, Martini AK, Bernd L (2002) Mantel transplant for defect reconstruction after resection of malignant bone tumors of the lower extremity [in German]. Unfallchirurg 105:120–127
51. Hierner R, Stock W, Wood MB, Schweiberer L (1992) Vascularized fibula transfer. A review [in German]. Unfallchirurg 95:152–159
52. Hierner R, Wood MB (1995) Comparison of vascularised iliac crest and vascularised fibula transfer for reconstruction of segmental and partial bone defects in long bones of the lower extremity. Microsurgery 16:818–826
53. Hillmann A, Hoffmann C, Gosheger G, Rodl R, Winkelmann W, Ozaki T (2003) Tumors of the pelvis: complications after reconstruction. Arch Orthop Trauma Surg 123:340–344
54. Hong A, Stevens G, Stalley P, Pendlebury S, Ahern V, Ralston A, Estoesta E, Barrett I (2001) Extracorporeal irradiation for malignant bone tumors. Int J Radiat Oncol Biol Phys 50:441–447
55. Hsu RW, Wood MB, Sim FH, Chao EY (1997) Free vascularised fibular grafting for reconstruction after tumour resection. J Bone Joint Surg Br 79:36–42
56. Ihara K, Doi K, Yamamoto M, Kawai S (1998) Free vascularized fibular grafts for large bone defects in the extremities after tumor excision. J Reconstr Microsurg 14:371–376
57. Ilizarov GA (1990) Clinical application of the tension-stress effect for limb lengthening. Clin Orthop Relat Res 8–26
58. Ilizarov GA, Deviatov AA (1969) Surgical lengthening of the shin with simultaneous correction of deformities [in German]. Ortop Travmatol Protez 30:32–37
59. Innocenti M, Ceruso M, Manfrini M, Angeloni R, Lauri G, Capanna R, Bufalini C (1998) Free vascularized growth-plate transfer after bone tumor resection in children. J Reconstr Microsurg 14:137–143
60. Innocenti M, Delcroix L, Manfrini M, Ceruso M, Capanna R (2004) Vascularized proximal fibular epiphyseal transfer for distal radial reconstruction. J Bone Joint Surg Am 86-A:1504–1511
61. Jarka DE, Nicholas RW, Aronson J (1998) Effect of methotrexate on distraction osteogenesis. Clin Orthop Relat Res 209–215
62. Jeon DG, Kim MS, Cho WH, Song WS, Lee SY (2007) Pasteurized autograft for intercalary reconstruction: an alternative to allograft. Clin Orthop Relat Res 456:203–210
63. Kapukaya A, Subasi M, Kandiya E, Ozates M, Yilmaz F (2000) Limb reconstruction with the callus distraction method after bone tumor resection. Arch Orthop Trauma Surg 120:215–218
64. Kawai A, Muschler GF, Lane JM, Otis JC, Healey JH (1998) Prosthetic knee replacement after resection of a malignant tumor of the distal part of the femur. Medium to long-term results. J Bone Joint Surg Am 80:636–647
65. Krieg AH, Davidson AW, Stalley PD (2007) Intercalary femoral reconstruction with extracorporeal irradiated autogenous bone graft in limb-salvage surgery. J Bone Joint Surg Br 89:366–371
66. Krieg AH, Hefti F (2007) Reconstruction with non-vascularised fibular grafts after resection of bone tumours. J Bone Joint Surg Br 89:215–221
67. Lammens J, Fabry G (1992) Reconstruction of bony defects using the Ilizarov "bone transport" technique. A preliminary report. Arch Orthop Trauma Surg 111:70–72
68. Lazar E, Rosenthal DI, Jupiter J (1993) Free vascularized fibular grafts: radiographic evidence of remodeling and hypertrophy. AJR Am J Roentgenol 161:613–615
69. Leung PC, Hung LK (1989) Bone reconstruction after giant-cell tumor resection at the proximal end of the humerus with vascularized iliac crest graft. A report of three cases. Clin Orthop Relat Res 101–105

70. Link MP, Goorin AM, Miser AW, Green AA, Pratt CB, Belasco JB, Pritchard J, Malpas JS, Baker AR, Kirkpatrick JA, et al (1986) The effect of adjuvant chemotherapy on relapse-free survival in patients with osteosarcoma of the extremity. N Engl J Med 314:1600–1606
71. Malawer MM, Chou LB (1995) Prosthetic survival and clinical results with use of large-segment replacements in the treatment of high-grade bone sarcomas. J Bone Joint Surg Am 77:1154–1165
72. Mankin HJ, Gebhardt MC, Jennings LC, Springfield DS, Tomford WW (1996) Long-term results of allograft replacement in the management of bone tumors. Clin Orthop Relat Res 86–97
73. McKee NH, Haw P, Vettese T (1984) Anatomic study of the nutrient foramen in the shaft of the fibula. Clin Orthop Relat Res 141–144
74. Meyers PA, Gorlick R, Heller G, Casper E, Lane J, Huvos AG, Healey JH (1998) Intensification of preoperative chemotherapy for osteogenic sarcoma: results of the Memorial Sloan-Kettering (T12) protocol. J Clin Oncol 16:2452–2458
75. Millett PJ, Lane JM, Paletta GA Jr (2000) Limb salvage using distraction osteogenesis. Am J Orthop 29:628–632
76. Minami A, Kasashima T, Iwasaki N, Kato H, Kaneda K (2000) Vascularised fibular grafts. An experience of 102 patients. J Bone Joint Surg Br 82:1022–1025
77. Minami A, Kato H, Iwasaki N (2002) Vascularized fibular graft after excision of giant-cell tumor of the distal radius: wrist arthroplasty versus partial wrist arthrodesis. Plast Reconstr Surg 110:112–117
78. Mittermayer F, Krepler P, Dominkus M, Schwameis E, Sluga M, Heinzl H, Kotz R (2001) Long-term followup of uncemented tumor endoprostheses for the lower extremity. Clin Orthop Relat Res 167–177
79. Moore JR, Weiland AJ, Daniel RK (1983) Use of free vascularized bone grafts in the treatment of bone tumors. Clin Orthop Relat Res 37–44
80. Moran SL, Shin AY, Bishop AT (2006) The use of massive bone allograft with intramedullary free fibular flap for limb salvage in a pediatric and adolescent population. Plast Reconstr Surg 118:413–419
81. Naggar L, Chevalley F, Blanc CH, Livio JJ (1993) Treatment of large bone defects with the Ilizarov technique. J Trauma 34:390–393
82. Ono H, Yajima H, Mizumoto S, Miyauchi Y, Mii Y, Tamai S (1997) Vascularized fibular graft for reconstruction of the wrist after excision of giant cell tumor. Plast Reconstr Surg 99:1086–1093
83. Ozaki T, Nakatsuka Y, Kunisada T, Kawai A, Dan'ura T, Naito N, Inoue H (1998) High complication rate of reconstruction using Ilizarov bone transport method in patients with bone sarcomas. Arch Orthop Trauma Surg 118:136–139
84. Pho RW (1979) Free vascularised fibular transplant for replacement of the lower radius. J Bone Joint Surg Br 61-B:362–365
85. Prevot J, Poncelet T, Lemelle JL, Lascombes P, Blanquart D, Membre H, Olive D (1988) Study of distraction osteogenesis in an animal body submitted to anticancer chemotherapy [in German]. Chir Pediatr 29:226–230
86. Restrepo J, Katz D, Gilbert A (1980) Arterial vascularization of the proximal epiphysis and the diaphysis of the fibula. Int J Microsurg 2:49
87. Rose PS, Shin AY, Bishop AT, Moran SL, Sim FH (2005) Vascularized free fibula transfer for oncologic reconstruction of the humerus. Clin Orthop Relat Res 438:80–84
88. Sabo D, Bernd L, Buchner M, Treiber M, Wannenmacher M, Ewerbeck V, Parsch D (2003) Intraoperative extracorporeal irradiation and replantation in local treatment of primary malignant bone tumors [in German]. Orthopade 32:1003–1012
89. Sabo D, Brocai DR, Eble M, Wannenmacher M, Ewerbeck V (2000) Influence of extracorporeal irradiation on the reintegration of autologous grafts of bone and joint. Study in a canine model. J Bone Joint Surg Br 82:276–282
90. Said GZ, el-Sherif EK (1995) Resection-shortening-distraction for malignant bone tumours. A report of two cases. J Bone Joint Surg Br 77:185–188
91. Schuind F, Burny F, Lejeune FJ (1988) Microsurgical free fibular bone transfer: a technique for reconstruction of large skeletal defects following resection of high-grade malignant tumors. World J Surg 12:310–317
92. Schwameis E, Dominkus M, Krepler P, Dorotka R, Lang S, Windhager R, Kotz R (2002) Reconstruction of the pelvis after tumor resection in children and adolescents. Clin Orthop Relat Res 220–235
93. Shaffer JW, Field GA, Wilber RG, Goldberg VM (1987) Experimental vascularized bone grafts: histopathologic correlations with postoperative bone scan: the risk of false-positive results. J Orthop Res 5:311–319

94. Shea KG, Coleman DA, Scott SM, Coleman SS, Christianson M (1997) Microvascularized free fibular grafts for reconstruction of skeletal defects after tumor resection. J Pediatr Orthop 17:424–432
95. Smeland S, Muller C, Alvegard TA, Wiklund T, Wiebe T, Bjork O, Stenwig AE, Willen H, Holmstrom T, Folleras G, Brosjo O, Kivioja A, Jonsson K, Monge O, Saeter G (2003) Scandinavian Sarcoma Group Osteosarcoma Study SSG VIII: prognostic factors for outcome and the role of replacement salvage chemotherapy for poor histological responders. Eur J Cancer 39:488–494
96. Spira E, Lubin E (1968) Extracorporeal irradiation of bone tumors. A preliminary report. Isr J Med Sci 4:1015–1019
97. Springfield D (1996) Autograft reconstructions. Orthop Clin North Am 27:483–492
98. Subasi M, Kapukaya A, Kesemenli C, Balci TA, Buyukbayram H, Ozates M (2001) Effect of chemotherapeutic agents on distraction osteogenesis. An experimental investigation in rabbits. Arch Orthop Trauma Surg 121:417–421
99. Sundaresh DC, Gopalakrishnan D, Shetty N (2000) Vascularised rib graft defects of the diaphysis of the humerus in children. A report of two cases. J Bone Joint Surg Br 82:28–32
100. Sys G, Uyttendaele D, Poffyn B, Verdonk R, Verstraete L (2002) Extracorporeally irradiated autografts in pelvic reconstruction after malignant tumour resection. Int Orthop 26:174–178
101. Taylor GI, Miller GD, Ham FJ (1975) The free vascularized bone graft. A clinical extension of microvascular techniques. Plast Reconstr Surg 55:533–544
102. Thoma A, Heddle S, Archibald S, Young JE (1988) The free vascularized anterior rib graft. Plast Reconstr Surg 82:291–298
103. Tsuchiya H, Abdel-Wanis ME, Sakurakichi K, Yamashiro T, Tomita K (2002) Osteosarcoma around the knee. Intraepiphyseal excision and biological reconstruction with distraction osteogenesis. J Bone Joint Surg Br 84:1162–1166
104. Tsuchiya H, Tomita K, Minematsu K, Mori Y, Asada N, Kitano S (1997) Limb salvage using distraction osteogenesis. A classification of the technique. J Bone Joint Surg Br 79:403–411
105. Tsuchiya H, Wan SL, Sakayama K, Yamamoto N, Nishida H, Tomita K (2005) Reconstruction using an autograft containing tumour treated by liquid nitrogen. J Bone Joint Surg Br 87:218–225
106. Tsukushi S, Nishida Y, Takahashi M, Ishiguro N (2006) Clavicula pro humero reconstruction after wide resection of the proximal humerus. Clin Orthop Relat Res 447:132–137
107. Uyttendaele D, De Schryver A, Claessens H, Roels H, Berkvens P, Mondelaers W (1988) Limb conservation in primary bone tumours by resection, extracorporeal irradiation and re-implantation. J Bone Joint Surg Br 70: 348–353
108. Vidyadhara S, Rao SK (2007) A novel approach to juxta-articular aggressive and recurrent giant cell tumours: resection arthrodesis using bone transport over an intramedullary nail. Int Orthop 31:179–184
109. Voggenreiter G, Ascherl R, Blumel G, Schmit-Neuerburg KP (1996) Extracorporeal irradiation and incorporation of bone grafts. Autogeneic cortical grafts studied in rats. Acta Orthop Scand 67:583–588
110. Wada T, Usui M, Isu K, Yamawakii S, Ishii S (1999) Reconstruction and limb salvage after resection for malignant bone tumour of the proximal humerus. A sling procedure using a free vascularised fibular graft. J Bone Joint Surg Br 81:808–813
111. Wada T, Usui M, Nagoya S, Isu K, Yamawaki S, Ishii S (2000) Resection arthrodesis of the knee with a vascularised fibular graft. Medium- to long-term results. J Bone Joint Surg Br 82:489–493
112. Walter M (1911) Resection de l'extremite inferieure du radius pour osteosarcome: greffe de l'extrémité supériuie du péroné. Bull Mem Soc Chir Paris 37:739–747
113. Weiland AJ, Phillips TW, Randolph MA (1984) Bone grafts: a radiologic, histologic, and biomechanical model comparing autografts, allografts, and free vascularized bone grafts. Plast Reconstr Surg 74:368–379
114. Winkelmann W (1999) Extremitätenerhalt bei malignen Knochentumoren. Dtsch Arztebl 96:A-1270/B-1085/C-1013. http://www.aerzteblatt.de/v4/archiv/artikel.asp?src=suche&id=17165. Cited 22 May 2008
115. Winkelmann WW (1992) Clavicula pro humero—a new surgical method for malignant tumors of the proximal humerus [in German]. Z Orthop Ihre Grenzgeb 130:197–201
116. Wood MB (1987) Upper extremity reconstruction by vascularized bone transfers: results and complications. J Hand Surg Am 12:422–427
117. Wood MB, Cooney WP 3rd, Irons GB Jr (1985) Skeletal reconstruction by vascularized

bone transfer: indications and results. Mayo Clin Proc 60:729–734
118. Wu KJ, Hou SX, Zhang WJ, Wang F, Guo JD, Sun DM, Zheng XY (2005) Vascularized pedicle iliac crest for the repair of bone and soft tissue defect of lower extremity [in German]. Zhonghua Wai Ke Za Zhi 43:784–787
119. Yadav SS (1990) Dual-fibular grafting for massive bone gaps in the lower extremity. J Bone Joint Surg Am 72:486–494
120. Yajima H, Tamai S, Mizumoto S, Ono H (1993) Vascularised fibular grafts for reconstruction of the femur. J Bone Joint Surg Br 75:123–128
121. Yamamoto N, Tsuchiya H, Tomita K (2003) Effects of liquid nitrogen treatment on the proliferation of osteosarcoma and the biomechanical properties of normal bone. J Orthop Sci 8:374–380
122. Yoshimura M, Shimamura K, Iwai Y, Yamauchi S, Ueno T (1983) Free vascularized fibular transplant. A new method for monitoring circulation of the grafted fibula. J Bone Joint Surg Am 65:1295–1301
123. Zaretski A, Amir A, Meller I, Leshem D, Kollender Y, Barnea Y, Bickels J, Shpitzer T, Ad-El D, Gur E (2004) Free fibula long bone reconstruction in orthopedic oncology: a surgical algorithm for reconstructive options. Plast Reconstr Surg 113:1989–2000
124. Zwipp H, Flory P, Berger A, Tscherne H (1989) Combination of cancellous bone grafts and free microvascular bone transplantation in large osseous defects [in German]. Handchir Mikrochir Plast Chir 21:235–245

Bone Sarcoma of the Spine   10

Klaus-Dieter Schaser*, I. Melcher*, A. Luzzati, and A. C. Disch

Abstract Primary malignant bone tumors of the vertebral column, i.e., bone sarcomas of the spine, are inherently rare entities. Vertebral osteosarcomas and chordomas represent the largest groups, followed by the incidence of chondro-, fibro-, and Ewing's sarcomas. Detailed clinical and neurological examination, complete radiographic imaging [radiographs, computed tomography (CT), magnetic resonance imaging (MRI)], and biopsy are the decisive diagnostic steps. Oncosurgical staging for spinal tumors can serve as a decision-guidance system for an individual's oncological and surgical treatment. Subsequent treatment decisions are part of an integrated, multimodal oncological concept. Surgical options comprise minimally invasive surgery, palliative stabilization procedures, and curative, wide excisions with complex reconstructions to attain wide or at least marginal resections. The most aggressive mode of surgical resection for primary vertebral column tumors is the total en bloc vertebrectomy, i.e., single- or multilevel en bloc spondylectomy. En bloc spondylectomy involves a posterior or combined anterior/posterior approach, followed by en bloc laminectomy, circumferential (360°) vertebral dissection, and blunt ventral release of the large vessels, intervertebral discectomy and rotation/en bloc removal of the vertebra along its longitudinal axis. Due to the complex interdisciplinary approach and the challenging surgical resection techniques involved, management of vertebral bone sarcomas is recommended to be performed in specific musculoskeletal tumor centers.

10.1
Introduction and Epidemiology

Primary malignant spinal bone tumors (exclusive plasmocytoma), i.e., vertebral sarcomas, are inherently rare entities among malignant bone tumors of the spine and account for 5%–10% of all primary osseous malignancies (Dreghorn et al. 1990; Boriani et al. 2000; Flemming et al. 2000; Kelley et al. 2007). In children, 60% of these tumors are found to be benign while 80% of the adult cases present with malignant lesions (Kelley et al. 2007). The most common site of malignant primary tumors is the thoracic spine, followed by sacral, lumbar, and cervical locations (Kelley et al. 2007). Out of the malignant primary tumors of the spine, approximately 25% represent sarcomas. Osteosarcomas (Imai et al. 2006; Murakami et al. 2006) represent the largest

Klaus-Dieter Schaser (✉)
Section for Musculoskeletal Tumor Surgery
Center for Musculoskeletal Surgery
Charité University Medicine Berlin
Augustenburger Platz 1
13353 Berlin, Germany
E-mail: klaus-dieter.schaser@charite.de

*Both authors contributed equally to that manscript

group, followed by the incidence of chondro- (Boriani et al. 2000; Lloret et al. 2006), fibro-, and Ewing sarcomas (Sharafuddin et al. 1992). Other histopathological sarcoma entities are very rare, and most publications on this subject are case reports or series (Nishida et al. 2002; Aflatoon et al. 2004; Kawashima et al. 2004; Hamlat et al. 2005; Sharma et al. 2006).

In contrast to spinal metastatic disease, which typically involves multiple sites, primary vertebral tumors should be considered in mostly young back-pain patients with solitary lesions. Their appearance and progression, however, can—like other primary and secondary vertebral column malignancies—result in early impairment of spinal stability and involvement of surrounding essential structures as well as systemic tumor spread, fatefully determining patients' short- and mid-term outcome. Deformities, instability, and pathological fractures, together with nerval root compression and irreversible myelon involvement, have the potential—at an early stage of disease—to cause severe restrictions in life quality and complete immobility. Due to the rapid development of diagnostic tools and imaging techniques in the last two decades, the detection of these entities has tremendously improved and allows early inclusion of affected patients into current multimodal therapy concepts. One key component of this multimodal approach is induction of neoadjuvant/adjuvant polychemotherapy. Despite sarcoma of the axial skeleton seems to have a decreased chemoresponsiveness versus limb sarcoma, the performance of adjuvant/neoadjuvant polychemo- and radiotherapy has enormously increased overall survival (Bielack et al. 1995). Together with chemo- and radiotherapy, surgical treatment continues to represent one principal and decisive therapeutic mainstay in spine sarcoma. From the surgical perspective, an indispensable precondition for maximal postoperative benefit—namely improved tumor-free survival and minimal complication rates—is an exact oncosurgical staging and a realistic evaluation of tumor extension based on predefined anatomical landmarks and established classification systems for vertebral neoplasms. Due to the topographic vicinity of the essential neurovascular structures such as the spinal cord, nerve roots, and large vessels, vertebral column sarcomas have long been considered to be either nonresectable by en bloc excision or at least very difficult to resect and attain tumor-free margins. Hence, most of these lesions have been treated by intralesional resection, which is known to be associated with intraoperative dissemination and persistence of tumor cells, tumor-derived blood loss, and consequently markedly increased risk for local recurrence and poor prognosis.

To reduce these drawbacks of intralesional surgery and to improve survival times, different techniques for wide resections at the spine, involving either en bloc total or hemilaminectomy followed by en bloc corporectomy and dorsoventral stabilization, have been developed. In the early 1980s, Stener and Roy-Camille et al. were the first to describe en bloc spondylectomy via a posterior approach (Stener 1971; Roy-Camille et al. 1990) after complete resection of the dorsal vertebral structures, resulting in an oncologically adequate resection for primary vertebral bone tumors.

10.2
Clinical Presentation

Even at an early stage of disease the majority of vertebral column sarcoma patients (over 90%) report localized or eradiating back pain that is, in every second patient, accompanied with neurological deficits (Kelley et al. 2007). They are caused by an equally distributed involvement of the spinal canal or the nerve roots. Patients show a wide range of pain sensations including minor localized bone pain, neuropathic pain syndromes, and pain resulting from biomechanical spinal instability (Sundaresan et al. 1991) leading to immobility. Less than 10% of all patients present with local swelling or a palpable mass.

10.3
Diagnostics and Radiographic Imaging

An early diagnostic approach involves a detailed anamnesis and clinical investigation including a clinical estimation of the affected spinal level by the preoperative neurological presentation. The neurological assessment includes explicit sensorimotor status and bladder and anal sphincter function; if necessary, it is completed by electrophysiological investigations. To standardize the neurological deficits, the Frankel classification is widely used (Davis et al. 1993):

A. Paraplegia (complete lesion)
B. Maintained sensibility
C. Motoric function without the ability to walk
D. Motoric function with the ability to walk
E. No deficits

In addition, initial imaging diagnostics involve local radiographs of the affected spinal regions. To detect the tumor dimensions and borders, especially in regard to extracompartmental invasion of the surrounding soft tissue, the spinal and nerval root canal, a magnetic resonance image (MRI) scan in combination with a contrast medium is indispensable and considered as a diagnostic standard (Ecker et al. 2005).

Computed tomography (CT) scans are of major interest for preoperative and intraoperative planning, in particular for assessment of the lesion's matrix (lytic or mineralized) (Green et al. 1996; Ilaslan et al. 2004b). Including two- and three-dimensional reconstructions, CT scans offer an excellent impression of bone structures enabling the specialist to estimate mechanical spinal stability. For the illustration of neighboring vessels (e.g., A. Adamkiewicz, aorta) CT angiography showed good results. Furthermore, CT-based navigation is increasingly attracting major interest in terms of tumor resection surgery, as CT-based navigation for tumor resection, as well as implant positioning (e.g., transpedicular screw placement), can effectively assist in both tumor resection and spinal reconstruction.

Positron emission tomography (PET) scans have shown—compared to the results achieved with MRI—equal results for the detection of spinal tumors (Schirrmeister et al. 2001). Because of its lesser availability and higher costs, it is not established in standardized diagnostic schemes. Rather it seems increasingly integrated in the staging procedure and detection of skip lesions or distant metastasis.

Additional staging comprises extraregional diagnostics with CT scans of the thorax, abdomen, and pelvis, and nuclide bone scans, which are eventually completed by native angiography to assess hypervascularized tumor entities with the possibility of preoperative embolization (Hess et al. 1997).

10.4
Role and Technique of Biopsy

The biopsy represents the final key step in the diagnostic process and should be not performed before after all local imaging studies, i.e., radiographs, CT and MRI, have been completed. This is essential as hematomas, cavities, and contrast medium enhancements resulting from the CT-guided fine needle or incision biopsy may mimic necrotic or liquid tumor substrates or tumor extension along the biopsy tract, which leads to inadequate diagnostic imaging. The primary objective of the biopsy is to obtain a representative vital tumor specimen. Nowadays much more than normal histological stainings are performed, since vital tissue is additionally needed for immunohistology, molecular biology, and ultrastructural and cytogenetic analysis. Thus, the tissue specimen must be large enough to cover these requirements. Furthermore, the surgeon has to clearly differentiate between necrotic, reactive, well-differentiated, and less-differentiated parts of the lesion, mostly based on the preoperative CT/MRI scans and the distinct contrast enhancement pattern.

Among the three traditional forms of biopsy, i.e., excision, fine needle, and incision biopsy, the fine needle biopsy (either under fluoroscopic or CT control) and incision biopsy are generally and mostly used for primary tumors of the osseous spine. Performance of excision biopsy seems only indicated for posterior benign lesions that have a pathognomonic radiographic pattern, e.g., osteoid osteoma.

CT-guided transpedicular fine needle biopsies have been shown to be safe in terms of injury to surrounding neurovascular and visceral structures. A CT-based trocar or needle biopsy also appears to be the least invasive and lteast contaminating biopsy technique (Jacobs 2006a, b). On the downside, apart from rarely reported complications such as pain, pneumothorax, and bleeding, fine needle biopsy is subject to sampling errors with either nondiagnostic tissue or undersized specimens that are too small for further evaluation. According to our experience and that of others, needle biopsy of the spine fails to provide the correct diagnosis or samples nondiagnostic tissue in up to 25% of all patients.

In particular, the incisional biopsies, as well as all other biopsy techniques, have to be performed strictly according to basic surgical principles (Weinstein 1989; Kornblum et al. 1998; Kang et al. 1999; Talac et al. 2002; Jacobs 2006a, b; Bancroft et al. 2007):

1. The biopsy incision and tract has to be planned and placed in consideration of the subsequent surgical approach for definitive resection, i.e., it can be excised with safe margins in total during definitive procedure. To consequently pursue this approach and to prevent known hazards of biopsy, many spine surgeons (including our team) deem it best that biopsy of primary spinal malignancies be performed by the treating physician, responsible for definitive resection rather than in the referring hospital.
2. Transverse incisions should be avoided.
3. Direct access, using the shortest way to the tumor without opening of other compartments, i.e., either transpedicularly or anteriorly, should be undertaken.
4. It is imperative to preserve contamination of the epidural space, which is an extracompartmental region (as it would be performed during laminectomy).
5. Large bone windows should be avoided in order to prevent resulting spinal instability or pathological fractures. During incisional biopsies, open bone cross-sections and surfaces that expose tumor tissue should be sealed with bone wax if possible.
6. Meticulous and hemostasis and spotless cauterization of small vessels is essential for prevention of postoperative hematoma, which would inevitably lead to tumor dissemination along fascial planes and muscles.
7. The gained tissue specimen should be carefully handled never crushed, distorted, or otherwise altered to preserve its macropathological aspect and morphology.
8. If available on site, a fresh frozen intraoperative histopathological evaluation should be performed to assure that vital and representative tumor tissue was obtained.

10.5 Oncosurgical Staging Systems of Primary Vertebral Tumors

Detailed and correct oncological and surgical staging of a primary vertebral column tumor includes anatomic localization and typing and grading of the lesion together with the presence or absence of distant metastases. It is made in order to help in predicting its clinical course and biological behavior. Correct surgical staging of the lesion is helpful for individual decision-making toward the approach and performance of the definitive resection.

10 Bone Sarcoma of the Spine

Table 10.1 Oncological staging system according to Enneking applied for primary malignant vertebral column tumors (modified from Jacobs WB 2006)

Stage	Description	Recommended management
Low grade (I)	No capsule, pseudocapsule with islands of tumor	Wide en bloc resection
IA	Within/confined to the vertebra	
IB	Paravertebral soft tissue invasion	
High grade (II)	Pseudocapsule infiltrated by tumor, islands of tumor are found remote from the original tumor mass (skip metastases)	Wide en bloc resection and (neo-)adjuvant therapy (polychemotherapy/radiation depending on tumor type)
IIA	Within/confined to the vertebra	
IIB	Paravertebral soft tissue invasion	
High grade (III) with distant metastases		Palliative surgery and adjuvant therapy, (polychemotherapy/radiation depending on tumor type)
IIIA	Within/confined to the vertebra	
IIIB	Paravertebral soft tissue invasion	

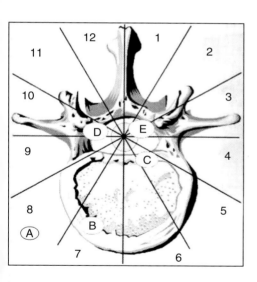

Fig. 10.1 The Weinstein–Boriani–Biagini (WBB) surgical staging system for primary spinal vertebral column tumors. In analogy to a clock face, the transverse plane of the vertebra is subdivided into 12 radiating zones. Numbered in a clockwise order, sector 1 is at the spinal process. In addition, the transverse section is compartmentalized into five concentric layers with: A being extraosseous paraspinal soft tissue; B, superficial intraosseous; C, deep intraosseous; D, invasion of the spinal canal with extradural tumor extension; and E, dural involvement/intradural tumor invasion. (Modified from Boriani et al. 1997; Jacobs WB 2006)

Application of the Enneking system to primary spinal column tumors has successfully been made (Boriani et al. 1997; Hart et al. 1997; Sundaresan et al. 2004; Jacobs 2006). Depending on tumor biology (low grade: type I; high grade: type II) and location of the tumor relative to anatomic compartments, the Enneking system divides malignant tumors into 6 stages (IA, IB, IIA, IIB, IIIA, and IIIB). This subclassification (Table 10.1) defines type A lesions as intracompartmental (confined to the vertebra/within the vertebra) and type B lesions as extracompartmental (extension beyond the cortex of the vertebral body).

After completion of all imaging studies, the establishment of the diagnosis, and the determination of oncological staging, surgical staging is then performed. The most widely used system for staging of primary benign and malignant spinal vertebral column tumors is the WBB (Weinstein–Boriani–Biagini) system, which has been validated in numerous previous studies (Boriani et al. 1997; Hart et al. 1997; Boriani et al. 2000; Bohinski and Rhines 2003; Jacobs 2006a, b). In a transverse plane the vertebra is divided analogously to the dial of a clock in 12 radiating zones (numbered 1–12 in a clockwise direction) with zone 1 at the spinal process. In addition, the transverse extension of the tumor is described in 5 concentric layers (A to E, i.e., from paravertebral extraosseous soft tissues to intradural tumor spread). The longitudinal extension of the tumor spread is assessed using the affected vertebral level (Boriani et al. 1997; Fig. 10.1).

Using that system, transversal tumor extension can be reliably described, e.g., involvement of one or both pedicles. Consequently, the feasibility of en bloc excision can be assessed. Therefore, this system provides a basic classification, which includes the specific anatomic conditions of the human spine, considers the rationale for en bloc excisions, and has been proved to be useful to plan surgical resections of vertebral column tumors.

Similar to the WBB system—but used less often and more in context with spinal metastases—is the surgical classification of vertebral tumors as devised by Tomita et al. (1997, 2006). According to the Tomita-surgical classification system, type I lesions are restricted to the vertebral body, type II extends from the body to the pedicle(s), type III is characterized by body-pedicle-lamina extension, type IV shows epidural tumor extension, type V tumors invade the paraspinal soft tissues, type VI involves 2–3 neighboring vertebrae, and type VII lesions stand for multiple skip lesions on several levels. Types I, II, and III are considered as intracompartmental, whereas type IV, V, and VI are extracompartmental.

10.6
Surgical Approaches

10.6.1
Posterior/Posterolateral Approach

To achieve curative tumor resections with wide surgical margins, especially in the case of non-metastatic primary malignancies, more radical surgical techniques have been established in order to minimize local recurrence and tumor cell contamination. This approach is an extension of the classical posterior approach as commonly used for palliative surgery in spinal metastases (Nicholls and Jarecky 1985; Bach et al. 1990; Schoeggl et al. 2002). This approach offers access to the more laterally located structures including transverse processes, facet joints, and the ribs. Through a costotransversectomy, the spinal canal can be exposed unilaterally or bilaterally. In cases of ventrally located lesions an en bloc spondylectomy (Roy-Camille et al. 1981; Stener 1989; Tomita et al. 1997)—as the most radical surgical option—can be performed. Even certain lesions with extracompartmental extension can be en bloc removed via this posterolateral approach (Fig. 10.2).

10.6.2
Anterior Approaches

In contrast to posterior approaches (Steinmetz et al. 2001) anterior procedures are associated with increased surgical stress and morbidity resulting from pre- and postoperative lung complications (Gokaslan et al. 1998). The additional or combined anterior approach during wide resection of vertebral column sarcoma can be indicated depending on stage/extension of the tumor and involvement of adjacent neurovascular, mediastinal, or visceral structures. The anterior approach can either precede or follow the posterior approach, depending on the thoracolumbar level

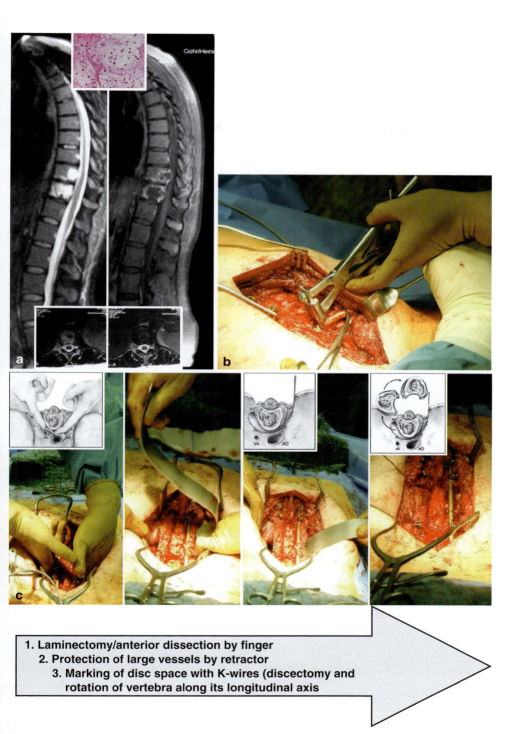

Fig. 10.2 A 43-year-old female patient with vertebral chondrosarcoma of the Th10/Th11. **a** MR images show involvement of two levels and tumor extension into the epidural space. Incisional biopsy revealed chondrosarcoma (inset:, histology). En bloc spondylectomy of two segments was performed via a posterolateral

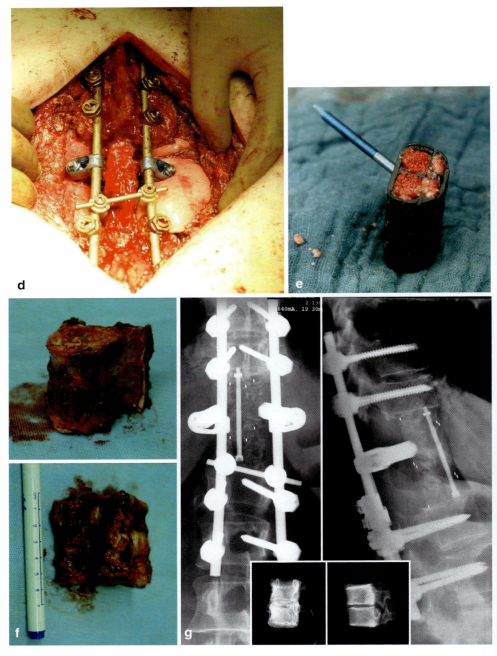

Fig. 10.2 (continued) approach and costotransversectomy (**b**). After laminectomy blunt dissection by finger of the anterior aspect of the both vertebrae from the ventral vessels was performed (**c**). After marking the disc spaces with K-wires for radiographic approval of the correctness, the vascular and pleural mediastinal structures were protected by specifically shaped retractors during discectomy. Finally, en bloc spondylectomy is performed by rotation of vertebra along its longitudinal axis; (insets: sequential schematic drawings of the procedure). Spinal reconstruction is completed by dorsal rods and crosslinks (**d**) and a carbon cage filled with autologous bone graft (**e**) is implanted for anterior vertebral body replacement. (**f**) Surgical specimen with postoperative radiographs (**g**)

of resection and on whether it is used for improved preparation/dissection or for spinal reconstruction after completed excision (Vrionis and Small 2003). The main advantage of the anterior approach is the easier preparation and bilateral ligation of segmental vessels. In addition, in case of large tumor expansion around or adjacent to anterior large vessels the anterior approach allows for direct visualization of the anterior tumor mass and its dissection from the vascular or visceral structures. In this context, separation of expansive, eccentric, or circumferential tumor from involved vascular (caval vein, aorta, renal arteries) or pulmonal structures with subsequent resection and replacement or lobectomies can only be approached in a safe and controlled way from anteriorly (Figs. 10.2 and 10.3; Roy-Camille et al. 1990; Boriani et al. 1997; Grunenwald et al. 2002; Mazel et al. 2003; Theodore and Dickman 2006; Gallia et al. 2007; Melcher et al. 2007).

Depending on the spinal level, anterior resections differ in technique and indication. For thoracic en bloc spondylectomy, a standard thoracotomy is performed depending on the pattern of tumor growth (eccentric, circumferential) and the spinal level involved (upper thoracic spine incl. Th5: right-sided; down to Th5: left-sided). Intubation with a double lumen tube eases the approach and exploration as well as the following anterior spinal reconstruction (e.g., tri-cortical bone grafts, expandable cage systems, etc.). The parietal pleura at the ventral aspect of the spine is incised in order to complete ligation of the segmental vessels. If needed, the esophagus or large vessels (or both) can be mobilized and retracted. The azygos vein can be ligated and resected en bloc with the vertebral specimen. Discectomy, which has been started from the posterior side at the levels corresponding to the resection, is easily performed. Anterior stabilization of the spine can then be realized using vertebral body replacement systems, or polyaxial or angular stable plate implants.

Approaches in the area of the thoracolumbar junction sometimes make it necessary to remove parts of the ipsilateral ribs and/or dissect parts of the diaphragm (thoraco-phrenico-lumbotomy).

In contrast to thoracic spondylectomy, lumbar en bloc excisions are not always feasible solely via a posterior approach. Contrary to thoracic spinal nerve roots, which may be transected without significant deficits in motor function, sacrificing nerve roots distant to L2 will markedly interfere with lower extremity motor function and impair ambulation. Therefore, rotation of the vertebra around its longitudinal axis is much more complicated and, in particular for multilevel en bloc excisions, not always possible via a single posterior approach. Consequently, for en bloc spondylectomy of middle to lower lumbar levels most authors recommend a combined (two staged) posterior and anterior approach (Boriani et al. 1996a; Murakami et al. 2001; Bohinski and Rhines 2003; Sundaresan et al. 2004; Theodore and Dickman 2006). Nevertheless, if sarcoma growth involves and extends to lumbar nerve roots transection and resection of nerve roots is necessary for oncological reasons in order to reach a wide to marginal resection.

The anterior approach may be performed in a retroperitoneal or transperitoneal exposure of the lumbar spine. Using one of these approaches, complete and safe controls of the vascular structures, and retraction of the aortocaval bifurcation and/or iliac vessels is allowed. Furthermore, the bilateral psoas muscle insertion at the lateral aspect of the vertebra can be subperiosteally elevated, and complete removal and replacement of the vertebral body is possible.

10.7
Surgical Strategies, Patient Selection, Treatment Decisions and Surgical Techniques

The optimum surgical treatment of musculoskeletal malignant tumors is a wide en bloc resection with appropriate margins. For modern surgical management of limb sarcoma this concept has become a *sine qua non*, and uncompromising attainment of tumor-free margins is expected to be a precondition for sufficient local and systemic tumor control. The practical implementation of this basic concept to the surgical therapy of primary vertebral column neoplasms is complicated by the topographic proximity and close relationship to the spinal cord, essential vascular and visceral structures. Thus, in the past surgical treatment mostly consisted of piecemeal resections and curettages via combined anterior–posterior approaches. However, such procedures, i.e., piecemeal removal, inevitably leads to local and systemic tumor cell dissemination and residual tumor tissue, thereby profoundly increasing the risk for local and systemic tumor recurrence.

Radical resections at the spine in terms of en bloc removal of the tumor together with the entire compartment (i.e., including the spinal cord), are usually not feasible. Recently, however, Murakami et al. (2001) have reported on the exceptional circumstance of complete segmental spine resection including the transected spinal cord in two patients with teleangiectatic osteosarcoma who had already complete and irreversible paralysis for at least 1 month.

According to Boriani et al. (1997) and Sundaresan et al. (2004) there are three major methods of en bloc resections of the spine: vertebrectomy, sagittal resections, and resections of the posterior arch. En bloc resection removal of the entire tumor in one piece, i.e., en bloc laminectomy followed by total en bloc vertebrectomy, is termed "en bloc spondylectomy" and is currently considered the most aggressive and favorable oncosurgical treatment concept of primary vertebral sarcoma (Stener 1971; Roy-Camille et al. 1981; Stener 1989; Boriani et al. 1996a; Boriani et al. 1997; Abe et al. 2000a; Krepler et al. 2002; Jacobs 2006; Theodore and Dickman 2006; Tomita et al. 2006).

10.8
Surgical Technique of En Bloc Spondylectomy/Total En Bloc Vertebrectomy

En bloc excision in terms of margin-free spondylectomy can be performed when the tumor extends to only one pedicle, i.e., is centrally located and confined only to zones 4–8 or 5–9 according to the WBB system. In this context, tumor extension to only the left pedicle/lamina, for instance, allows for contralateral right hemilaminectomy and subsequent careful passage of the dural sac through that "hemilaminectomy gap."

En bloc excision of the vertebra can be performed via a single approach from posterior, using an extended posterolateral approach or through a combined anterior (transthoracal, transperitoneal/retroperitoneal) and posterior approach. The decision about which surgical approach is ideal for each individual patient depends on spinal level (lumbar/thoracic) and the exact part of the vertebra involved (anterior/posterior), intra/extracompartmental tumor growth, involvement of the dural sac or large vessels, and the surgeon's familiarity with the approach (Theodore and Dickman 2006).

In view of the fact that wide total en bloc spondylectomy of one or even more spinal segments is a stressful and risky procedure ("surgical tour de force"), careful patient selection and identification of appropriate surgical candidates is a precondition for a good outcome. Therefore, a realistic evaluation of the disease stage, tumor burden, and general state of the patient and the honest and realistic assessment about whether a wide or at least marginal resection can be reached is of vital importance in order to justify the risk for the patient. Ideal candidates for total spondylectomy are patients with solitary primary vertebral column tumors (preferably intracompartmental) without metastatic disease, which show no intradural invasion and do not encase the aorta, vena cava, or mediastinal structures (e.g., esophagus). Exceptional cases of primary vertebral column tumors with aortocaval or dural involvement are reported in which en bloc spondylectomy is accompanied by great vessel or dura resection with subsequent vascular prosthetic replacement or dural reconstruction (Biagini et al. 2002; Biagini et al. 2003; Krepler et al. 2003).

10.8.1
Resection Technique

The patient is placed in a prone position on a radiolucent special spine table. After dorsomedian skin incision, the paraspinal muscles are detached from the spinous processes and the laminae, as well as the facet joints. However, in cases with extracompartmental tumor manifestation/extension an overlying soft tissue layer is left untouched. Midline incision should be long enough, i.e., one or two levels longer than the segments needed for spinal instrumentation in order to reach sufficient lateral exposure (Disch et al. 2007b; Melcher et al. 2007). The dorsal approach can be extended laterally if en bloc excision of paraspinal soft tissues, the chest wall, or ribs together with the vertebrectomy is necessary. In the thoracic spine the dorsal parts of ribs adjacent to the costotransverse joint are resected (minimum 5–8 cm) in order to reach access to the ventral aspect of the affected vertebrae. En bloc laminectomy is performed when tumor growth did not extend into the laminae, as judged from coronar MRI/CT scans. In case of tumor invasion in either one of the laminae, hemilaminectomy of the unaffected side is recommended. Open cut cross-sections and bone surfaces are immediately sealed with bone wax. Intervertebral disc spaces adjacent to the spondylectomy segment(s) are marked by K-wire inserted in the annulus fibrosus, and the correctness of the spinal level/segment(s) to be excised is checked using an image intensifier. Intervertebral dissection of the neighboring disc spaces and of the posterior and partially anterior longitudinal ligaments is performed carefully using a specific chisel-like dissector, rongeur, or scissor. The resection of the anterior column of the affected vertebrae is preceded by gentle and blunt digital dissection in the interface between the anterior aspect of the vertebral body and the pleura ("subpleural space"), aorta as well as the iliopsoas muscle in the thoracic and lumbar spine, respectively.

Separation of aorta, cava vein, and lungs from the anterior aspect of the vertebral segment(s) and their release in the craniocaudal plane represents the most demanding and challenging step of the operation. During this maneuver the azygos vein is at risk of injury and may cause severe and—from the posterior approach—difficult-to-control bleeding. After complete release of the anterior aspect of the vertebral body from the pleura, a vertebral spatula is inserted in the subpleural space for protection of the great vessels during dissection of the intervertebral disc. In the thoracic spine, nerve roots can be transected and ligated near to the dural sac if root infiltration by the extracompartmental tumor is present. The segmental intercostal/lumbar vessels are ligated on both sides. Intraoperatively multiple frozen specimens can be sent to the histopathological evaluation to exclude tumor infiltration and to determine the status of resection margins.

Before segmental resection of the vertebral body is completed, unilateral posterior instrumentation (CT-based navigation of pedicle screws) is performed in order to reach stability of the spine. Due to total loss of spinal osseous spinal continuity resulting from en bloc spondylectomy, at least two vertebral levels above and below the spondylectomy level should be fixed. Experimental studies of our group have shown that long posterior fixation most effectively increases stiffness and biomechanical stability of the reconstruction (Disch et al. 2007a). After gentle dissection of the spinal cord from the surrounding epidural venous plexus and the ligamentous tissue in the spinal canal using a thin nerve dissector, the entire vertebra(e) is (are) mobilized step by step followed by meticulous bipolar coagulation of bleeding branches of the venous plexus. Finally, the vertebra is rotated along its longitudinal axis in the direction opposite to the unilateral instrumentation without compression or injury of the spinal cord, leading to a circumferential decompression of the spinal cord and a segmental total en bloc vertebrectomy. The rotation procedure for en bloc removal of the vertebrae but also former discectomy is made easier by temporarily and slightly distracting (not overdistracting!) the spine segment using the unilateral internal fixator/pedicle screw system. Distraction is then reversed in compression after vertebral body replacement implants have been placed.

10.8.2
Technique: Spinal Reconstruction

After spondylectomy the cartilage from the end plates is removed for exposure and direct contact of the cortical vertebral surface to the vertebral body replacement implant and bone graft. For vertebral body replacement we either use an expandable titanium cage or a connected composite carbon fiber cage (Trabis in OstaPek), both filled with autologous cancellous bone graft and/or bone substitute (Figs. 10.2 and 10.3). After central placement of the vertebral body replacement implant, the dorsal instrumentation is completed by the second rod and either the cage is expanded or compression is applied to the anterior vertebral body replacement system. Crosslinking rods connect the two dorsal connection rods in order to increase rotational stability. Remaining cancellous bone is grafted to the posterolateral aspect for spondylodesis. If the posterolateral exposure allows a sufficient approach, an additional ventral angular stable plate system between the neighboring healthy vertebrae can be implanted (Fig. 10.3).

10.9
Current Management of Individual Primary Malignant Vertebral Column Tumors

Primary malignant tumors of the vertebral column tumors are rare entities and account (excluding plasmocytoma and lymphoma) only for approx. 6% of all primary neoplasms of the mobile spine (Abdu and Provencher 1998). Chordoma is the most frequent nonlymphoproliferative tumor of the spine with predominant cervical and sacral manifestation. Involvement of the thoracolumbar spine is observed in less than 30% of all manifestations in the axial skeleton (Boriani et al. 1996b; Sundaresan et al. 2004). Classic, common primary sarcomas include osteosarcoma, Ewing's sarcoma, chondrosarcomas, and some mediastinal or retroperitoneal soft tissue sarcomas involving the spine (Abdu and Provencher 1998; Flemming et al. 2000; Sundaresan et al. 2004; Boriani et al. 2006; Jacobs 2006). Within the multimodal treatment concept, surgery remains the mainstay of treatment together with preceding and/or following polychemotherapy and radiation, depending on the underlying tumor type. Due to improved surgical techniques and the advanced developments of new chemotherapy protocols, survival and local control continue to improve (Ferrari and Palmerini 2007).

10.9.1
Osteosarcoma

Osteosarcoma is the most nonhematologic primary malignant bone tumor. Although its management has been extensively documented in the appendicular skeleton, the descriptions of vertebral osteosarcoma, which accounts for less then 4% of all osteosarcoma cases, are mainly limited to case series and reports (Barwick et al. 1980; Ilaslan et al. 2004b). Furthermore, among all primary malignant tumors of the vertebral

10 Bone Sarcoma of the Spine

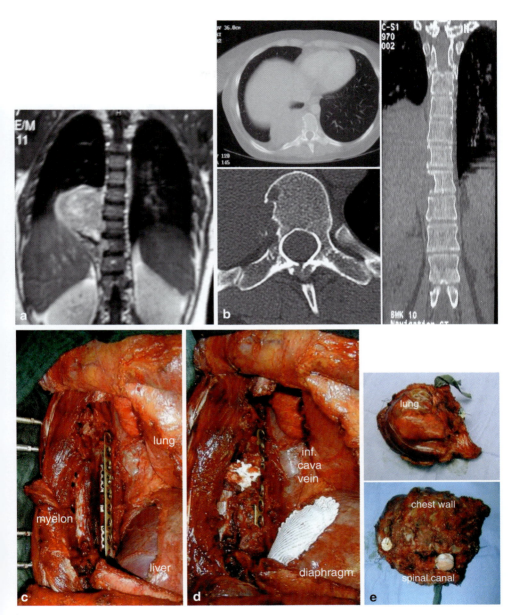

Fig. 10.3 MR images (**a**) and CT scans (**b**) of a 32-year-old female patient with leiomyosarcoma of the costovertebral junction involving the spine (Th9, 10, 11), the chest wall, the lower lung lobe, and the diaphragm. Wide resection with en bloc excision of Th9–11, lower right lung lobe, parts of the diaphragm, and chest wall in one piece. Intraoperative view after completed resection (**c**) and reconstruction (**d**) using an expandable cage and an angular stable plate, Gore-Tex patch for diaphragm repair and autologous bone graft for spondylodesis. **e** Surgical specimen. Radiograph (**f**) and clinical images (**g**) at 18 months after surgery

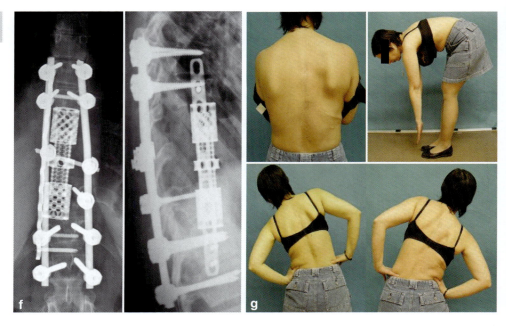

Fig. 10.3 (continued)

column it accounts for only 5%. Patients with hereditary retinoblastoma are reported to have a high risk of secondary tumor manifestation, which occurs in more than 50% of cases as osteosarcoma. In addition, osteosarcoma may arise more commonly than average in patients with preexisting Paget's disease of bone, enchondromatosis, hereditary multiple exostoses, and fibrous dysplasia (Sundaresan et al. 2004). Peak incidence of classic osteosarcoma is known to occur during adolescence, with a second peak occurring during late adulthood in response to radiation exposure, after a 5- to 20-year latency period. Vertebral osteosarcoma patients seem to have an older age at presentation, with an average patient age in the fourth decade. Spinal osteosarcoma can arise in all vertebral levels; however, predilective levels include the lumbar spine (Flemming et al. 2000). Characteristically, osteosarcoma is eccentrically located in the vertebral body with possible extension to the posterior structures. Pathological fracture due to vertebral osteosarcoma is observed in up to 90% of cases. Radiographic appearance and CT/MRI findings strictly depend on the matrix composition. The majority of vertebral osteosarcoma is typically densely mineralized and has an osteoblastic matrix, frequently appearing dark in all MRI sequences. In our experience osteosarcomas have the potential to change their matrix composition depending on the response to neoadjuvant polychemotherapy. Often there seems to occur an increased sclerosis of the lesion in patients with a good response. Nuclide bone scan or PET–CT scans are helpful to diagnose skip, satellite, and multifocal/multisegmental lesions. Clinically, patients with vertebral osteosarcoma become symptomatic with pain, and neurologic symptoms are present in nearly 80% of all patients (Barwick et al. 1980; Jacobs 2006) at the point of initial presentation.

Currently, effective treatment of vertebral osteosarcoma should be performed by a combination of neoadjuvant polychemotherapy and total en bloc spondylectomy. According to the experience of the osteosarcoma study group, postoperative radiotherapy may improve survival in selected patients (Ozaki et al. 2002). Depending on the spinal level, multisegmental extension, and involvement of visceral or vascular structures, a combined anterior and posterior approach may be necessary (Fig. 10.4). In view of local and systemic tumor control and due to reduced intraoperative tumor cell dissemination, a wide en bloc excision is expected to be associated with the best chance of tumor-free survival (Weinstein and McLain 1987; Sundaresan et al. 1988; Stener 1989; Roy-Camille et al. 1990; Boriani et al. 1996a; Takaishi et al. 1996; Boriani et al. 1997; Tomita et al. 1997; Flemming et al. 2000; Krepler et al. 2002; Ozaki et al. 2002; Talac et al. 2002; Bohinski and Rhines 2003; Krepler et al. 2003; Sundaresan et al. 2004; Melcher et al. 2007).

10.9.2
Ewing Sarcoma

Ewing sarcoma is the most common primary malignant vertebral column tumor in children. Despite metastatic involvement of the spine it is frequently observed in patients with metastasized and relapsing disease; the incidence for primary vertebral thoracolumbar Ewing tumors is only 0.9%, and that increases to 3.5% if the sacrum is included (Flemming et al. 2000; Ilaslan et al. 2004a; Sundaresan et al. 2004; Marco et al. 2005; Jacobs 2006). Most of the patients become symptomatic with pain or neurological deficits (56%–94%) (Sundaresan et al. 2004; Jacobs 2006). However, in contrast to osteosarcoma, there are sometimes systemic symptoms at the point of presentation with fever and increased levels of lactate dehydrogenase (LDH) and leukocyte count. The spinal Ewing sarcoma typically presents between ages 10 and 30 years and is usually centered in the vertebral body. Extension of the tumor mass in the soft tissue and posterior elements is frequently seen, possibly leading to spinal cord or nerve root compression with early onset of neurological symptoms. Spinal Ewing sarcoma most commonly affects the sacrum, followed by thoracic and lumbar levels. Cervical cases are rarely seen (Sharafuddin et al. 1992; Grubb et al. 1994). In contrast to osteosarcoma, there is no second peak of incidence in adults after a long latency period following irradiation. Radiographic appearance is variable with mostly permeative moth-eaten irregular lytic bone destruction (Flemming et al. 2000; Ilaslan et al. 2004a; Sundaresan et al. 2004; Marco et al. 2005; Jacobs 2006). In addition, osseous expansion with sclerotic features or vertebra plana secondary to pathologic fracture and collapse may also be present (Papagelopoulos et al. 2002; Ilaslan et al. 2004a). MRI and CT scans often and typically reveal a large paraosseal soft tissue tumor portion, which usually downsizes during chemotherapy in responding patients. About 20% of all patients become initially symptomatic with metastatic disease. There continues to be controversy, however, about whether metastatic status in any way affects the overall prognosis (Villas and San Julian 1996; Venkateswaran et al. 2001).

Ewing sarcoma is sensitive to both chemotherapy and radiation. Systemic polychemotherapy is currently accepted as representing the primary and most important step of treatment. The multimodal treatment approach with initial polychemotherapy has led to the fact that more than half of the patients with solitary lesions can be cured. There is a continuing controversy about the role of radiation and/or surgery for local control. Using radiotherapy alone, local control rates range from 55% to 90% (Pilepich et al. 1981a, b; Sundaresan et al. 2004). However, extraskeletal Ewing sarcoma and primitive neuroectodermal tumors involving the spinal column seem to be associated with a less favorable prognosis (Harimaya et al. 2003). A more recent study of nonmetastatic spinal Ewing sarcoma patients undergoing systemic polychemo-

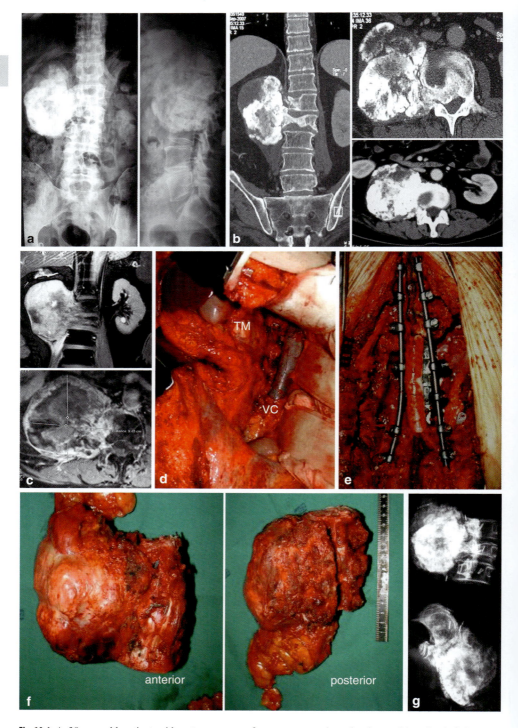

Fig. 10.4 A 39-year-old patient with osteosarcoma of Th12/L1/L2. Radiographs (**a**), CT scans (**b**), and MR images (**c**) demonstrate the large extracompartmental tumor extension closely reaching the inferior cava vein and the left renal vessels. After neoadjuvant polychemotherapy the patient was treated by wide resection,

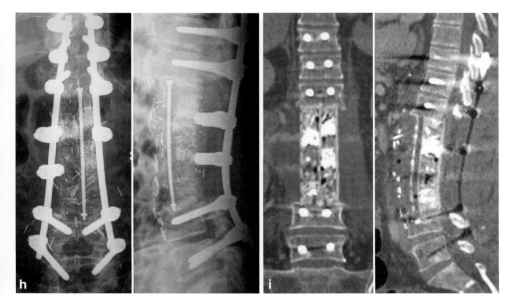

Fig. 10.4 (continued) i.e., three level–en-bloc spondylectomy (Th12-L2) via a combined anterior–posterior approach. The anterior approach (**d**) was used first to release the inferior cava vein (VC) and the renal vessels and to dissect extensive tumor mass (TM) from the retroperitoneal/visceral structures. Thereafter the posterior approach and en bloc excision was performed with anterior/posterior stabilization using anterior carbon cage and standard posterior stabilization (**e**). Surgical specimen (**f, g**) with resection margins (R0). Postoperative radiographs (**h**) and CT scans (**i**)

therapy and radiation for definitive local control demonstrates disease-free survival rates of only 49% and 36% at 5- and 10-years, respectively (Marco et al. 2005). One possible reason for these relatively deflated results may be the fact that none of the included patients was treated by en bloc spondylectomy, i.e., with a wide or marginal resection. In this context the authors discuss a residual persistence of viable tumor cells within the radiated site (Marco et al. 2005). Comparing results for radiotherapy versus surgical excision following initial polychemotherapy for definitive local control in patients with Ewing sarcoma of the extremities or trunk reveals higher survival rates after surgical excision (Bacci et al. 2004a). Pursuing this approach, Tomita et al. (1997) as well as Boriani et al. (1996a) have performed en bloc excision on more than 20 patients with primary vertebral bone tumors (5 of them having been Ewing sarcoma patients) and no local recurrence within an adequate follow-up period. Possibly, the combination of polychemotherapy with en bloc spondylectomy may further improve overall oncological treatment outcome, in particular in patients with poor response to, or residual disease after, radiation and/or polychemotherapy.

There is less controversy about the role of surgery for patients with progressive neurological compromise or structural deformity in response to underlying vertebral Ewing sarcoma (Sharafuddin et al. 1992; Jacobs 2006). However, given the radio- and chemosensitivity of Ewing sarcoma, the benefits and risks should be critically balanced and calculated whether or not in those patients rapid induction of polychemotherapy or radiation can also effectively arrest and reverse neurological compromise. Nevertheless, if absolutely necessary due to impending paraplegia or progressive sensorimotor deficits, an emergency laminectomy has to be performed. Decompressive laminectomy should be followed by dorsal instrumentation and stabilization in order to prevent postlaminectomy kyphosis and spinal instability.

10.9.3
Chondrosarcoma

Among all skeletal sites, only approximately 10% of all chondrosarcomas originate from the mobile spine, most commonly affecting the thoracic and lumbar segments in patients older than 30–40 years (Boriani et al. 2000; Sundaresan et al. 2004). Chondrosarcoma can arise primarily from the vertebral bone or derive secondarily from preexisting osteochondroma with malignant transformation (Flemming et al. 2000; Jacobs 2006). Most of the vertebral chondrosarcomas are slowly growing low-grade lesions that only occasionally become symptomatic with spinal cord compression and neurological compromise. Typically radiographic features include signs of bone destruction with central chondroid and calcified mineralization (Lloret et al. 2006). More often than in Ewing sarcoma or osteosarcoma, the posterior elements are involved, sometimes causing a palpable mass (Shives et al. 1989). CT scans and MR imaging studies usually confirm the chondroid composition with mixed lytic-flocculent calcified matrix and further evaluate the extent of spinal cord or vascular involvement. According to clinical and oncological experience, chondrosarcomas are resistant to chemotherapy and radiation, leaving surgical excision as the mainstay of treatment (Takaishi et al. 1996; York et al. 1999a; Boriani et al. 2000; Flemming et al. 2000; Sundaresan et al. 2004; Jacobs 2006).

Boriani et al. (2000) have demonstrated that the risk of intralesional surgery is associated with a risk of local recurrence of nearly 100%. To the contrary, en bloc excision causes a marked decrease in local tumor relapse ranging from 0% to 22% (Shives 1989; York et al. 1999c; Boriani et al. 2000; Jacobs 2006). Consequently, complete surgical excision—whenever possible by en bloc spondylectomy—should be the therapeutic target (Fig. 10.2).

10.9.4
Chordoma

Chordoma is the most frequent nonlymphoproliferative tumor of the vertebral column, with thoracolumbar spinal involvement of nearly 30% of all manifestations in the axial skeleton (Boriani et al. 1996b; Sundaresan et al. 2004). Histogenetically, chordoma derives from the primitive notochord and can therefore occur along the entire neural axis, predominantly presenting in the sacrococcygeal and cervical (particularly C2) region, followed by lumbar and thoracic segments. Typically, chordoma develops in patients older than 40 years of age with a slight preference for males. In most patients chordoma becomes symptomatic with slowly progressive nonspecific low back pain. Depending on the spinal level or sacral involvement, 30%–50% of all patients develop neurological deficits with weakness, radiculopathy, or rectal dysfunction (Healey and Lane 1989).

Imaging findings typically reveal osteolytic vertebral destruction in the midline of the affected vertebral body. Despite the fact that nucleus pulposus is the only anatomic derivative of the primitive notochord in the adult spine, chordoma does not develop in these structures but directly in the vertebral body. In MR images and CT scans, chordomas appear lobulated, often with a large soft tissue portion. From imaging findings these lesions sometimes closely resemble a mucinous carcinoma or a chondroid, cartilage-like myxoid tumor with a semifluid pattern. Clinically, CT scans and MRI have enormous importance to evaluating the topographic relationship of the tumor to the dural sac, nerve roots, large vessels, and rectum. In particular on T2-weighted images a possible tissue plane between the tumor and the above-mentioned structures can be seen (Sundaresan et al. 2004; Boriani et al. 2006).

Current studies and our own experience also suggest that chordomas, which are traditionally considered to be low-grade lesions, have a considerable tendency for distant metastasis in different organs, including the spine in up to 40% of all patients (Sundaresan et al. 1987; Krol et al. 1989; Bergh et al. 2000; Sundaresan et al. 2004; Boriani et al. 2006). Chordomas are characterized by a marked propensity for local recurrence and tumor cell seeding after intralesional resections or even along the tract after open biopsy. In this context and in view of the known resistance of this tumor to conventional radiotherapy and chemotherapy, margin-free en bloc excision/spondylectomy at the initial presentation—when technically feasible—seems the only adequate approach to reach oncologically sufficient long-term local and systemic control (Fig. 10.5). Although shown only in very few cases with limited follow-up, there are some reports for en bloc resection of chordoma in cervical spine (Fujita et al. 1999; Currier et al. 2007; Leitner et al. 2007). According to our experience, intraoperative application of 2D and 3D CT-based navigation is an enormous relief during en bloc resection, in particular for sacral manifestation (Fig. 10.5), as there is a real gain in anatomic orientation during surgery (Stöckle et al. 2003). A database for CT-based navigation can additionally be fused with MRI images, allowing further visualization and navigation of associated soft tissue tumor portions.

Due to the slowly growing behavior and an often large size at presentation mostly in the challenging upper cervical or sacral region, many lesions have been frequently intralesionally resected. In those patients with chordoma unsuitable for en bloc resection, a combined multimodal therapy consisting of surgery (extracapsular intralesional resection; Boriani et al. 1996b), specific irradiation (high-energy proton-beam therapy; Catton et al. 1996; Munzenrider and Liebsch 1999; Park et al. 2006; Rutz et al. 2007), and chemotherapy (Casali et al. 2004; Casali et al. 2007; Orzan et al. 2007) is expected to improve local control when compared to intralesional surgery alone.

10.10
Nonsurgical Treatment Options

10.10.1
Radiation

Apart from Ewing sarcomas, all other bone sarcomas show only a weak to moderate response to any kind of radiation therapy. The low sensitivity to radiation therapy underscores the importance of radical, en bloc excision. Osteosarcoma is regarded as relatively radioresistant. Older studies demonstrated only poor results of radiotherapy for vertebral osteosarcomas with dead of disease in most of the patients (Barwick et al. 1980; Shives et al. 1986). More recent studies indicate an improved local control in more than 70% of all patients using combined photon–proton radiotherapy in a 3D planning (Hug et al. 1995). These results are supported by Ozaki et al. who also found that postoperative radiation may exert beneficial influence on local and systemic control (Ozaki et al. 2002). Chondrosarcoma and chordoma are also rather radioresistant. At present adjuvant postoperative radiation seems to increase local control when combined with radical resections. Shives and colleagues as well as Boriani et al. did not find a statistically significant benefit from postoperative radiotherapy (Shives et al. 1989; Boriani et al. 2000). However, York et al. demonstrated for spinal chondrosarcoma a significant effect of radiotherapy in terms of increased disease-free interval and survival (York et al. 1999a). For chordoma, postoperative adjuvant radiation also was shown to increase the postoperative disease-free survival (York et al. 1999b; Hug and Slater 2000). In Ewing sarcoma

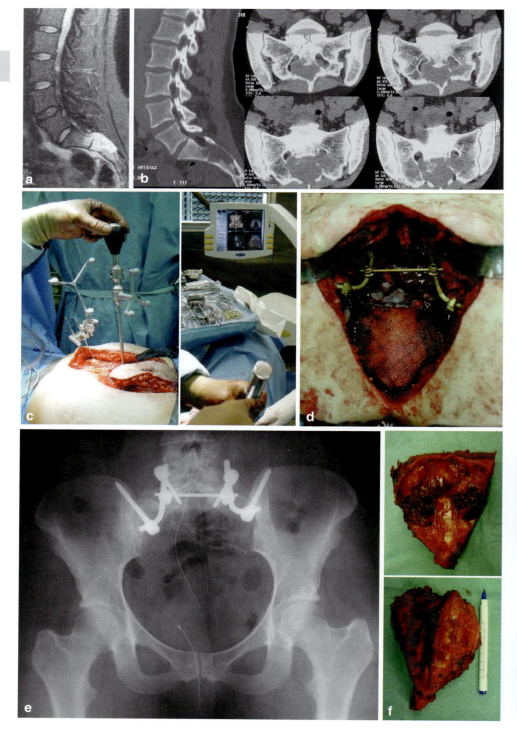

Fig. 10.5 MR image (**a**) and CT scans (**b**) of a 34-year-old female patient with sacral chordoma involving S1–S5 segments. CT-based navigation-assisted resection (**c**) of the sacrectomy (caudal parts of S1–S5) sparing the S1 nerve root right. Spinopelvic stabilization was performed using bilateral lumboiliacal distraction spondylodesis (**d**). Postoperative pelvic radiograph (**e**) and surgical specimen (**f**)

patients, radiation plays a specific role and can be a part of the multimodal treatment concept (Pilepich et al. 1981a; Sharafuddin et al. 1992; Grubb et al. 1994; Villas and San Julian 1996; Barbieri et al. 1998; Ilaslan et al. 2004a). Barbieri et al. reported a 5-year survival rate of 44% with radiation and chemotherapy for definitive local control in 28 patients suffering from vertebral Ewing sarcoma. In this context Marco et al. confirm these results with 49% disease-free survival at 5 years. The authors propose to combine wide en bloc resection together with radiochemotherapy to further improve local and systemic control (Marco et al. 2005).

10.10.2
Chemotherapy

Response to chemotherapy and resection margins are the main predictors for local and distant disease control in sarcomas of the bone (Picci et al. 1994; Bielack et al. 1995;, 1996). Threefold local recurrences were reported for patients with minor response to common treatment schemes. Actually, different international chemotherapy protocols are under investigation (e.g., EurAmOS, Euro-EWING) offering the possibility to achieve comparable outcome results even with individualized regimes regarding age, initial response, and entity.

10.10.3
Embolization

Transarterial embolization of primary and secondary tumors of the skeletal system has developed into a safe and very effective method. Preoperative application to vertebral column tumors is an effective adjuvant therapy tool for preoperative devascularization showing tumor mass reduction, reduced perioperative bleeding, and better overall outcome (Hess et al. 1997; Brado et al. 1998; Radeleff et al. 2006). Even in sarcomas with an overall minor bleeding tendency compared to some secondary tumor entities, e. g., metastases of renal cell- or thyroid cancers (Manke et al. 2001; Smit et al. 2000), the preoperative use is recommended.

10.10.4
Pain Management

Tumor-associated pain sensations derive from different aspects of the malignant disease ranging from direct involvement of neural structures to biomechanical spinal instability. Apart from central- and periphery-acting analgesics, treatment strategies in an interdisciplinary approach to pain reduction comprise preoperative embolization (Brado et al. 1998; Radeleff et al. 2006), high dose corticosteroids in the case of neurological deficits (Ushio et al. 1977; Delattre et al. 1989), bisphosphonates for suppression of osteoclast-induced bone degradation (Neville-Webbe et al. 2002), or radiation therapy. Installation of pre- or intraoperative peri-/epidural catheters with controlled drug application is a major part of interventional pain management (Sloan 2004). In addition, oncologically orientated psychotherapy and the appropriate application of adjuvant drugs (Lussier et al. 2004; Fallon and McConnell 2006) are a part of a comprehensive therapy.

10.11
Complications

Direct intraoperative and postoperative mortality rates are—regarding the extensive type of surgery—relatively low (Boriani et al. 1996a; Abe et al. 2000b; Talac et al. 2002; Melcher et al. 2007). Possible intraoperative complications include the entire range of well-known complications known to be associated with spinal surgery. However, due to the demanding and challenging procedure of en bloc spondylectomy with extended approaches, including circumferential 360° dissection of the vertebral segment, there is an increased risk of large vessel injury, dural tears, and nerve root damage. Furthermore, this type of surgery is usually accompanied by moderate to major blood loss and the need for appropriate volume management, and erythrocyte and plasma substitution. In particular, intraoperative anesthesiological management requires substantial experience. During dissection and en bloc excision, large cancellous bone surfaces may be exposed, and epidural veins are often subject to diffuse bleeding. Therefore, the supine position with a free abdomen (reduced pressure in the inferior cava vein) and a hypotensive anesthesia during this period is known to reduce intraoperative blood loss.

Overall, postoperative complications can be divided into severe and slight events. Severe complications comprise pneumonia, pulmonal embolia, coagulation disturbances, cardiac decompensation, paraplegia, urosepsis, kyphotic deformity derived from implant failure, wound infection, and osteomyelitis. Slight postoperative complications are superficial wound healing disturbances, intestinal atonia, and temporary peripheral sensorimotor deficits.

10.12 Prognosis

Primary malignant lesions of the spine show—depending on time of diagnosis, the achieved resection margins, and the resulting local recurrence rates—varying outcomes. Radical resection of metastatic free osteosarcoma combined with adjuvant and neoadjuvant chemotherapy results in a 5-year survival between 55% and 65% (Kempf-Bielack et al. 2005). Multimodal therapy in spinal Ewing sarcoma leads to a 5-year survival of approximately 60% (Sharafuddin et al. 1992; Weber 2002; Bacci et al. 2004b; Ilaslan et al. 2004a; Marco et al. 2005; Ferrari et al. 2007). Outcomes in chondrosarcoma seem solely related to achieved resection results. Patients with negative tumor-free margins show recurrence rates between 0% and 25% (Boriani et al. 1996a, 2000; Talac et al. 2002; Melcher et al. 2007). Incomplete resection, either microscopically or macroscopically, however, leads to local recurrence rates from 50% to 100% (Boriani et al. 2000; Talac et al. 2002). Local relapse is directly related to poor survival. Average time to death in patients suffering from local recurrence is shorter than 18 months (Talac et al. 2002) and 80%–90% will die before midterm follow-up (Boriani et al. 2000; Talac et al. 2002). Patients free of local disease show survival times exceeding 4 years (Boriani et al. 2000; Talac et al. 2002; Melcher et al. 2007). Overall prognosis in chordoma patients continues to be poor with death in 63% of all cases, and 5- and 10-year survival rates of 50% and 28%, respectively (Sundaresan et al. 1979, 1987, 2004; Healey and Lane 1989; Bjornsson et al. 1993; York et al. 1999b; Boriani et al. 2006; Jacobs 2006). More recent results indicate moderate improvement of disease-free survival with estimated 5-, 10-, 15-, and 20-year survival rates of 84%, 64%, 52%, and 52%, respectively (Bergh et al. 2000).

References

Abdu WA, Provencher M (1998) Primary bone and metastatic tumors of the cervical spine. Spine 23:2767–2777

Abe E, Sato K, Murai H, Tazawa H, Chiba M, Okuyama K (2000a) Total spondylectomy for solitary spinal metastasis of the thoracolumbar spine: a preliminary report. Tohoku J Exp Med 190:33–49

Abe E, Sato K, Tazawa H, Murai H, Okada K, Shimada Y, Morita H (2000b) Total spondylectomy for primary tumor of the thoracolumbar spine. Spinal Cord 38:146–152

Aflatoon K, Staals E, Bertoni F, Bacchini P, Donati D, Fabbri N, Boriani S, Frassica FJ (2004) Hemangioendothelioma of the spine. Clin Orthop Relat Res 418:191–197

Bacci G, Ferrari S, Longhi A, Donati D, Barbieri E, Forni C, Bertoni F, Manfrini M, Giacomini S, Bacchini P (2004a) Role of surgery in local treatment of Ewing's sarcoma of the extremities in patients undergoing adjuvant and neoadjuvant chemotherapy. Oncol Rep 11:111–120

Bacci G, Forni C, Longhi A, Ferrari S, Donati D, De Paolis M, Barbieri E, Pignotti E, Rosito P, Versari M (2004b) Long-term outcome for patients with non-metastatic Ewing's sarcoma treated with adjuvant and neoadjuvant chemotherapies. 402 patients treated at Rizzoli between 1972 and 1992. Eur J Cancer 40:73–83

Bach F, Larsen LB, Rohde K, Borgesen SE, Gjerris F, Boge-Rasmussen T, Agerlin N, Rasmussen B, Stjernholm P, Sorensen PS (1990) Metastatic spinal cord compression: occurrence, symptoms, clinical presentations and prognosis in 398 patients with spinal cord compression. Acta Neurochir (Wien) 107:37–43

Bancroft LW, Peterson JJ, Kransdorf MJ, Berquist TH, O'Connor MI (2007) Compartmental anatomy relevant to biopsy planning. Semin Musculoskelet Radiol 11:16–27

Barbieri E, Chiaulon G, Bunkeila F, Putti C, Frezza G, Neri S, Boriani S, Campanacci M, Babini L (1998) Radiotherapy in vertebral tumors. Indications and limits: a report on 28 cases of Ewing's sarcoma of the spine. Chir Organi Mov 83:105–111

Barwick KW, Huvos AG, Smith J (1980) Primary osteogenic sarcoma of the vertebral column: a clinicopathologic correlation of ten patients. Cancer 46:595–604

Bergh P, Gunterberg B, Remotti F, Ryd W, Meis-Kindblom JM (2000) Prognostic factors in chordoma of the sacrum and mobile spine: a study of 39 patients. Cancer 88:2122–2134

Biagini R, Casadei R, Boni F, Mascari C, Sturiale C, Bortolotti C, Boriani S, Gamberini G, Di Fiore M, Mercuri M (2002) Spondylectomy (thoracolumbar spine) combined with dural resection for bone tumor: surgical technique. Chir Organi Mov 87:97–101

Biagini R, Casadei R, Boriani S, Erba F, Sturale C, Mascari C, Bortolotti C, Mercuri M (2003) En bloc vertebrectomy and dural resection for chordoma: a case report. Spine 28:E368–372

Bielack SS, Delling G, Göbel U, Kotz R, Ritter J, Winkler K (1995) Osteosarcoma of the trunk treated by multimodal therapy: experience of the Cooperative Osteosarcoma study group (COSS). Med Pediatr Oncol 24:6–12

Bielack SS, Kempf-Bielack B, Winkler K (1996) Osteosarcoma: relationship of response to preoperative chemotherapy and type of surgery to local recurrence. J Clin Oncol 14:683–684

Bjornsson J, Ebersold MJ, Laws ER (1993) Chordoma of the mobile spine. A clinicopathologic analysis of 40 patients. Cancer 71:735–740

Bohinski RJ, Rhines LD (2003) Principles and techniques of en bloc vertebrectomy for bone tumors of the thoracolumbar spine: an overview. Neurosurg Focus 15:E7

Boriani S, Biagini R, De Iure F, Bertoni F, Malaguti MC, Di Fiore M, Zanoni A (1996a) En bloc resections of bone tumors of the thoracolumbar spine. A preliminary report on 29 patients. Spine 21:1927–1931

Boriani S, Chevalley F, Weinstein JN, Biagini R, Campanacci L, De Iure F, Piccill P (1996b) Chordoma of the spine above the sacrum. Treatment and outcome in 21 cases. Spine 21:1569–1577

Boriani S, Weinstein JN, Biagini R (1997) Primary bone tumors of the spine. Terminology and surgical staging. Spine 22:1036–1044

Boriani S, De Iure F, Bandiera S, Campanacci L, Biagini R, Di Fiore M, Bandello L, Picci P, Bacchini P (2000) Chondrosarcoma of the mobile spine: report on 22 cases. Spine 25:804–812

Boriani S, Bandiera S, Biagini R, Bacchini P, Boriani L, Cappuccio M, Chevalley F, Gasbarrini A, Picci P, Weinstein JN (2006) Chordoma of the mobile spine: fifty years of experience. Spine 31:493–503

Brado M, Hansmann HJ, Richter GM, Kauffmann GW (1998) Interventional therapy of primary and secondary tumors of the spine [in German]. Orthopade 27:269–273

Casali PG, Stacchiotti S, Tamborini E, Crippa F, Gronchi A, Orlandi R, Ripamonti C, Spreafico C, Bertieri R, Bertulli R, Colecchia M, Fumagalli E, Greco A, Grosso F, Olmi P, Pierotti MA, Pilotti S (2004) Imatinib mesylate in chordoma. Cancer 101:2086–2097

Casali PG, Sangalli C, Olmi P, Gronchi A (2007) Chordoma. Curr Opin Oncol 19:367–370

Catton C, Bell R, Laperriere N, Cummings B, Fornasier V, Wunder J (1996) Chordoma: long-term follow-up after radical photon irradiation. Radiother Oncol 41:67–72

Currier BL, Papagelopoulos PJ, Krauss WE, Unni KK, Yaszemski MJ (2007) Total en bloc spondylectomy of C5 vertebra for chordoma. Spine 32:E294–299

Davis LA, Warren SA, Reid DC, Oberle K, Saboe LA, Grace MG (1993) Incomplete neural deficits in thoracolumbar and lumbar spine fractures. Reliability of Frankel and Sunnybrook scales. Spine 18:257–263

Delattre JY, Arbit E, Thaler HT, Rosenblum MK, Posner JB (1989) A dose response study of dexamethasone in a model of spinal cord compression caused by epidural tumor. J Neurosurg 70:920–925

Disch AC, Luzzati A, Melcher I, Schaser KD, Feraboli F, Schmoelz W (2007a) Three-dimensional stiffness in a thoracolumbar en-bloc spondylectomy model: a biomechanical in vitro study. Clin Biomech (Bristol, Avon) 22:957–964

Disch AC, Melcher I, Luzatti A, Haas NP, Schaser KD (2007b) Surgical technique of en bloc spondylectomy for solitary metastases of the thoracolumbar spine [in German]. Unfallchirurg 110:163–170

Dreghorn CR, Newman RJ, Hardy GJ, Dickson RA (1990) Primary tumors of the axial skeleton. Experience of the Leeds Regional Bone Tumor Registry. Spine 15:137–140

Ecker RD, Endo T, Wetjen NM, Kraus WE (2005) Diagnosis and treatment of vertebral column metastases. Mayo Clin Proc 80:1177–1186

Fallon M, McConnell S (2006) The principles of cancer pain management. Clin Med 6:136–139

Ferrari S, Palmerini E (2007) Adjuvant and neoadjuvant combination chemotherapy for osteogenic sarcoma. Curr Opin Oncol 19:341–346

Ferrari S, Bertoni F, Palmerini E, Errani C, Bacchini P, Pignotti E, Mercuri M, Longhi A, Cesari M, Picci P (2007) Predictive factors of histologic response to primary chemotherapy in patients with Ewing sarcoma. J Pediatr Hematol Oncol 29:364–368

Flemming DJ, Murphey MD, Carmichael BB, Bernard SA (2000) Primary tumors of the spine. Semin Musculoskelet Radiol 4:299–320

Fujita T, Kawahara N, Matsumoto T, Tomita K (1999) Chordoma in the cervical spine managed with en bloc excision. Spine 24:1848–1851

Gallia GL, Sciubba DM, Bydon A, Suk I, Wolinsky JP, Gokaslan ZL, Witham TF (2007) Total L-5 spondylectomy and reconstruction of the lumbosacral junction. Technical note. J Neurosurg Spine 7:103–111

Gokaslan ZL, York JE, Walsh GL, McCutcheon IE, Lang FF, Putnam JB, Wildrick DM, Swisher sG, Abi Said d, Sawaya R (1998) Transthoracic vertebrectomy for metastatic spinal tumors. J Neurosurg 89:599–609

Green R, Saifuddin A, Cannon S (1996) Pictorial review: imaging of primary osteosarcoma of the spine. Clin Radiol 51:325–329

Grubb MR, Currier BL, Pritchard DJ, Ebersold MJ (1994) Primary Ewing's sarcoma of the spine. Spine 19:309–313

Grunenwald DH, Mazel C, Girard P, Veronesi G, Spaggiari L, Gossot D, Debrosse D, Caliandro R, Le Guillou JL, Le Chevalier T (2002) Radical en bloc resection for lung cancer invading the spine. J Thorac Cardiovasc Surg 123:271–279

Hamlat A, Saikali S, Gueye EM, Le Strat A, Carsin-Nicol B, Brassier G (2005) Primary liposarcoma of the thoracic spine: case report. Eur Spine J 14:613–618

Harimaya K, Oda Y, Matsuda S, Tanaka K, Chuman H, Iwamoto Y (2003) Primitive neuroectodermal tumor and extraskeletal Ewing sarcoma arising primarily around the spinal column: report of four cases and a review of the literature. Spine 28:E408–412

Hart RA, Boriani S, Biagini R, Currier B, Weinstein JN (1997) A system for surgical staging and management of spine tumors. A clinical outcome study on giant cell tumors of the spine. Spine 22:1773–1782

Healey JH, Lane JM (1989) Chordoma: a critical review of diagnosis and treatment. Orthop Clin North Am 20:417–426

Hess T, Kramann B, Schmidt E, Rupp S (1997) Use of preoperative vascular embolization in spinal metastasis resection. Arch Orthop Trauma Surg 116:279–282

Hug EB, Slater JB (2000) Proton radiation therapy for chordomas and chondrosarcomas of the skull base. Neurosurg Clin N Am 11:627–638

Hug EB, Fitzek MM, Liebsch NJ, Munzenrider JE (1995) Locally challenging osteo- and chondrogenic tumors of the axial skeleton: results of combined proton and photon radiation therapy using three-dimensional treatment planning. Int J Radiat Oncol Biol Phys 31:467–476

Ilaslan H, Sundaram M, Unni KK, Dekutoski MB (2004a) Primary Ewing's sarcoma of the vertebral column. Skeletal Radiol 33:506–513

Ilaslan H, Sundaram M, Unni KK, Shives TC (2004b) Primary vertebral osteosarcoma: imaging findings. Radiology 230:697–702

Imai R, Kamada T, Tsuji H, Tsujii H, Tsuburai Y, Tatezaki S (2006) Cervical spine osteosarcoma treated with carbon-ion radiotherapy. Lancet Oncol 7:1034–1035

Jacobs WB (2006a) Oncologic classification of vertebral neoplasms. In: Dickman C, Fehlings MG, Gokaslan ZL (eds) Spinal cord and spinal column tumors. Principles and practice. Thieme Medical Publishers, New York, pp 24–40

Jacobs WB (2006b) Primary vertebral column tumors. In: Dickman C, Fehlings MG, Gokaslan ZL (eds) Spinalcord and spinal column tumors. Principles and practice. Thieme Medical Publishers, New York, Stuttgart, pp 369–389

Kang M, Gupta S, Khandelwal N, Shankar S, Gulati M, Suri S (1999) CT-guided fine-needle aspiration biopsy of spinal lesions. Acta Radiol 40:474–478

Kawashima H, Ishikawa S, Fukase M, Ogose A, Hotta T (2004) Successful surgical treatment of angiosarcoma of the spine: a case report. Spine 29:E280–283

Kelley SP, Ashford RU, Rao AS, Dickson RA (2007) Primary bone tumours of the spine: a 42-year survey from the Leeds Regional Bone Tumour Registry. Eur Spine J 16:405–409

Kempf-Bielack B, Bielack SS, Jurgens H, Branscheid D, Berdel WE, Exner GU, Gobel U, Helmke K, Jundt G, Kabisch H, Kevric M, Klingebiel T, Kotz R, Maas R, Schwarz R, Semik M, Treuner J, Zoubek A, Winkler K (2005) Osteosarcoma relapse after combined modality therapy: an analysis of unselected patients in the Cooperative Osteosarcoma Study Group (COSS). J Clin Oncol 23:559–568

Kornblum MB, Wesolowski DP, Fischgrund JS, Herkowitz HN (1998) Computed tomography-guided biopsy of the spine. A review of 103 patients. Spine 23:81–85

Krepler P, Windhager R, Bretschneider W, Toma CD, Kotz R (2002) Total vertebrectomy for primary malignant tumours of the spine. J Bone Joint Surg Br 84:712–715

Krepler P, Windhager R, Toma CD, Kitz K, Kotz R (2003) Dura resection in combination with en bloc spondylectomy for primary malignant tumors of the spine. Spine 28:E334–338

Krol G, Sze G, Arbit E, Marcove R, Sundaresan N (1989) Intradural metastases of chordoma. AJNR Am J Neuroradiol 10:193–195

Leitner Y, Shabat S, Boriani L, Boriani S (2007) En bloc resection of a C4 chordoma: surgical technique. Eur Spine J 16:2238–2242

Lloret I, Server A, Bjerkehagen B (2006) Primary spinal chondrosarcoma: radiologic findings with pathologic correlation. Acta Radiol 47:77–84

Lussier P, Huskey AG, Portenoy RK (2004) Adjuvant analgesics in cancer pain management. Oncologist 9:571–591

Manke C, Bretschneider T, Lenhart M, Völk M, Link J, Feuerbach S (2001) Spinal metastases from renal cell carcinoma: effect of preoperative particle embolization on intraoperative blood loss. AJNR Am J Neuroradiol 22:997–1003

Marco RA, Gentry JB, Rhines LD, Lewis VO, Wolinski JP, Jaffe N, Gokaslan ZL (2005) Ewing's sarcoma of the mobile spine. Spine 30:769–773

Mazel C, Grunenwald D, Laudrin P, Marmorat JL (2003) Radical excision in the management of thoracic and cervicothoracic tumors involving the spine: results in a series of 36 cases. Spine 28:782–792

Melcher I, Disch AC, Khodadadyan-Klostermann C, Tohtz S, Smolny M, Stockle U, Haas NP, Schaser KD (2007) Primary malignant bone tumors and solitary metastases of the thoracolumbar spine: results by management with total en bloc spondylectomy. Eur Spine J 16:1193–1202

Munzenrider JE, Liebsch NJ (1999) Proton therapy for tumors of the skull base. Strahlenther Onkol 175[Suppl 2]:57–63

Murakami H, Kawahara N, Abdel-Wanis ME, Tomita K (2001) Total en bloc spondylectomy. Semin Musculoskelet Radiol 5:189–194

Murakami H, Tomita K, Kawahara N, Oda M, Yahata T, Yamaguchi T (2006) Complete segmental resection of the spine, including the spinal cord, for telangiectatic osteosarcoma: a report of 2 cases. Spine 31:E117–122

Neville-Webbe H, Holen IL, Coleman RE (2002) The anti-tumor activity of bisphosphonates. Cancer Treat Rev 28:305–319

Nicholls PG, Jarecky TW (1985) Evaluate posterior decompression by laminectomy for malignant tumors of the spine. Clin Orthop Relat Res 201:210

Nishida J, Kato S, Shiraishi H, Ehara S, Sato T, Okada K, Shimamura T (2002) Leiomyosarcoma of the lumbar spine: case report. Spine 27:E42–46

Orzan F, Terreni MR, Longoni M, Boari N, Mortini P, Doglioni C, Riva P (2007) Expression study of the target receptor tyrosine kinase of Imatinib mesylate in skull base chordomas. Oncol Rep 18:249–252

Ozaki T, Flege S, Liljenqvist U, Hillmann A, Delling G, Salzer-Kuntschik M, Jurgens H, Kotz R, Winkelmann W, Bielack SS (2002) Osteosarcoma of the spine: experience of the Cooperative Osteosarcoma Study Group. Cancer 94:1069–1077

Papagelopoulos PJ, Currier BL, Galanis E, Grubb MJ, Pritchard DJ, Ebersold MJ (2002) Vertebra plana caused by primary Ewing sarcoma: case report and review of the literature. J Spinal Disord Tech 15:252–257

Park L, Delaney TF, Liebsch NJ, Hornicek FJ, Goldberg S, Mankin H, Rosenberg AE, Rosenthal DI, Suit HD (2006) Sacral chordomas: impact of high-dose proton/photon-beam radiation therapy combined with or without surgery for primary versus recurrent tumor. Int J Radiat Oncol Biol Phys 65:1514–1521

Picci P, Sangiorgi L, Rougraff BT, Neff JR, Casadei R, Campanacci M (1994) Relationship of chemotherapy-induced necrosis and surgical margins to local recurrence in osteosarcoma. J Clin Oncol 12:2699–2705

Pilepich MV, Vietti TJ, Nesbit ME, Tefft M, Kissane J, Burgert EO, Pritchard D (1981a) Radiotherapy and combination chemotherapy in advanced Ewing's Sarcoma-Intergroup study. Cancer 47:1930–1936

Pilepich MV, Vietti TJ, Nesbit ME, Tefft M, Kissane J, Burgert O, Prichard D, Gehan EA (1981b) Ewing's sarcoma of the vertebral column. Int J Radiat Oncol Biol Phys 7:27–31

Radeleff B, Eiers M, Lopez-Benitez R, Noeldge G, Hallscheidt P, Grenacher L, Libicher M, Zeifang F, Meeder PJ, Kauffmann GW, Richter GM (2006) Transarterial embolization of primary and secondary tumors of the skeletal system. Eur J Radiol 58:68–75

Roy-Camille R, Saillant G, Bisserie M, Judet T, Hautefort E, Mamoudy P (1981) Total excision of thoracic vertebrae (author's transl) [in French]. Rev Chir Orthop Reparatrice Appar Mot 67:421–430

Roy-Camille R, Saillant G, Mazel CH, Monpierre H (1990) Total vertebrectomy as treatment of malignant tumors of the spine. Chir Organi Mov 75:94–96

Rutz HP, Weber CD, Sugahara S, Timmermann B, Lomax AJ, Bolsi A, Pedroni E, Coray A, Jermann M, Goitein G (2007) Extracranial chordoma: outcome in patients treated with function-preserving surgery followed by spot-scanning proton beam irradiation. Int J Radiat Oncol Biol Phys 67:512–520

Schirrmeister H, Glatting G, Hetzel J, Nussle K, Arslandemir C, Buck AK, Dziuk K, Gabelmann A, Reske SN, Hetzel M (2001) Prospective evaluation of the clinical value of planar bone scans, SPECT, and (18)F-labeled NaF PET in newly diagnosed lung cancer. J Nucl Med 42:1800–1804

Schoeggl A, Reddy M, Matula C (2002) Neurological outcome following laminectomy in spinal metastases. Spinal Cord 40:363–366

Sharafuddin MJ, Haddad FS, Hitchon PW, Haddad SF, el-Khoury GY (1992) Treatment options in primary Ewing's sarcoma of the spine: report of seven cases and review of the literature. Neurosurgery 30:610–618

Sharma H, Mehdi SA, MacDuff E, Reece AT, Jane MJ, Reid R (2006) Paget sarcoma of the spine: Scottish Bone Tumor Registry experience. Spine 31:1344–1350

Shives TC, Dahlin DC, Sim FH, Pritchard DJ, Earle JD (1986) Osteosarcoma of the spine. J Bone Joint Surg Am 68:660–668

Shives TC, McLeod RA, Unni KK, Schray MF (1989) Chondrosarcoma of the spine. J Bone Joint Surg Am 1989:1158–1165

Sloan PA (2004) The evolving role of interventional pain management in oncology. J Support Oncol 2:491–500, 503

Smit JW, Vielvoye GJ, Goslings BM (2000) Embolization for vertebral metastases of follicular thyroid carcinoma. J Clin Endocrinol Metab 85:989–994

Steinmetz MP, Mekhail A, Benzel EC (2001) Management of metastatic tumors of the spine: strategies and operative indications. Neurosurg Focus 11:1–6

Stener B (1971) Total spondylectomy in chondrosarcoma arising from the seventh thoracic vertebra. J Bone Joint Surg Br 53:288–295

Stener B (1989) Complete removal of vertebrae for extirpation of tumors. A 20-year experience. Clin Orthop Relat Res 245:72–82

Stöckle U, Schaser K, Melcher I, Haas NP (2003) CT and fluoroscopy based navigation in pelvic surgery [in German]. Unfallchirurg 106:914–920

Sundaresan N, Galicich JH, Chu FC, Huvos AG (1979) Spinal chordomas. J Neurosurg 50:312–319

Sundaresan N, Huvos AG, Krol G, Lane JM, Brennan C (1987) Surgical treatment of spinal chordomas. Arch Surg 122:1479–1482

Sundaresan N, Rosen G, Huvos AG, Krol G (1988) Combined treatment of osteosarcoma of the spine. Neurosurgery 23:714–719

Sundaresan N, Digiacinto GV, Hughes JE, Cafferty M, Vallejo A (1991) Treatment of neoplastic spinal cord compression: results of a prospective study. Neurosurgery 29:645–650

Sundaresan N, Boriani S, Rothman A, Holtzman R (2004) Tumors of the osseous spine. J Neurooncol 69:273–290

Takaishi H, Yabe H, Fujimura Y, Suzuki N, Toyama Y (1996) The results of surgery on primary malignant tumors of the spine. Arch Orthop Trauma Surg 115:49–52

Talac R, Yaszemski MJ, Currier BL, Fuchs B, Dekutoski MB, Kim CW, Sim FH (2002) Relationship between surgical margins and local recurrence in sarcomas of the spine. Clin Orthop Relat Res 397:127–132

Theodore N, Dickman C (2006) Complete spondylectomy for the excision of spinal neoplasms. In: Dickman C, Fehlings MG, Gokaslan ZL (eds)

Spinal cord and spinal column tumors. Principles and practise. Thieme Medical Publishers, New York, Stuttgart, p 523–536

Tomita K, Kawahara N, Baba H, Tsuchiya H, Fujita T, Toribatake Y (1997) Total en bloc spondylectomy. A new surgical technique for primary malignant vertebral tumors. Spine 22:324–333

Tomita K, Kawahara N, Murakami H, Demura S (2006) Total en bloc spondylectomy for spinal tumors: improvement of the technique and its associated basic background. J Orthop Sci 11:3–12

Ushio Y, Posner R, Kim JH, Shapiro WR, Posner JB (1977) Treatment of experimental spinal cord compression by epidural neoplasm. J Neurosurg 47:422–429

Venkateswaran L, Rodriguez-Galindo C, Merchant TE, Poquette CA, Rao BN, Pappo AS (2001) Primary Ewing tumor of the vertebrae: clinical characteristics, prognostic factors, and outcome. Med Pediatr Oncol 37:30–35

Villas C, San Julian M (1996) Ewing's tumor of the spine: report on seven cases including one with a 10-year follow-up. Eur Spine J 5:412–417

Vrionis FD, Small J (2003) Surgical management of metastatic spinal neoplasms. Neurosurg Focus 15:1–8

Weber KL (2002) Current concepts in the treatment of Ewing's sarcoma. Expert Rev Anticancer Ther 2:687–694

Weinstein JN (1989) Surgical approach to spine tumors. Orthopedics 12:897–905

Weinstein JN, McLain RF (1987) Primary tumors of the spine. Spine 12:843–851

York JE, Berk RH, Fuller GN, Rao JS, Abi-Said D, Wildrick DM, Gokaslan ZL (1999a) Chondrosarcoma of the spine: 1954 to 1997. J Neurosurg 90:73–78

York JE, Kaczaraj A, Abi-Said D, Fuller GN, Skibber JM, Janjan NA, Gokaslan ZL (1999b) Sacral chordoma: 40-year experience at a major cancer center. Neurosurgery 44:74–79

York JE, Walsh GL, Lang FF, Putnam JB, McCutcheon IE, Swisher SG, Komaki R, Gokaslan ZL (1999c) Combined chest wall resection with vertebrectomy and spinal reconstruction for the treatment of Pancoast tumors. J Neurosurg 91:74–80

Computer-Assisted Pelvic Tumor Resection: Fields of Application, Limits, and Perspectives

Sebastian Fehlberg, Sebastian Eulenstein, Thomas Lange, Dimosthenis Andreou, and Per-Ulf Tunn

Abstract The treatment of malignant tumors involving the pelvic area is a challenging problem in musculoskeletal oncology due to the complex pelvic anatomy and the often large tumor size at presentation. The use of navigation systems has effectively increased surgical precision aiming at optimal preservation of pelvic structures without compromising oncologic outcome by means of improved visibility of the surgical field, and enabling intraoperative display and 3D reproduction of preoperatively determined pelvic osteotomy and resection levels. In the following sections, current developments in computer-assisted pelvic surgery are reviewed and possible fields of application, as well as limitations of navigation systems, are discussed.

Sebastian Fehlberg (✉)
Department of Orthopedic Oncology
Sarkomzentrum Berlin-Brandenburg
Helios Klinikum Berlin-Buch
Schwanebecker Chaussee 50
13125 Berlin, Germany
E-mail: Sebastian.fehlberg@helios-kliniken.de

11.1 Introduction

Tumors involving the pelvic area represent one of the most difficult challenges in musculoskeletal oncology. Approximately 6%–15% of all primary malignant bone tumors involve the pelvis (Price and Jeffree 1977; Campanacci and Capanna 1991); chondrosarcoma, osteosarcoma, and Ewing's sarcoma are the most common diagnoses (Bacci et al. 2003; Ozaki et al. 2003a, b; Pring et al. 2001). The bony pelvis is also a frequent site of metastasis for numerous other malignancies, including kidney, prostate, breast, lung, thyroid, and bladder carcinomas (Wingo et al. 1995; Yasko et al. 2007).

Pelvic bone tumors are often large at presentation and can invade important anatomical structures, including the iliac vessels, the femoral and sciatic nerve, or the pelvic viscera. Furthermore, tumors of the iliac bone can invade the sacral bone and the sacral nerve roots (Ozaki et al. 2003a, b; Court et al. 2006). Multimodal approaches for the treatment of primary malignant pelvic bone tumors include resection with clear surgical margins, if necessary with medial surgical margin extension into the sacrum, in order to reduce local recurrence rates and improve overall survival (Yang et al. 1995; Kawai et al. 1998a, b; Kollender et al. 2000; Sucato et al. 2000).

In recent years, an increasing number of patients are being treated with limb-salvage surgery rather than mutilating procedures (Pant et al. 2001; Tunn et al. 2003), aiming at an improved function and quality of life without compromising the quality of surgical margins (Ozaki et al. 2003a, b; Kollender et al. 2000; Wirbel et al. 2001; Pring et al. 2001; Hoffmann et al. 2006). However, the demanding three-dimensional (3D) configuration of the pelvic anatomy, tumor size, structural alterations following neoadjuvant treatment, lack of experience, and attendant morbidity of a pelvic resection result in inadequate (contaminated or intralesional) surgical margins in 12%–75% of the cases, with a local recurrence rate between 70% and 80% for these patients (Kawai et al. 1998a, b; Sucato et al. 2000; Wirbel et al. 2001; Pring et al. 2001; Fuchs et al. 2002; Court et al. 2006). It is the art of surgery to find a compromise between required radicality and optimal preservation of pelvic structures. Therefore, intraoperative visualization and 3D observation of preoperative determined pelvic osteotomies and resection levels are necessary. Computer navigation systems have effectively improved the precision of musculoskeletal surgery. Although computer-assisted surgery has been used for more than two decades for cranial biopsies and tumor resections, this technology is relatively new in trauma and orthopedic surgery (Schlöndorff 1998). Since computed tomography (CT)-based navigation was introduced into spine surgery for pedicle screw insertion in 1993, the technique has been used in several areas such as cup replacement in hip arthroplasty, total knee replacement, reconstructive surgery, and tumor surgery (Steinmann et al. 1993; Amiot et al. 1995; Dessenne et al. 1995). The first CT-based computer-assisted osteotomy of the bony pelvis was performed by Langlotz et al. in 1995. Patients with symptomatic acetabular dysplasia underwent a computer-assisted periacetabular osteotomy, aiming at an improved execution of the required cuts and a 3D visualization of the reorientation of the liberated acetabular fragment (Langlotz et al. 1997, 1998, 2002). In 2004 Hüfner et al. were the first to use computer-navigated chisels to perform computer-assisted osteotomies in patients with sacral tumors, enabling a 3D observation of the spatial relationship of the chisel to the tumor (Hüfner et al. 2004). Krettek et al. expanded this technique, additionally using a computer-assisted K-wire insertion to visualize the preoperatively planned osteotomy levels during the resection of a periacetabular tumor (Krettek et al. 2004).

A further approach was introduced by Wong et al. in 2007. Due to the absence of commercially available navigation platforms for pelvic bone resection, he adapted a navigation platform for pedicle screw insertion to the spine to assist the planning and execution of pelvic bone resection. After attaching the navigation tracker to a conventional diathermy handle, he used the needle point as an "end-effector" to visualize the tumor extent in the virtual CT images displayed on the navigation monitor, thus identifying clear surgical margins, which were simultaneously marked on the bone surface with the diathermy needle. After also identifying and marking the preoperatively planned resection levels, the diathermy burn-in points were joined to form the resection line (Wong et al. 2007a, b).

In the following sections, current developments in computer-assisted pelvic surgery are reviewed and possible fields of application, as well as limitations of navigation systems, are discussed.

11.2 Navigation Procedures

The term computer-assisted surgery summarizes approaches that aim to improve visibility of the surgical field and increase spatial accuracy when carrying out surgical actions. To achieve these goals, the bony anatomy being operated on is linked with a display of the operating field, often based on radiologic images obtained preoperatively or intraoperatively. The link is established using several anatomical landmarks and points registered during the operation, which are correlated to the virtual images. Besides the image-based systems, image-free navigation systems are also available (Bowersox et al. 1997). Due to the diversity of tumor presentation in the pelvic bones, only image-based (CT- or MRI-based) navigation is of use for tumor resections. An image-based navigation system consists of an imaging modality, a tracking or position sensing system to track the location of an instrument, and a hardware and software platform for the registration process and visualization of the operating field (Nolte and Beutler 2004; Fig. 11.1).

11.2.1 Preoperative Imaging and Segmentation

By definition, an image-based navigation system requires a preoperatively acquired imaging modality such as CT or magnetic resonance imaging (MRI), in order to generate a precise 3D anatomical model of the region of interest (Richenberg and Hansell 1998). The so-called segmentation of pelvic structures is the most challenging part of 3D modeling. Segmentation is the process in which each voxel (volume element) of the image data (e.g., CT or MRI) is assigned (labeled) to a specific tissue—bone, muscle, nerve, vessel, tumor, etc. A prevalent method to segment the bone structure is the threshold algorithm (Fig. 11.2).

Based on this process, it is possible to automatically generate tissue surfaces consisting of triangle meshes by the efficient marching cube algorithm (Lorensen and Cline 1987). These meshes can display on the monitor a view from different directions (surface rendering). The accuracy and quality of these 3D models is mainly affected by the scanning parameters, particularly by slice thickness and spacing, while the time required to

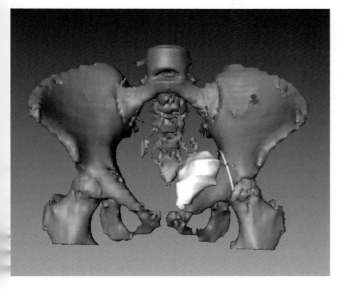

Fig. 11.1 CT-based 3D reconstruction of the pelvis of a 17-year-old female patient with Ewing's sarcoma of the pelvis

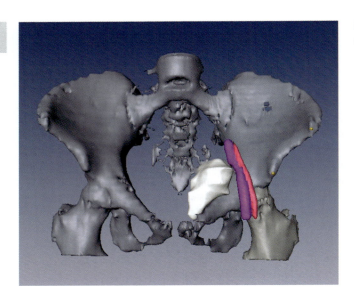

Fig. 11.2 Fusion of CT and MRI data to visualize the pelvic vessels

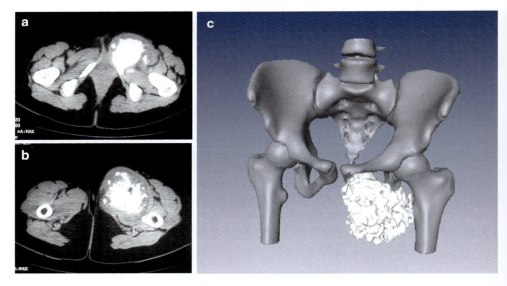

Fig. 11.3 a, b Chondrosarcoma of the left ischium and pubis in a 15-year-old female patient. **c** 3D reconstruction of the pelvis

complete the reconstruction can vary significantly, depending on the efficiency of the available graphic edition tool (Ney et al. 1991). Further enhancements of the 3D model can be achieved by volume rendering, a technique enabling tissue density to be incorporated in the 3D model (Figs. 11.3 and 11.4).

11.2.2
Tracking Systems

The heart of a navigation system is a tracking system, also called position-sensoring system or localizer. It consists of one or several sensors attached to a surgical instrument, which is

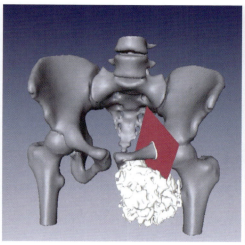 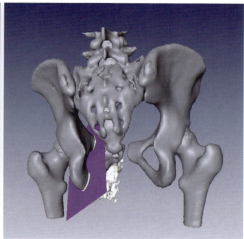

Fig. 11.4 The ventral (pubic) and dorsal (ischial) osteotomy planes are defined preoperatively

tracked by a device calculating the position and orientation of the sensors. The most common tracking systems for medical instruments are either optical, employing mostly infrared light-reflecting spheres, e.g., Polaris (Northern Digital Industries, Waterloo, ON, Canada), or electromagnetic (Kai et al. 1998; Bottland et al. 1997; Khadem et al. 2000; Amiot et al. 2000). Although electromagnetic tracking systems do not need a free line of sight between the field generators and the sensors, optical tracking systems are widely used because of their higher accuracy and a lower liability to malfunction against ferromagnetic and electromagnetic fields (Schicho et al. 2005). Various tracking systems are currently utilized for computer-assisted pelvic tumor resections, using either passive infrared light-reflecting spheres (Fehlberg et al. 2006; Reijnders et al. 2007) or active infrared light-emitting diodes (Hüfner et al. 2004; Krettek et al. 2004; Stöckle et al. 2004; Wong et al. 2007a, b; Fig. 11.5).

Before commencing surgery, the computer-navigated instruments have to be calibrated in order for their geometry and shape to be defined in the coordinate system of the navigator. So far, tracked chisels, conventional diathermy handles, and drills have been used for computer-assisted pelvic tumor resections (Fig. 11.6).

11.2.3
Intraoperative Patient-to-Image Registration

Intraoperative registration aims at providing a one-to-one correspondence between the surgical object and the virtual, often 3D, model, allowing for the location of the end-effectors to be integrated in the virtual representation. Furthermore, in order to compensate for possible movements of the navigator, the surgical object, or both during surgical actions, local coordinate systems need to be established on the surgical objects by attaching so-called dynamic referencing bases (DRBs), holding three or more optical markers (Fig. 11.7).

A wide variety of registration concepts, associated algorithms, and hardware exists (Simon and Lavallée 1998). In conventional navigation systems only rigid transformations, i.e., inflexible mappings of each point in the virtual display to its anatomically corresponding point in the operating field, are determined, using preoperatively defined anatomical landmarks or attached

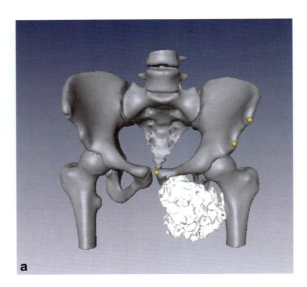

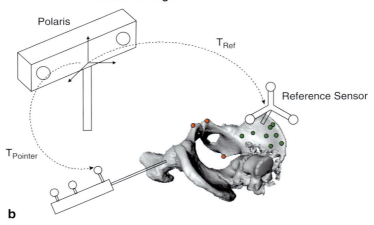

Fig. 11.5 a Three anatomical landmarks, to be used intraoperatively for point matching, are also defined preoperatively. **b** The optical tracking system, using passive, infrared light-reflecting spheres for intraoperative point matching and surface registration

artificial (fiducial) markers, which then have to be identified during the operation with a tracked pointer—a process called paired point matching. Given that the position of the landmarks identified on the patient may vary slightly compared to the position of their predefined counterparts on the virtual images, this approach is less than fully satisfactory. Despite the need for an additional invasive procedure, the best registration results have been achieved with bone-mounted fiducial markers (Maurer et al. 1997). In computer-assisted surgery of the pelvis only Hüfner et al. have used such a marker; titan pins were implanted into the iliac crest under local anesthesia prior to the preoperative CT scan and data segmentation (Hüfner et al. 2004).

11 Computer-Assisted Pelvic Tumor Resection

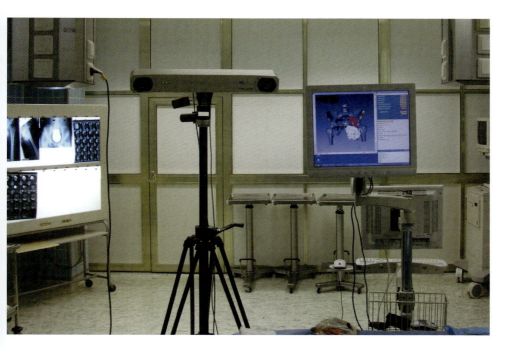

Fig. 11.6 The osteotomy planes are identified during the operation with a tracked chisel with the aid of the virtual 3D model

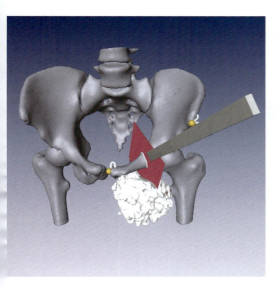

Fig. 11.7 Surface registration after attaching the DRB to the spina iliaca anterior superior

To increase the accuracy of registration and simplify manipulations, several surface-matching techniques have been introduced (Bächler et al. 2001; Glozman et al. 2001; Sugano et al. 2001), during which the surgeon needs to acquire intraoperatively a defined number of variable points on the patient, while a computer algorithm employs the complete model to locate the corresponding points. In computer-assisted resection of pelvic tumors, the identification of anatomical landmarks, usually involving the promontorium, the spina iliaca anterior superior/inferior, or the symphysis, precedes surface registration, most commonly along the iliac crest. Both the predefined anatomical landmarks and the dynamic referencing base should be located outside the resection area. Hüfner et al. reported a case of intraoperative loosening of a DRB, necessitating the repetition of registration after refixation of the DRB (Hüfner et al. 2004).

11.2.4
Intraoperative Visualization

After the calibration and registration process have been completed, the spatial relations and the movements of the calibrated instruments in the region of interest can be visualized in real-time on the monitor (Fig. 11.8).

A standard approach utilizes several 2D slices of the preoperative CT or MRI as a multiplanar image display, while 3D surface models can be additionally employed to provide a better overview. Visualization methods are one of the most active fields of research (Figs. 11.9 and 11.10).

11.3
Fields of Application

Computer-assisted surgery can be widely applied in patients with primary and secondary bone tumors of the pelvis, aiming at an improved accuracy of surgical manipulations to ensure the required radicality of the surgical procedure, while allowing for optimal preservation of pelvic structures. It thereby follows that the technique can play a role only in limb-salvage surgery—with curative or palliative intent—and not in ablative procedures.

Pelvic resection are classified into four types according to Enneking and Dunham; iliac (T1), acetabular (T2), pubis or ischium (T3), and sacral (T4). Combinations of these resections, with or without high femoral resection (H1), are also possible. The additional resection of the gluteal muscles in a T1 resection is distinguished as T1A, while the inclusion of the hip joint in a T2 resection as T2A (Enneking and Dunham 1978; Enneking et al. 1990). The reconstruction of the resulting bone defect is challenging and depends on the location and extent of bone resection. Yet not every defect needs to be reconstructed; this generally applies in small T1 resections, if the

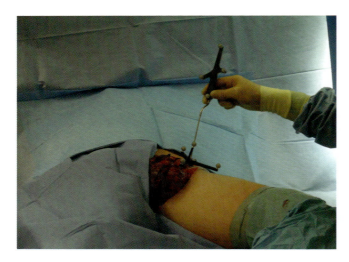

Fig. 11.8 Infrared camera and real-time monitor display of the osteotomy planes

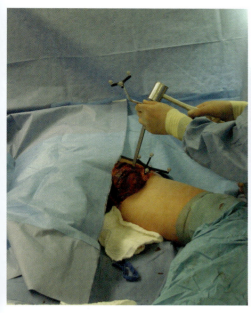
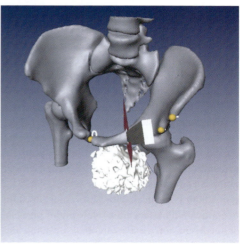

Fig. 11.9 The osteotomy is performed with a tracked chisel under visual control of the chisel position in relation to the predefined planes in real-time

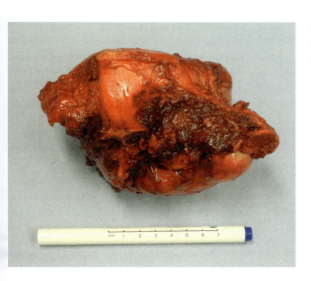

Fig. 11.10 Anatomical specimen after computer-assisted surgery; histology showed clear surgical margins (R0 resection)

pelvic ring remains closed, and in T3 resections. T1, T4, and combinations of T1 and T4 resections are best treated by means of biologic reconstruction using autologous bone grafts or custom-made pelvic endoprostheses. Hip trans- location can provide an alternative to pelvic endoprostheses for T2 resections.

The first published case reports regarding computer-assisted pelvic tumor resection came from a German group and included tumors infiltrating the sacrum (Hüfner et al. 2004; Krettek et al. 2004). Since a partial sacral resection can result in instability, while an iatrogenic lesion of the neural roots may impair the patient's quality of life due to incontinence and sexual dysfunction, it was critical to ensure the quality of surgical actions. With the aid of a navigation system, the tumors were removed with clear margins, while critical anatomical structures not infiltrated by the tumor could be preserved (Hüfner et al. 2004).

Computer-assisted surgery is particularly useful in resections of pediatric malignant bone tumors in the acetabular region, where accurate manipulations may lead to preservation of the joint, without compromising patient safety (Fehlberg et al. 2006; Wong et al. 2007 a, b). A further field of application has been the treatment of primary or recurrent soft tissue sarcomas invading the sacral or iliac cortex (Hüfner et al. 2004; Reijnders et al. 2007). In the cases published so far, however, the navigation system was only used to identify and reproduce the predetermined osteotomy levels with a computer-navigated chisel or by means of a computer-assisted K-wire insertion (Krettek et al. 2004; Hüfner et al. 2004; Reijnders et al. 2007). Furthermore, in cases where custom-made hemipelvic prostheses are to be implanted, navigation systems can ensure accurate fitting (Krettek et al. 2004; Wong et al. 2007 a, b). In our own setting we have used computer-navigated chisels only for identification and observation of preoperative determined pelvic and sacral osteotomies (Fehlberg et al. 2006).

11.4
Clinical Results

A review of available literature shows that in all published cases of computer-assisted pelvic tumor resection the predefined osteotomy planes could be successfully identified during the operation, while histology confirmed that the planned surgical margins were achieved. Up to date, no local recurrences have been detected in follow-up (Hüfner et al. 2004; Krettek et al. 2004; Stöckle et al. 2004; Fehlberg et al. 2006; Reijnders et al. 2007; Wong et al. 2007a, b). In our own pilot series, 13 consecutive patients underwent computer-assisted pelvic bone resection, including 6 patients with primary malignant bone tumor, 6 patients with bone metastasis, and 1 patient with soft tissue sarcoma (Fehlberg et al. 2006). The following pelvic resection types were performed; T1 ($n=2$), T1A ($n=2$), T2 ($n=4$), T3 ($n=4$), and T4 ($n=1$) (Enneking 1966; Enneking et al. 1990). Surgical margins were negative for 12 patients, while 1 patient with bone metastasis underwent resection with planned positive margins to allow for an improved functionality of the limb, due to limited prognosis; to improve local control, the patient received adjuvant radiation therapy.

The accuracy of the performed osteotomies can be evaluated using several methods. Some authors compare the results of the postoperative CT scans with the preoperative images used to plan the resection. However, in patients where a custom-made pelvic prosthesis was implanted, data analysis revealed that the quality of the postoperative scans was inadequate. In these cases the accuracy of the performed resection can be verified during the operation by documenting the correct fitting of the custom-made implant, or postoperatively with a simple X-ray (Wong et al. 2007a, b; Fig. 11.11).

In our series of patients, we found a median deviation of 3.3 mm between the planned and the performed osteotomy levels, comparing not only CT images, but also the reconstructed 3D models. Several possible causes have been suggested to explain this deviation. First, the surgeon might fail to exactly identify the planned osteotomy levels, most likely as a result of small, undetectable discrepancies during registration. Alternatively, spatial factors during the operation could render the planned osteotomies impossible to realize. What is more, upon completion of the

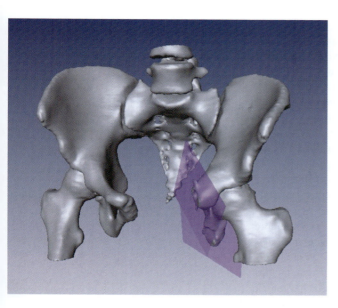

Fig. 11.11 A postoperative CT-based 3D model of the pelvis. The preoperatively planned and intraoperatively realized osteotomy planes are displayed

first osteotomy, the bones of the now open pelvic ring become slightly movable to each other, especially in younger patients where an additional loosening of the iliosacral joint is more likely. This in turn may lead to a minor expansion of the pelvis, preventing an exact comparison of the preoperative with the postoperative data. Given the quality of the surgical margins, this small deviation appears to have no clinical relevance; however, this aspect should be examined in larger trials.

11.5 Limits and Perspectives

Considering the lack of commercially available navigation platforms for pelvic applications, the preoperative process, including image processing, segmentation, and planning of the osteotomy levels, is rather time-consuming with current navigation systems. On the other hand, a learning curve seems to apply for intraoperative registration, while improved intraoperative orientation when using navigation systems could lead to a reduction of operation time (Wong et al. 2007a, b).

Further improvements are conceivable regarding the tracking systems. A significant disadvantage of the currently used optical tracking systems, compared to electromagnetic devices, consists in the fact that the former need a free line of sight. This can be a serious drawback for surgeries performed in small operating rooms due to possible restrictions in surgeon positioning. On the other hand, accuracy, the main handicap of electromagnetic devices, has been significantly improved in the new generation of systems of this type, enabling them to track very small sensor coils inserted in needles or catheters in the interior of the body (Schicho et al. 2005).

Registration, a process required for CT-based navigation technologies, is often a time-consuming process, related to most of the accuracy issues. A more convenient alternative could be a technique based on laser surface scans, where laser-projected infrared spots are identified with an infrared camera of a navigation system. By rapidly acquiring a high number of surface points (i.e., 100,000 points in only a few seconds), very accurate registrations can be achieved (Marmulla et al. 2004). However, soft tissue movements or inadequately dissected bone surfaces can significantly decrease the accuracy of the technique. Reijnders et al. advocated the use of fiducial markers (e.g., small titan screws, beryllium markers, etc.) to improve accuracy in pelvic tumor surgery (Reijnders et al. 2007), while Salehi and Ondra have demonstrated that no more than four fiducial markers are necessary to calibrate the system with a maximal deviation of 1.5 mm (Salehi and Ondra 2000).

A further development consists in data fusion from various imaging modalities to obtain more complex reconstructions and a higher accuracy. For example, fusing MR images with intraoperative ultrasound displays or CT angiographies could improve outcome in soft tissue navigation (Schlaier et al. 2004; Chopra et al. 2007). Computer-assisted soft tissue surgery has already been successfully applied in the treatment of gunshot and shrapnel injury (Mosheiff et al. 2004); nevertheless, the main challenge in the development of navigation platforms for soft tissue surgery is to solve the problem of tissue deformation. Two different approaches are possible; either to employ an intraoperative imaging modality to obtain an up-to-date image in the operating room, or to measure points of surfaces of anatomical structures directly in the OR and perform a nonrigid registration algorithm to compensate for the deformations (Carter et al. 2005).

The introduction of stereoscopic 3D displays, resulting in better depth perception, could lead to improvements in intraoperative visualization. Another promising approach is the use of augmented reality by merging real-world images and computer-generated virtual models to a common, real-time visualization. Available platforms vary between head-mounted or monitor displays, as well as optical see-through or video see-through devices. Augmented reality systems have already been applied in neuronavigation (Azuma 1997; Wirtz et al. 1998) and in interventional radiology (Fichtinger et al. 2004).

Summary

The value of navigation systems in musculoskeletal surgery has been established in both experimental and clinical settings. The main goal of this technique is to reduce the need for mutilating procedures, aiming at an improved limb function and quality of life without compromising the oncologic outcome. CT- and MRI-based computer-assisted surgery enables the accurate detection and realization of the preoperatively defined osteotomy levels, although commercially available navigation systems for pelvic applications have yet to be developed. Further clinical trials are required to evaluate the impact on long-term limb salvage, local recurrence, and overall survival rates.

References

Amiot LP, Labelle H, De Guise JA, Sati M, Brodeur P, Rivard CH (1995) Computer-assisted pedicle screw fixation. A feasibility study. Spine 20:208–1212

Amiot LP, Lang K, Putzier M, Zippel H, Labelle H (2000) Comparative results between conventional and computer-assisted pedicle screw installation in the thoracic, lumbar and sacral spine. Spine 25:606–614

Azuma RT (1997) A survey of augmented reality. Presence Teleoperator Virtual Environments. 6: 355–385

Bacci G, Ferrari S, Mercuri M, Longhi A, Giacomini S, Forni C, Bertoni F, Manfrini M, Barbieri E, Lari S, Donati D (2003) Multimodal therapy for the treatment of nonmetastatic Ewing's sarcoma of pelvis. J Pediatr Hematol Oncol 25:118–124

BacciG, FerrariS, Mercuri M, et al.: Multimodal therapy for the treatment of nonmetastatic Ewing's sarcoma ofpelvis. J Pediatr Hematol Oncol 2003; 25:118-124.

Bächler R, Bunke H, Nolte LP (2001) Restricted surface matching: numerical optimization and technical evaluation. Comput Aided Surg 6:143–152

Bottland M, Marsh JL, Brown TD (1997) Accuracy of screw displacement axis detection by DC electromagnetic motion tracking. Oral presentation for the departments of Orthopedic Surgery and Biomedical Engineering, University of Iowa, February 1997

Bowersox JC, Bucholz RD, Delp SL (1997) Excerpts from the final report for the Second International Workshop on Robotics and Computer Assisted Medical Interventions. Comput Aided Surg 2:69–101

Campanacci M, Capanna R (1991) Pelvic resections: the Rizzoli Institute experience. Orthop Clin North Am 22:65–86

Carter TJ, Sermesant M, Cash DM, Barratt DC, Tanner C, Hawkes DJ (2005) Application of soft tissue modelling to image-guided surgery. Med Eng Phys 27:893–909

Chopra SS, Hünerbein M, Eulenstein S, Lange T, Schlag PM, Beller S (2007) Development and validation of a three dimensional ultrasound based navigation system for tumor resection. Eur J Surg Oncol 34:456–461

Court C, Bosca L, Le Cesne A, Nordin JY, Missenard G (2006) Surgical excision of bone sarcomas involving the sacroiliac joint. Clin Orthop Relat Res 451:189–194

Dessenne V, Lavallée S, Julliard R, Orti R, Martelli S, Cinquin P (1995) Computer assisted knee anterior cruciate ligament reconstruction: first clinical tests. J Image Guid Surg 1:59–64

Enneking WF (1966) Local resection of malignant lesions of the hip and pelvis. J Bone Joint Surg Am 48:991–1007

Enneking WF, Dunham WK (1978) Resection and reconstruction for primary neoplasms involving the innominate bone. J Bone Joint Surg 60A:731–746

Enneking WF, Dunham WK, Gebhardt M, Malawar M, Pritchard D (1990) A system for the classification of skeletal resections. Chir Organi Mov 75[1 Suppl]:217–240

Fehlberg S, Lange T, Eulenstein S, Schlag PM, Tunn PU (2006) Navigationsgestützte Resektion maligner Knochentumoren des Beckens. Onkologe 12:152–157

Fichtinger G, Deguet A, Masamune K, Fischer G, Iordachita I, Balogh E, Masamune K, Taylor RH, Fayad LM, de Oliveira M, Zinreich SJ (2004) Needle insertion in CT scanner with image overlay—cadaver studies. In: Medical image computing and computer assisted intervention (MICCAI). vol 3217. Lecture notes in computer science (LNCS). Springer, Heidelberg Berlin New York, pp 795–803

Fuchs B, O'Connor MI, Kaufman KR, Padgett DJ, Sim FH (2002) Iliofemoral arthrodesis and pseudarthrosis: along-term functional outcome evaluation. Clin Orthop Relat Res 397:29–35

Glozman D, Shoham M, Fischer A (2001) A surface matching technique for robot-assisted registration. Comput Aided Surg 6:259–269

Hoffmann C, Gosheger G, Gebert C, Jürgens H, Winkelmann W (2006) Functional results and quality of life after treatment of pelvic sarcomas involving the acetabulum. J Bone Joint Surg Am 88:575–582

Hüfner T, Kfuri M, Galanski M, Bastian L, Loss M, Pohlemann T, Krettek C (2004) New Indications for computer-assisted surgery—tumor resection in the pelvis. Clin Orthop Relat Res 426:219–225

Kai J, Shiomi H, Sasama T, Sato Y, Inoue T, Tamura S, Inoue T (1998) Optical high-precision three-dimensional position measurement system suitable for head motion tracking in frameless stereotactic radiosurgery. Comput Aided Surg 3:257–263

Kawai A, Healey JH, Boland PJ, Lin PP, Huvos AG, Meyer PA (1998a) Prognostic factors for patients with sarcomas of the pelvic bones. Cancer 82:851–859

Kawai A, Huvos AG, Meyers PA, Healey JH (1998b) Osteosarcoma of the pelvis: oncologic results of 40 patients. Clin Orthop Relat Res 348:196–207

Khadem R, Yeh CC, Sadeghi-Tehrani M, Bax MR, Johnson JA, Welch JN, Wilkinson EP, Shahidi R (2000) Comparative tracking error analysis of five different optical tracking systems. Comput Aided Surg 5:98–107

Kollender Y, Shabat S, Bickels J, Flusser G, Isakov J, Neuman Y, Cohen I, Weyl-Ben-Arush M, Ramo N, Meller I (2000) Internal hemipelvectomy for bone sarcomas in children and young adults: surgical considerations. Eur J Surg Oncol 26:398–404

Krettek C, Geerling J, Bastian L (2004) Computer aided tumor resection in the pelvis. Injury 35[Suppl 1]:SA79–83

Langlotz F, Stucki M, Bächler R (1997) The first twelve cases of computer assisted periacetabular osteotomy. Comput Aided Surg 2:317–326

Langlotz F, Bächler R, Berlemann U, Nolte LP, Ganz R (1998) Computer assistance for pelvic osteotomies. Clin Orthop Relat Res 354:92–102

Langlotz F, Hinsche AF, Smith RM (2002) Hip and pelvic osteotomies. In: Di Gioia AM, Jaramaz B, Picard F, Nolte LP (eds) Hip and knee surgery—navigation, robotics, and computer assisted surgical tools. Oxford University Press, Oxford

Lorensen WE, Cline HE (1987) Marching cubes: a high resolution 3D surface construction algorithm. Proc ACM SIGGRAPH 21:163–169

Marmulla R, Lüth T, Mühling J, Hassfeld S (2004) Automated laser registration in image-guided surgery: evaluation of the correlation between laser scan resolution and navigation accuracy. Int J Oral Maxillofac Surg 33:642–648

Maurer CR, Fitzpatrick JM, Wang MY, Galloway RL, Maciunas RJ (1997) Registration of head volume images using implantable fiducial markers. IEEE Trans Med Imaging 16:447–462

Mosheiff R, Weil Y, Khoury A, Liebergall M (2004) The use of computerized navigation in the treatment of gun shot and shrapnel injury. Comput Aided Surg 9:39–43

Ney DR, Fishman EK, Magid D, Robertson DD, Kawashima A (1991) Three-dimensional volumetric display of CT data: effect of scan parameters upon image quality. J Comput Assist Tomogr 15:875–885

Nolte L, Beutler T (2004) Basic principles of CAOS. Injury 35[Suppl 1]:SA6–A16

Ozaki T, Flege S, Kervic M, Lindner N, Maas R, Delling G, Schwarz R, von Hochstetter AR, Salzer-Kuntschik M, Berdel WE, Jürgens H, Exner GU, Reichardt P, Mayer-Steinacker R, Ewerbeck V, Kotz R, Winkelmann W, Bielack SS (2003a) Osteosarcoma of the pelvis: experience of the Cooperative-Osteosarcoma Study Group. J Clin Oncol 21:334–341

Ozaki T, Rodl R, Grosheger G, Hoffmann C, Poremba C, Winkelmann W, Lindner L (2003b) Sacral infiltration in pelvic sarcomas: joint infiltration analysis II. Clin Orthop Relat Res 407:152–158

Pant R, Moreau P, Ilyas I, Paramasivan ON, Younge D (2001) Pelvic limb-salvage surgery for malignant tumors. Int Orthop 24:311–315

Price CH, Jeffree GM (1977) Incidence of bone sarcoma in SW England, 1946–1974, in relation to age, sex, tumour site and histology. Br J Cancer 36:511–522

Pring ME, Weber KL, Unni K, Sim FH (2001) Chondrosarcoma of the pelvis: a review of sixty-four cases. J Bone Joint Surg 83A:1630–1642

Salehi SA, Ondra SL (2000) Use of internal fiducial markers in frameless stereotactic navigational systems during spinal surgery: technical note. Neurosurgery 47:1460–1462

Reijnders K, Coppes MH, van Hulzen ALJ, Gravendeel JP, van Ginkel RJ, Hoekstr HJ (2007) Image guided surgery: new technology for surgery of soft tissue and bone sarcomas. J Cancer Surg 33:390–398

Richenberg JL, Hansell DM (1998) Image processing and spiral CT of the thorax. Brit J Radiol 71:708–716

Schicho K, Figl M, Donat M, Birkfellner W, Seemann R, Wagner A, Bergmann H, Ewers R (2005) Stability of miniature electromagnetic tracking systems. Phys Med Biol 50:2089–2098

Schlaier JR, Warnat J, Dorenbeck U, Proescholdt M, Schebesch KM, Brawanski A (2004) Image fusion of MR images and real-time ultrasonography: evaluation of fusion accuracy combining two commercial instruments, a neuronavigation system and a ultrasound system. Acta Neurochir (Wien) 146:271–277

Schlöndorff G (1998) Computer assisted surgery: historical remarks. Comput Aided Surg 3:150–152

Simon DA, Lavallée S (1998) Medical imaging and registration in computer-assisted surgery. Clin Orthop Relat Res 354:17–27

Steinmann JC, Herkowitz HN, El-Kommos H, Wesolowsko DP (1993) Spinal pedicle fixation: confirmation of an image-based technique for screw placement. Spine 18:1856–1861

Sucato DJ, Rougraff B, McGrath BE, Sizinski J, Davis M, Papandonatos G, Green D, Szarzanowicz T, Mindell ER (2000) Ewing's sarcoma of the pelvi: long-term survival and functional outcome. Clin Orthop Relat Res 193–201

Sugano N, Sasama T, Sato Y, Nakajima Y, Nishii T, Yonenobu K, Tamura S, Ochi T (2001) Accuracy evaluation of surface-based registration methods in a computer navigation system for hip surgery performed through a posterolateral approach. Comput Aided Surg 6:195–203

Tunn PU, Delbrück H, Schlag PM (2003) Ablative Verfahren bei der operativen Behandlung maligner Knochentumoren. Orthopäde 32:955–964

Wingo PA, Tong T, Bolden S (1995) Cancer statistics, 1995. CA Cancer J Clin 45:8

Wirbel RJ, Schulte M, Mutschler WE (2001) Surgical treatment of pelvic sarcomas: oncologic and functional outcome. Clin Orthop Relat Res 190–205

Wirtz CR, Knauth M, Hassfeld S, Tronnier VM, Albert FK, Bonsanto M, Kunze S (1998) Neuronavigation—first experiences with three different commercially available systems. Zentralbl Neurochir 59:14–22

Wong KC, Kumta SM, Chiu KH, Antonio GE, Unwin P, Leung KS (2007a) Precision tumour resection and reconstruction using image-guided computer navigation. J Bone Joint Surg Br 89:943–947

Wong KC, Kumta SM, Chiu KH, Cheung KW, Leung KS, Unwin P, Wong MC (2007b) Computer assisted pelvic tumor resection and reconstruction with a custom-made prosthesis using an innovative adaptation and its validation. Comput Aided Surg 12:225–232

Yang RS, Eckhardt JJ, Eilber FR, Rosen G, Forscher CA, Dorey FJ, Kelly CM, al-Shaikh R (1995) Surgical indications for Ewing's sarcoma of the pelvis. Cancer 76:1388–1397

Yasko A, Rutledge J, Lewis VO, Lin PP (2007) Disease- and recurrence-free survival after surgical resection of solitary bone metastases of the pelvis. Clin Orthop Relat Res 459:128–132

Pulmonary Metastasectomy for Osteosarcoma: Is It Justified?

Klaus-Dieter Diemel, Heinz-Jürgen Klippe, and Detlev Branscheid

Abstract Lung metastases are found in up to 30% of patients with osteosarcoma. Survival rates up to 45% are possible in interdisciplinary concepts, i.e. studies with aggressive surgical approach and (neo-) adjuvant chemotherapy. To elucidate these concepts concerning pulmonary metastasectomy, existing studies are reviewed and our own results are presented. *Methods:* Studies with the main topic in pulmonary metastases in osteosarcoma were reviewed. They overlook a period of 70 years and a total of more than 10,000 osteosarcoma patients and about 1,800 patients with pulmonary metastases. Studies have been reviewed concerning surgical concepts, prognostic factors and survival outcome. Our own results in 85 patients operated on for pulmonary metastases in 164 operations are presented and surgical procedures, prognostic factors and outcome are discussed. *Results:* About 1,800 patients with pulmonary metastases are presented in the reviewed studies from 1939 to 2007. There is a surprising consistency concerning surgical techniques, historically changing with the introduction of stapling machines and laser surgery. Survival rates between 30% and 40% also show a certain consistency in interdisciplinary studies, with a range from 11% to 63% in all studies. The main prognostic factor affecting survival is complete surgical remission (CSR). It shows high significance particularly in studies with large numbers of patients. Time of metastatic presentation, and number and localization of metastases show significance more infrequently. Our own series focusses on overall survival rate (48%) and the importance of CSR as a prognostic factor ($p<.001$). *Conclusion:* Pulmonary metastasectomy is mandatory for long-termsurvival in patients with pulmonary metastases in osteosarcoma. This does not depend on the metastatic stage or the number of operations needed to achieve CSR, which is the main prognostic factor for survival. Bilateral surgery is necessary in most patients; minimally invasive techniques should not be used routinely.

12.1
History of Osteosarcoma and Pulmonary Metastasectomy

Starting with Galen (second century A.D.) and throughout nearly 2000 years the term "sarcoma" was used for growths of "fleshy structure".

Klaus-Dieter Diemel (✉)
Department of General Thoracic Surgery
Krankenhaus Grosshansdorf, Hamburg
Wöhrendamm 80
22927 Großhansdorf, Germany
E-mail: k.diemel@pulmosurgery.de

The distinction of different types of sarcomas first developed at the turn of eighteenth to nineteenth century, e.g. in the early classification by Abernethy (1764–1831). Boyer (1807) coined the term "osteosarcoma" to characterize malignant primary bone tumours. For secondary malignant growth, the term metastasis together with an early concept of tumour spread by blood vessel invasion was proposed by Récamier (1829). With the development of histopathological techniques by Müller and Virchow, the term sarcoma was fixed to connective tissue growth. The incidence of osteosarcoma in childhood and youth was recognized quite early and the marked formation of pulmonary metastases was well known (Eve 1883).

Concerning chest malignancies, the two possible ways of tumour spread, at first from chest wall to lung, like in breast cancer (Macewen 1886), or the opposite way, like in lung cancer (Walshe 1846), were already known. Seydel (1909) published an early review on the operability on lung and pleura tumours classifying them into three groups: metastatic tumours, tumours invading the lung from extrapulmonary sources and primary lung tumours. With regards to the then knowledge of cancer growth, it is not surprising that in early onset of chest surgery, chest wall operations prevailed and metastasis surgery preceded lung surgery for several decades. Table 12.1 gives a summary of early reports on chest wall and lung surgery.

Weinlechner (1882) reported the first operation with excision of three unilateral metastases of a child's head-sized chest wall tumour (Fig. 12.1). Parham (1898) gives a detailed review and case analyses of 46 cases of osteosarcoma, according to the then used histological classification. Quénu and Longuet (1898) presented 34 cases of "thoracotomies pénétrantes et intrapleurales" with markedly favourable results. In 19 cases of osteosarcoma, 4 patients (21%) died, and in 15 cases of enchondroma 5 patients (33%) died, in contrast to Seydel (1909) reporting an overall mortality of 53%.

After World War II the surgical know-how won during decades in tuberculosis surgery could be applied to the growing demand of cancer and metastases surgery. Furthermore, beginning in the 1950s, surgical techniques turned more towards lung tissue-sparing procedures (see Sect. 12.5.2, Techniques in Pulmonary Resection).

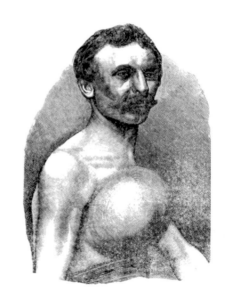

Fig. 12.1 Chest wall metastasis reported by Weinlechner (1882)

1855	C. Sédillot	France	1 case
1882	K. Weinlechner	Austria	1 case
1883	U. Krönlein	Switzerland	1 case
1898	F.W. Parham	USA	2 cases, review of 98 cases
1898	Quénu and Longuet	France	34 cases

Table 12.1 Early studies in chest wall and lung surgery

Table 12.2 Early reports on surgery in lung metastases

1921/1937	W. Röpke	Germany
1926	G. Divis	Czechoslovakia
1927	A.T. Edwards	United Kingdom
1930	F. Torek	USA
1933	E.D. Churchill	USA

Whereas pulmonary metastasectomy in the 1920s and 1930s had been most often single case reports (Table 12.2), from then on, more collective statistics were published focussing on pulmonary metastasectomy, even in osteosarcoma. Thomford et al. (1965) report on 221 thoracotomies in 205 metastases patients, 41 of them sarcomas and 9 osteosarcomas. Two important developments in pulmonary metastasectomy began: first, the insight in resectability of multiple metastases, as reported by Mannix (1953), which created an approach of maximal radicality and it was confirmed as probably the right way by Martini et al. (1971) and Morton et al. (1973). Following was the discussion of known and unforeseen bilaterality of metastases. Takita and colleagues' (1977) report thereby favoured the bilateral approach by sternotomy as the more radical surgical approach, although this position remains under discussion still today.

Without doubt, these above-mentioned publications opened the door towards the modern surgical concept of pulmonary metastasectomy, more and more as part of interdisciplinary concepts with chemotherapy and immunotherapy.

12.2 Thoracic Surgery Becomes Important Part of Interdisciplinary Concepts

In many institutions in Europe and the United States, the resection of pulmonary metastases had become a standard procedure since the 1950s. Surgical techniques had evolved into parenchyma-sparing resections, and operations in general had become less hazardous. These factors led to a broader spectrum of surgical indications, particularly for the resection of metastases. The benefit of metastasectomy, i.e. a surgical therapy of generalizing malignancies, had been controversial for a long time. The natural lack of prospective double-blind studies led to large cohort of studies established by specialized cancer centres and international registers of lung metastases. These studies demonstrated the benefit of metastasectomy in more than 5,000 patients with carcinogenic or sarcomatous primary tumours (Pastorino et al. 1997), especially in osteosarcomas (Bielack et al. 2002). However, osteosarcomas present a rare disease not comparable to the incidence of colon cancer, breast and lung cancer, etc. For this reason, the reports of systematically treating pulmonary metastases of osteosarcoma began with small studies.

Early reports came from Morrow using 16 clinical records from 1939 to 1978 (Morrow et al. 1980) completing an earlier report of Edlich et al. (1966) that represented a single centre experience of 40 years with pulmonary metastases, renewed in the following papers with increasing numbers of cases (Saltzman et al. 1993; Thompson et al. 2002) from the University of Minnesota. Another long period of observation that focussed on osteosarcoma is reported from the Memorial Sloan-Kettering Cancer Center (Marcove et al. 1975; Martini et al. 1971; Meyers et al. 1993). Other institutions also published series with a few patients per year in single centres (Table 12.3).

Despite long observation periods, the recruitment of patients operated on for pulmonary metastases in most single-centre studies does not exceed 5 patients per year to date. However, these studies tellingly demonstrate the increasing success in therapy of a rare disease and the consecutive need of a larger numbers of patients to evaluate the effectiveness of surgical therapy, particularly under consideration of frequently changing chemotherapy protocols.

Table 12.3 Studies in pulmonary metastases of OS: single-centre experiences and national databases with long observation periods from oncologic (O), surgical/orthopaedic (S), thoracic surgical (T) or radiologic (R) departments

Reference	Dept.	Time period	Length (yrs)	All OS-pts	OS-pts. with PM	OS-PM operated n	Prognostic factors defined?	% Survival (years)	Institution or database
Single institution experiences									
Morrow et al. 1980[a]	S	1939–78	40	-	16	16	Yes	36 (5)	University of Minnesota, USA
Saltzman et al. 1993[a]	S	1977–92	16	-	29	27	n.i.	24 (5)	
Thompson et al. 2002	S	1982–97	16	85	40	29	Yes	43 (4)	
Marcove et al. 1975	S	1969–71	3	145	-	22 rel	n.i.	31(5)ltr, 0 untr.	Mem. Sloan-Kettering Cancer Center, New York, USA
Martini et al. 1971	S	1965–70	6	-	22	22	Yes	45 (3)	
Meyers et al. 1993	O	1975–84	10	342	62	19 pr	Yes	Not differentiated	
Meyer et al. 1987	O	1968–84	17	175	74	6 pr, 39 rel	Yes	38 (5)	St. Jude Children´s Hosp.
Kaste et al. 1999	R	1977–97	21	215	31	21 pr	Yes	29 (5)	Memphis, USA
Goorin et al. 1984	O	1972–81	10	93	32	26 rel	Yes	40 (.)	Faber-Cancer-Institute, USA
Huth and Eilber 1989	S	1974–86	13	255	77	51	Yes	17 (10)	UCLA School of Med., USA
Carter et al. 1991	T	1977–83	7	111	43	25	Yes	20 (5)	Birmingham, UK
Ward et al. 1994	S	1981–90	10	111	53	36	Yes (mv)	36 (5)	UC, Los Angeles, USA
Bacci et al. 1998	O	1986–91	6	188	44	28	n.i.	17 (5)	Rizzoli, Bologna, I
Antunes et al. 1999	T	1989–97	9	198	58	31	n.i.	61 (3)	Universidade Coimbra, P
Briccoli et al. 2005	S	1980–2001	22	1,418	267	94 recurr	Yes (mv)	37 (5)	Rizzoli, Bologna, I
Pfannschmidt et al. 2006	T	1997–2001	5	-	21	21	Yes	34,2 (5)	Heidelberg Univ., D
Harting et al. 2006	S	1980–2000	21	272	131	93	Yes	22,6 (5)	Univ. Texas, Houston, USA

12.2.1 From Single-Centre Experience to Large Databases

It became a new approach to create larger multi- or single-centre studies based on national databases as realized, for example, in Japan, Italy and Germany in the early 1980s. The Italian databases reported on 789 patients recruited between 1983 and 1999 (Bacci et al. 2006) by the Rizzoli Institute in Bologna. The German–Austrian–Swiss Osteosarcoma study group COSS reported on 1,702 patients from between 1980 and 1998 (Bielack et al. 2002). Both groups enabled the evaluation of subgroups as primary metastatic patients (Kager et al. 2003), patients with tumour relapse (Kempf-Bielack et al. 2005), and patients with pulmonary metastases (synchronously metastasizing) and pulmonary relapse (metachronously metastasizing) at different dates of diagnosis, as in the Japanese database (Tsuchiya et al. 2002).

Creating statistically significant results, large interdisciplinary studies such as the COSS studies showed an increasing survival for osteosarcoma patients under combined pre- and postoperative chemotherapy (with enhancing drug combinations) and aggressive surgical strategies. Since the first statistical evidence of long-term survival after metastasectomy appeared, pulmonary (and other) metastasectomies have become part of an overall interdisciplinary concept (Bielack et al. 2002).

12.3 Evaluating the Patient with Pulmonary Metastases

For successfully establishing interdisciplinary studies, specialists in each faculty are necessary to guarantee each patient the maximum number of therapy options. Therefore, reference institutions for diagnostics and therapy have been created in all protocols of interdisciplinary osteosarcoma research. The organization of most study groups is located in departments of oncology or paediatric oncology. The indications about surgery to perform when are established in a multidisciplinary approach and can be adjusted promptly to the patient's needs. Radiological findings are reconfirmed with specialized radiologists and surgeons, and operations are performed in orthopaedic, thoracic and other surgical reference centres. Figure 12.2 demonstrates a regular therapy pattern in patients with newly detected osteosarcoma.

Concerning pulmonary metastasectomy, two main questions have to be answered after the basic indication for a lung resection is established by the study protocol:

1. Will a complete surgical remission be possible or at least as likely to be viable as not?
2. Will the patient regain pulmonary and life quality postoperatively?

12.3.1
Computed Tomography of the Lung

Computed tomography (CT) scans for preoperative diagnostics are most suitable assessing the probability of complete surgical remission, as they are the essential tool for detecting pulmonary nodules at any date in the therapeutic course. Pulmonary screening with CT scan is one of the first routine diagnostics in patients presenting with osteosarcoma, at least since the beginning of the CT era. At that time (in the 1980s), the dramatically improving quality of diagnosis was reported from all authors presenting their data. Further improvement was observed with the technical evolution of the CT scanners. Although currently the use of 16 (or more) line CT scans gives a very good impression of number, size and localization of pulmonary nodules, their predictive value needs is under discussion (Kayton et al. 2006). Nevertheless, it is most important to evaluate the scans by a second radiologist and the thoracic surgeon who will operate on the patient. The surgeon's participation becomes still more important for the discrimination of postoperative alterations and relapsing metastases after one or more thoracotomies.

12.3.2
SPECT and PET Scans

Additional diagnostic input is reported in few studies from the ^{99m}Tc-SPECT, which shows a poor sensitivity but good specificity and good positive predictive value most notably in patients with preceding operations and extensive altered radiological findings. Pevarski et al. (1998) found this technique predictive of small lesions that had been overseen in standard CT scans.

Concerning positron emission tomography (PET) scans, our own experience with a few cases shows some similarities to the above-mentioned quality of the SPECT technique. If there will be a place for diagnosing metastases with PET, it has yet to be evaluated. It is easily imaginable that we will see diagnostic benefits in patients with preceding operations or metastatic findings that extend beyond the borders of lung parenchyma.

Functional lung testing is a preoperative routine required for every patient who will undergo lung resection. Its evaluation depends on the surgeon's experience calculating the extent of resection for complete surgical remission. The delay since chemotherapy and the application of chemotherapy drugs that might be hazardous to lung integrity intraoperatively or postoperatively have to be considered also.

12 Pulmonary Metastasectomy for Osteosarcoma: Is It Justified?

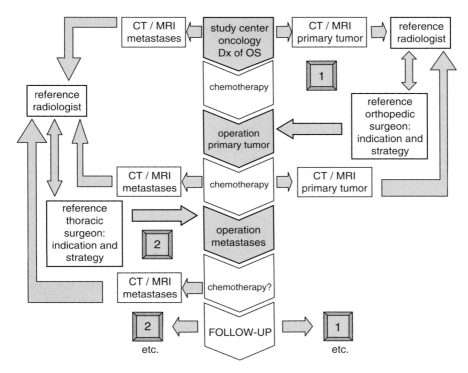

Fig. 12.2 The clinical path of diagnoses and therapies with the *central column* focussed on chemotherapy, surrounded by recurring circles of primary tumour care (*1*) and pulmonary metastases care (*2*). An equivalent to *circle 2* is also applied in the care of other metastases with the need of other reference surgeons

12.4
Prognostic Factors and Their Impact for Pulmonary Metastasectomy

Describing prognostic factors is an inherent part of all studies evaluating the outcome of osteosarcoma patients. There is an interest in the risk of developing metastases, which has become an investigational domain of molecular biological studies (Khanna et al. 2000; Tofuku et al. 2006; Gordon et al. 2007; Koshkina et al. 2007). However, most studies investigating the outcome of patients with primary or relapsing metastases of osteosarcoma have aimed at specifying one or more prognostic factors concerning the influence of metastatic modalities and therapies on survival.

Concerning pulmonary metastases, three main groups of factors have been analysed, as covered in the following sections.

12.4.1
Factors Correlating to Modalities and Therapies of the Primary Tumour

The factor most frequently discussed is the histological response of the primary tumour as well as surgical complete remission. This factor is well documented in large series (Bacci et al. 2006; Kempf-Bielack et al. 2005). Bacci et al. (2006) find an increased rate of recurrence (29.2%) in patients with poor histological response, but this is not significant. In contrast, bad response in the group of all investigated osteosarcoma patients ($n=789$) doubles the risk of death. Kempf-Bielack et al. (2005) also do not report statistical significance of histological response for patients with pulmonary relapse ($n=481$) in contrast to all patients of this group ($n=1,702$) with a 2.57-fold risk of death (Bielack et al. 2002) after bad histological response. In the 202 patients with primary pulmonary metastases out of this group, this factor does not even reach univariate relevance (Kager et al. 2003).

12.4.2
Factors Concerning the Time of Presentation of Metastases

The disease free interval (DFI) from primary surgery to the date of development of metastases is the most often investigated time-related factor. Morrow et al. (1980) report a 5-year DFI to be a prognostic factor. Thompson et al. (2002), evaluating the later experience from Minneapolis, confirms this with an increasing risk to survive of .8 per year. The Sloan-Kettering experience also has no significance for DFI (Meyers et al. 1993). In large sample studies, the DFI remains in statistical irrelevance (Bielack et al. 2002; Bacci et al. 2006), whereas, when exclusively focussing on pulmonary tumour relapse, the DFI shows a certain impact (Kempf-Bielack et al. 2005). An interesting grouping of DFI results is from the study of the Japanese Musculoskeletal Oncology Group: Tsuchiya et al. (2002) report 248 patients with metastases who show significantly variant survival according to the date of appearance during the therapy course.

12.4.3
Factors Concerning Properties of Metastases and Surgical Remission

Properties of metastases and the metastasing pattern have been investigated in all reviewed studies revealing prognostic factors. The most common focus is the number of metastases resected. For long time this factor was the most common reason to assume inoperability. The results concerning properties of metastases and the impact of surgical remission are shown in Table 12.4. Although in most studies these factors play an important role, their statistical evidence is under discussion (see below).

12.5
Techniques in Pulmonary Metastasectomy

12.5.1
Operative Approach to the Metastatic Lung

Bilaterality of pulmonary metastases is a frequent phenomenon in osteosarcoma patients. Therefore, a bilateral operative approach has been discussed since the early reports of pulmonary metastasectomy (Takita et al. 1977; Johnston 1983). All reports consistently state that an occult bilateral involvement takes places in a certain number of patients. This seems to be an unforeseeable factor, despite exhaustive radiological diagnostics. The CT scan, which dramatically improved the detection of pulmonary nodules in the late 1970s, before that time had an enormous lack of imaging resolution and therefore a poor predictive value for the detection of particular nodules. With the development of 16- to 64-line (and more) CT scanners today, this factor has improved significantly. Nevertheless, there is still a discrepancy between radiological and intraoperative findings concerning the numbers of nodules and their localization, particularly in the contralateral side. On this background—that complete surgical remission might be a statistically relevant factor of survival—the strategy of the operative approach and the impact of hidden bilaterality have to be discussed.

In our own series, the thoracic approach was by sternotomy in 47 (55%) of 85 first-line operations and in 7 (16%) of the 44 first redo

Table 12.4 Studies in pulmonary metastases of OS: evaluated risk factors affecting survival after pulmonary metastasectomy

	Patients operated	Age	Gender	Pulmonary metastasectomy (p)	Disease-free interval (p)	Number of nodules (p)	Metastatic size and extent (p)	Bilaterality (p)	Complete surgical remission (p)	Tumour necrosis
Martini et al. 1971	22			+(.)		+(.)			+++(.)	
Morrow et al. 1980[a]	16				>5 yrs (.)		Extent +			
Putnam et al. 1983	39				(.014)	>3 (.0003)			++(.002)	
Goorin et al. 1984	26				>1yr N.S.	N.S.			+++(<.001)	
Meyer et al. 1987 (mv)	45		Male (.002)		>1yr N.S.	>6 (.0056)		+(.058)		
Huth et al. 1989	51			++(.)						
Carter et al. 1991	25				N.S.	N.S.	Lobes (.04)	N.S.		
Meyers et al. 1993	19	>21 (.04)						+(.03)	+++(<.001)	
Saltzman et al. 1993[a]	27				>2 yrs. (.05)	>3 N.S.	1–2 cm N.S.			
Ward et al. 1994 (mv)	36				N.S.	<4 (.047)		+(.04)	+++(<.001)	>90% (.01)
Kaste et al. 1999 (mv)	21	N.S.	N.S.			>3 (.0009)	Lobes (.04)	N.S.		
Thompson et al. 2002	29					>3 (.04)	Size N.S.			
Tsuchiya et al. 2002 (mv)	248			+++(.001)	4 gr. (.001)					

(continued)

Table 12.4 (continued)

	Patients operated	Age	Gender	Pulmonary metastasectomy (p)	Disease-free interval (p)	Number of nodules (p)	Metastatic size and extent (p)	Bilaterality (p)	Complete surgical remission (p)	Tumour necrosis
Kager et al. 2003 (mv)	145					>1 (.012)			+++ (.003)	
Briccoli et al. 2005 (mv)	94				3%/yr (.)	+ (.046)				
Pfannschmidt et al. 2005	21					N.S.			++ (.004)	
Kempf-Bielack et al. 2005 (mv)[b]	N.Sp.			+++ (.001)	>18 μ (.01)	+++ (.001)	PIDis (.001)	+++ (.001)	+++ (.0001)	
Harting et al. 2006	93				1 yr (.001)	N.S.	PIDis N.S.	+ 8.02		
Diemel et al. 2007	85				N.S.				++ (.01)	>98% (.04)

Abbreviations: (.), significance level unavailable; gr., groups; Lobes, involvement of more than one lung lobe; mv, established by multivariate analysis; N.Sp., not specified; N.S., not reaching $p<.5$; μ, months; p, significance level of applied statistics; PIDis, pleural disruption; yr(s), year(s)

[a] Indicates studies not exclusively focussed on osteosarcoma metastases

[b] Study analysing all types of osteosarcomic metastases with 373 patients with lung-only metastases and 436 patients with lung metastases overall

operations, as it was a staged double-sided thoracotomy in 8 (9%) of first-line and 24 (55%) of the first redo operations.

12.5.2
Techniques in Pulmonary Resection

Pulmonary metastasectomy in most cases means resecting single pulmonary nodules located near the pleura. Initially the procedure was suggested only to enucleate these lesions. The technique created the familiar term "berry picking" to describe this form of operation. Early on, the original form of "berry picking" was given up in favour of small extraanatomic resections, the so-called "wedge-resections", for the oncological reason of clean resection margins (Mannix 1953). These wedge-resections describe a simple but oncologically secure operation technique for a few metastases in first-line operations.

However, with increasing numbers of nodules or increasing frequency of thoracotomies the surgical challenge grows. All oncological resections abate the lung tissue volume and with that, respiratory reserves and life quality. Pulmonary metastasectomy, even when carried out with simple surgical manoeuvres (at first), demands a surgeon's mastery in sparing lung tissue. Furthermore, the resection of centrally located nodules adhering to or invading pulmonary vessels or bronchial structures already requires good thoracic surgical training and familiarity with reconstructive techniques as well as with modern technologies such as laser surgery, an innovative technique providing excellent radicality and results in the resection of central metastases with a 1,318-nm Ndyn:YAG laser.

The number of redo operations in patients with osteosarcoma is frequent for several reasons, but chiefly because the main surgical goal is complete surgical remission in metastasectomy (Kempf-Bielack et al. 2005). Furthermore, patients may still benefit with long-term survival from complete remission in the fourth or fifth redo operation (Briccoli et al. 2005). In these redo operations, the metastasizing patterns change from simple resection of peripheral nodules to more extended resections. As demonstrated below, in our own results the most common extensions concern the chest wall and the pericardium.

On this account, all thoracic surgical and bronchological interventional standards have their place in pulmonary metastasectomy: from wedge resections up to laser resections and extended chest wall replacement. All procedures and the different approaches to the lung will be discussed in detail.

12.5.2.1
Bronchological Manoeuvres

Although endobronchial problems in osteosarcoma metastases are rare (Heitmiller et al. 1993; Mogulkoc et al. 1999) bronchological competence is anticipated not only by pulmonologists but also in thoracic surgeons. Bronchoscopy (most often rigid) combined with laser resection, being an effective procedure to free metastatically blocked airways, can be exclusively a palliative therapy. Nevertheless, there is no loss of lung tissue, and quality of life improves dramatically. If there is a statistical effect about prolonging life, it is unknown for these rare and singular cases.

12.5.2.2
Wedge Resections (Small Extraanatomic Segmental Resections)

Before the era of using stapling devices, the resection of solitary nodules was performed by clamping the lung parenchyma around the metastasis, cutting out the clamped material by knife or scissors and sewing the resulting defect with a running suture (Fig. 12.3a, b). This technique has been abandoned in most operating rooms favouring stapling devices available in many sizes and applications. Thus, pulmonary resection has become safer and quicker, and the frequency of postoperative air leaks has diminished considerably (Diemel et al. 2006). On the other hand, the extent of each portion of resected lung parenchyma might be a little larger than in conventional clamp resections (Fig. 12.4a, b) when metastases show an unfavourable location or distance to pleura. This matters most when large numbers of metastases must be resected. Moreover, metastasectomies, particularly in osteosarcoma patients, may have to be redone or done bilaterally. When faced with these factors, especially in first-line operations aiming to use a parenchyma-sparing operation, wedge resection techniques are indicated.

12.5.2.3
Anatomical Resections (Anatomical Segmentectomies, Lobectomies, Pneumonectomies)

Two conditions in pulmonary metastases may demand anatomical resections: (1) large-sized solitary metastases situated in the hilus of a lung lobe or the entire lung or (2) the miliary involvement of the whole lobe. Pneumonectomies are rare resections in metastasectomy, regarded as indicated only in cases of singular metastases, which extend themselves through or around the hilus. Miliary-affected whole lungs must be seen as very critical as subject for pneumonectomy because of the possibly bilateral involvement that would counter the principle of radicality.

In some cases an anatomical segmentectomy might be a good and radical procedure for centrally localized metastases. In contrast to wedge resections, an anatomical segmentectomy can handle this problem due to its greater reach into the hilus (Fig. 12.5). However, anatomical segmentectomies assume more thoracic surgical competence than wedge resections or uncomplicated lobectomies.

Martini et al. (1971) report on 59 thoracotomies, including 6 lobectomies in 22 patients, while Briccoli et al. (2005) showed an increasing part of anatomic resections in the redo operations in 94 patients (first redo) and 23 patients (second redo). Our own results have shown a total of 21 anatomic resections in 162 operations for pulmonary metastases.

12.5.2.4
Bronchoplastic Procedures

A valuable technique providing good lung parenchyma sparing is a bronchoplastic procedure, in which resections of bronchial segments with or without lung tissue are followed by anastomotic reconstruction. By this means, an extensive loss of lung tissue can be avoided. Producing good results in bronchoplastic operations means respecting bronchial blood supply, creating tension-free anastomoses and covering anastomoses with living materials such as musculature and pericardial or pleural flaps (Vogt-Moykopf et al. 1986). Bronchoplastic procedures are irreplaceable in treating metastatic lesions, which affect lobar or large segmental bronchi.

12.5.2.5
Laser Resections

The most revolutionary modification in pulmonary metastasectomy followed the introduction of the Nd:YAG laser (Branscheid et al. 1992). This made possible combining excellent oncological radicality with the lung tissue-sparing effects of the former "berry picking". Greater numbers of metastases were resectable without the need for resecting a whole lobe. Furthermore, centrally located lesions were resectable with resection of lung tissue only. The laser enabled surgeons to resect metastases located in vascular bifurcations or deep in the lung parenchyma (Fig. 12.6). With increasing experience the complications of bleeding and persisting air leakages became increasingly marginal.

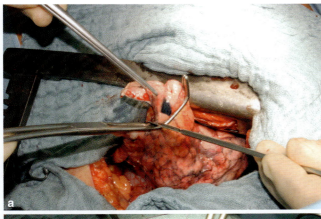
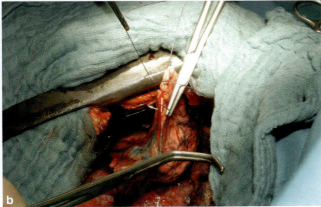

Fig. 12.3 a, b Pulmonary wedge resection over clamp (**a**) and closure by running suture (**b**)

The most important evolution within the laser technology itself was the creation of a Nd:YAG laser with a wave length of 1,318 nm. It is an optimized tool concerned with the water resorption coefficient of the lung and involves fewer complications in air leakage and concurrently it establishes the possibility of wider resection extents (Rolle et al. 2006).

12.5.2.6
Extrapulmonary Extensions

In contrast to most first-line resections of pulmonary metastases, non-pulmonary structures of the thorax are involved increasingly in redo operations. Despite the fact that there is little reported on this subject in most studies from oncological specialists, there is a clear tendency manifesting in our own series. With an increasing number of operations, there is a rising demand to resect metastases invading the chest wall and pericardium, and even vertebral bodies or central vessels of the lung. This fact affects the strategy of redo operations: chest wall resections with plastic reconstructions or resections with stabilization of the vertebral column have to be planned, possibly in interdisciplinary teams. Furthermore, bronchoplastic and angioplastic procedures are gaining importance because these extended resections become more hazardous concerning cardiopulmonary function postoperatively. The amount and character of resect extensions are infrequently reported. Briccoli

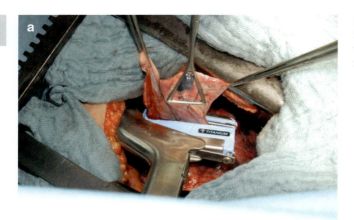
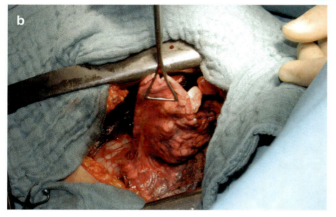

Fig. 12.4 a, b Pulmonary wedge resection with a stapling device with replaceable stapling magazines

et al. (2005) show for redo operations a relative increase in anatomical resections but do not comment on it. Table 12.5 lists the extensions experienced in our series.

12.6
Our Own Results

In 1978 the first children with osteosarcoma metastases were operated on in our institution according to the protocol of the COSS-77 study. This protocol was designed as an adjuvant chemotherapy protocol (Winkler et al. 1982) and led to the following neo-adjuvant protocol, the COSS-80 study. For institutional reasons, paediatric thoracic surgery was abandoned in mid 1980s and re-established 1993, and from 1997 our institution became a reference centre for thoracic surgery in the follow-up COSS-96 study. For this reason, there is unfortunately no uninterrupted COSS data from the mid 1970s to today.

From 1993 to 2006, 93 patients were operated on for primary or relapsing metastases of osteosarcoma. Of the patients, 46 had one redo operation, 17 had two redo operations, 4 patients had three, and 2 patients had four redo operations. Altogether, 164 operations were performed in these patients. At the moment of writing, 8 patients (2 of whom had two operations)

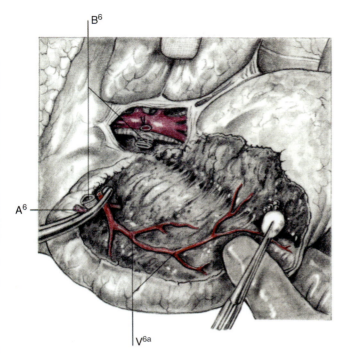

Fig. 12.5 Anatomical segmentectomy of S6: blunt dissection along the intersegmental vein (*V6a*). Resection of the entire segment with bronchial dissection and separate closure

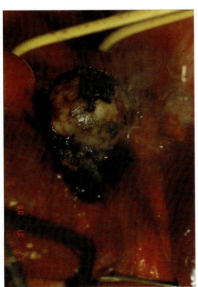

Fig. 12.6 Metastasis in the pulmonary arterial bifurcation, uncovered by laser before complete laser resection, which was possible without residual metastatic tissue. (Pulmonary artery slung by loop ligature)

were out of follow-up with unknown status. These patients are excluded; we will report on 85 patients with a total of 152 operations.

In total, 85 patients had first-line operations, 44 had one redo-operation, 17 had two redo-operations, 4 had three redo-operations, and 2 had four redo-operations. The thoracic approach was a sternotomy in 47 (55%) of 85 first-line operations and in 7 (16%) of the 44 first redo operations, as it was a staged double-sided thoracotomy in 8 (9%) of first-line and in 24 (55%) of the first redo operations. There were no additional re-sternotomies in the redo operations (up to four in 2 patients). In the case of sternotomy, both lungs had been investigated and operated on.

Of the 85 patients, 49 were operated on for primary metastases, and 36 patients presented with pulmonary relapse after first-line treatment.

The most frequent surgical procedure was a wedge resection, which usually was carried out as multiple wedge resections. In the first operations,

Table 12.5 Operative extensions necessary to achieve complete surgical remission in 85 patients and 152 operations. For lung resections see Table 6

Resection with Nd:YAG-Laser	51
Bronchoplastic procedures	7
Angioplastic procedures	16
Pericardial resections	36
Chest Wall Resections	30
With reconstruction	21
Resections of vertebral bodies (partial)	6
Diaphragm	13
Mediastinal metastases	12
Metastases of mamma	4
Left-sided adrenalectomy	1
Right hemihepatectomy	1

anatomical resections were infrequent, but the incidence increased in the following redo operations. In 5 patients, intraoperative situ showed inoperability because of miliary metastases in 3 patients and extensive mediastinal infiltration in 2 of them. Three patients did not achieve complete surgical remission, and 4 patients showed no metastatic growth at all in the resected nodules (Table 12.6).

From the 85 patients with a first-line operation (2 patients incomplete resection, 1 patient unresectable), 50 relapsed, 17 died, and 18 are alive and free of disease (FOD); 44 patients who relapsed had a second resection (1 patient with incomplete resection, 3 patients unresectable), and 19 of them relapsed, 14 died and 11 are alive (FOD). Regarding the 19 patients who relapsed, 17 had a third operation, of whom 6 relapsed again, 6 died (3 incomplete resections) and 5 are alive (FOD). The 4 patients who relapsed had a fourth resection, of whom 2 relapsed, 1 died (incomplete resection) and 1 is alive (FOD). The two patients who relapsed had a fifth operation, one with complete resection, who is now living 16 months free of disease, and the other patient died 12 weeks after the operation involving incomplete resection (see flowchart, Fig. 12.7).

Statistical analysis was carried out with SPSS (SPSS 16.0 Statistical Software, SPSS Inc., Chicago), using descriptive and cross table analyses and computing Kaplan-Meier survival estimates with log rank (95% confidence intervals) comparisons.

The actuarial survival of all patients without comparing metastases subgroups was 84.6% for 24 months and 71.8% for 36 months, and the actuarial 5-year survival was 49.7% (Fig. 12.8).

Mean follow-up for all patients is 51.7 (SE 4.42) months, follow-up of the yet living 46 patients is 60.14 (SE 6.98) months, while mean follow-up from diagnosis to pulmonary relapse in all patients is 41.76 (2–121.5) months.

Comparing the metastases subgroups, there was a tendency towards a better survival in patients with pulmonary relapse vs patients with primary metastases (Fig. 12.9). However, this difference did not reach a significant level ($p<.48$).

Comparing the extent of metastasectomy, a tendency towards an increasing amount of operative extensions could be observed with the increasing number of redo operations, predominantly chest wall and pericardium resections. Furthermore, in some chest wall or other metastases in close proximity to the lung, an extremely rapid growth had been casually observed. Figures 12.10 and 12.11 show the course of a 24-year-old woman who experienced a pulmonary relapse after pulmonary metastasectomy 4.5 years ago. Besides pulmonary re-metastases, left-sided chest wall involvement had to be resected. During thoracic exploration, the structure, initially suspected to be pericardial (Fig. 12.10, arrow), showed an intrapericardial metastasis, originating from the right-sided pericardial fold on the inferior caval outflow. As resection of this metastasis via left-sided thoracotomy (by reasons of chest wall replacement, Fig. 12.10, circle) was too hazardous for caval injury, a following operation with extracorporal circulation stand-by was planned. The patient recovered very slowly,

Extended (intrapericardial) pneumonectomies	5
Lobectomies with and without extension	6
Bilobectomies	2
Anatomical segmentectomies	8
No complete surgical remission in the lung (CSR)	8
No metastases after resection of suspicious nodules	4

Table 12.6 Anatomical resections performed in 85 patients in 152 operations. For other extensions, see Table 5

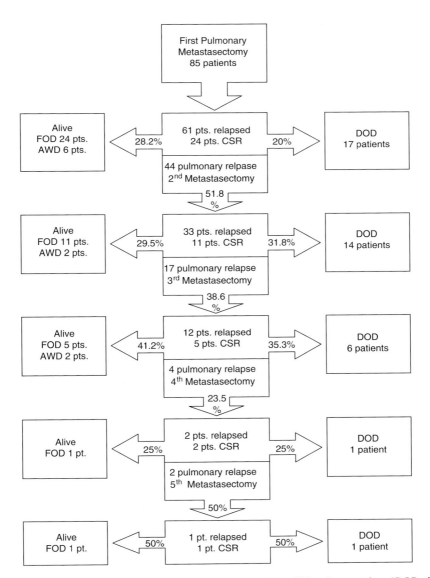

Fig. 12.7 Patients' outcome from first operation (metastasectomy) to fifth redo operation. (*DOD*, dead of disease; *FOD*, free of disease; *AWD*, alive with disease)

and the redo operation had to be delayed: 4 weeks postoperatively, an increasing left heart failure was reported. A CT scan showed the intrapericardial mass having grown considerably (Fig. 12.11), and the patient died before an emergency operation could be performed.

12.7 Discussion

12.7.1 The Reviewed Studies

In this review, a wide experience in treating osteosarcoma patients was collected comprising a time interval of about 70 years and more than 10,000 patients. Nevertheless, most studies show relatively few patients treated and even smaller numbers of patients treated with pulmonary metastases. A critical problem comparing the different studies relates to the interdisciplinary approach, which now is widely accepted in osteosarcoma therapy. For this reason, therapy is multifactorial and, furthermore, is changing multifactorially. Concerning oncological therapy, a wide variety of chemotherapy protocols has been used with different drug combinations and different concepts of adjuvancy or neo-adjuvancy, both factors influencing therapy of the primary tumour as well as metastases therapy. This is observed in many studies, which are conducted over a long period. Furthermore, most studies focus on osteosarcoma or metastases therapy from the point of view of (paediatric) oncologists or orthopaedic surgeons, and few reports exist from thoracic surgeons (Carter et al. 1991; Antunes et al. 1999; Pfannschmidt et al. 2005). This leads to a variety of descriptions of surgical procedures, ranging from "thoracotomy was performed" up to detailed information about the surgical manoeuvres.

The outcome of osteosarcoma patients in the studies of each generation, however, is well comparable. The overall survival of osteosarcoma

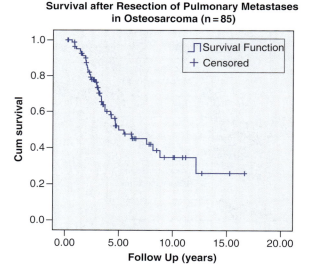

Fig. 12.8 Overall survival (Kaplan-Meier) in 85 patients with pulmonary metastases from the date of first operation

Survival after Resection of Primary Metastases and Pulmonary Relapse in Osteosacroma

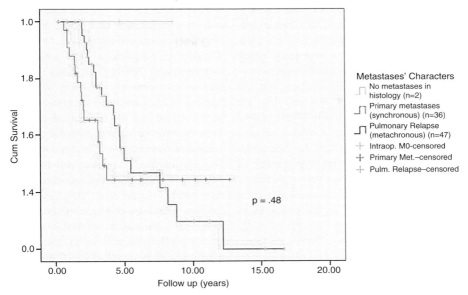

Fig. 12.9 Overall survival (Kaplan–Meier) in 85 patients with pulmonary metastases from the date of first operation presenting with metastases ($n=36$) or with pulmonary metastatic relapse($n=47$, pulmonary relapse only at time of presentation)

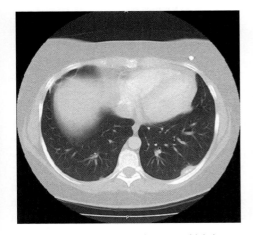

Fig. 12.10 Pericardial metastatic mass which intraoperatively was shown to be attached to the right infracardial caval angle. Resection from left-sided thoracotomy proved too risky by reason of uncontrollable bleeding. Right-sided thoracotomy was planned

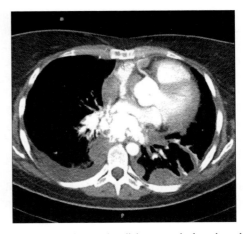

Fig. 12.11 The intrapericardial mass had enlarged 4 weeks after left-sided thoracotomy. Left ventricle failure occurred and the patient died of heart failure before an emergency operation could be done

patients in interdisciplinary concepts has widely exceeded the 50% margin and reached 80% under beneficial circumstances, whereas survival in metastasizing patients remains poor. Besides some very low survival rates, which probably derive from the era of inconsequent or lacking application of chemotherapy, survival rates show levels between 30% and 45% for 5 years. Some authors previously have discussed prognostic factors to avoid burdening surgical therapy or defining subgroups for aggressive therapy protocols. Concerning the therapy of pulmonary metastases there are only a few factors worthy of discussion here. The second part of this discussion addresses surgical principles in pulmonary metastasectomy.

12.7.2
Risk Factors Affecting Survival After Pulmonary Metastasectomy

The interest in defining risk factors that affect survival after pulmonary resection is widespread and has been reported since the first studies from early in the last century. However, the number of patients investigated in the subgroup of osteosarcoma with pulmonary metastases is very small. Single-centre studies have recruited 0.4 to 4.7 patients per year, and even national databases such as COSS, MIOS, and JMSOG, and national centres such as the Rizzoli Institute in Bologna, Italy could increase recruitment to 12–19 patients per year (see Table 12.3). Many studies report on prognostic factors that certainly reach statistical significance, but the study power remains poor because of the small numbers. Therefore, consequences from establishing prognostic factors remain difficult for statistical reasons (Bentzen 2001). Table 12.4 provides an overview of a selection of studies in patients with pulmonary metastases from 1971 to now, covering the chemotherapy era.

Complete surgical remission (CSR) is one of the most frequently investigated factors, depending highly on the number of nodules resected (or to be resected), the necessary extent of surgery and the completeness of surgical manoeuvres. From the first study (Martini et al. 1971) seen in this context, complete surgical remission has been evaluated. Although it seems not easy at first to determine completeness of resection, both radiological and histological radicality have been assessed and show statistical consistency. There has never been inconsistency about whether a patient without complete resection will survive. This phenomenon is documented in the latest studies with large numbers regarding all metastatic patients (Kager et al. 2003; Tsuchiya et al. 2002) or subgroups of patients (Kempf-Bielack et al. 2005; Briccoli et al. 2005), and it was already evaluated significant in one of the first statistically drawn evaluations (Putnam et al. 1983). Briccoli et al. (2005) do not explicitly evaluate the statistics concerning CSR, but using a large number (267) of metastasectomies they state that CSR is the precondition to survive, consistent with Tsuchiya et al. (2002) who had 248 patients. Statistical significance is (if given) in the range of .001 in most studies. Nevertheless, some doubts concerning the confirmation of completeness in radicality must be allowed. Surgical radicality always depends on a surgeon's operation report, and histological radicality can only confirm or deny positive resection margins. Therefore, radiological control of surgical radicality conducted by CT scans is essential. The quality of CT scans has improved enormously in the last 10 years, and hence the number of nodules detected has risen. It is unknown how reliable radiological control might have been 10 or 20 years ago.

Furthermore, there is no evidence about whether there is an increasing radicality in surgery from the early studies to now. Most studies with large numbers of patients have been conducted under the guidance of oncologists or paediatric oncologists (Bielack et al. 2002; Bacci et al. 2006). Therefore, it is not surprising that surgical details are often missing.

Comparing some early studies (up to the 1980s) with some modern studies and our own data, there is the impression that today fewer patients are declared inoperable, resection extents have become wider, and larger numbers of metastases have become resectable, at least partly as a merit of laser surgery.

The number of metastases has been a matter of interest since the study of Putnam et al. (1983) who described a decrease in survival with more than three metastases. They used a survival curve comparison using the Gehan–Wilcoxon test, which showed statistical significance when between three and four nodules are resected. Usually, the cut-off point for the number of nodules is not described. One study dealing with all types of pulmonary metastases resected by laser surgery used a statistical model to determine critical levels (Branscheid et al. 1992). Although in most studies the cut-off point changes between "more than one" (Kager et al. 2003) and six nodules or more (Meyer et al. 1987), larger studies confirm a correlation between an increasing number of nodules and decreased survival, as they do for the extent of metastasizing: pleural disruption (Kempf-Bielack et al. 2005), involvement of more than one lobe (Carter et al. 1991; Kaste et al. 1999) and the presence of bilateral metastases show statistical impact in some studies. However, for all these risk factors, studies also exist that deny statistical significance. This might be due to the small numbers in some studies and different statistical methods. Comparisons are computed with log rank tests on the one side and progressive regressions on the other side.

Nevertheless, suggestions that a larger or more aggressive mass of metastases influence survival are serious. It remains unclear whether the reason for this effect is found in the larger tumour burden, or if we should be concerned about tumours of different levels of aggressiveness.

The latter might be supported by some studies describing the disease-free interval (DFI) as a significant risk factor. Most often, the cut-off is set at 12 months after diagnosis or surgery. Studies investigating primary metastases (synchronous) versus pulmonary relapse (metachronous) do not produce different survival rates (Goorin et al. 1984; Meyer et al. 1987; Kaste et al. 1999; Briccoli et al. 2005). Significance is high in a single-centre experience with the cut-off at 12 or 18 months (Harting et al. 2006), as well as in two database investigations (Kempf-Bielack et al. 2005; Tsuchiya et al. 2002) that highly rate the importance of DFI and the fact that not performing metastasectomy is associated with a fivefold increase in the risk of death. Tsuchiya et al. (2002) find DFI subgroups affecting survival: group 1 presenting with metastases, group 2 developing metastases under first-line chemotherapy, group 3 developing metastases under adjuvant chemotherapy after surgery, and group 4 developing metastases after treatment has finished. Group 4 shows the best survival ($p<.0001$) after metastasectomy, followed by group 1. Hence, no different survival between these groups was seen in patients who for several reasons did not undergo metastasectomy ($n=15$). Good histological response in group 1 and group 4 showed significant impact on survival ($p<.0001$). This effect is not as evident in group 4 as in the others; however, 5-year survival after bad response was 20%–40% in group 4 (relapse after completed therapy).

12.7.3
Surgical Approach for Pulmonary Metastasectomy

Considering that incomplete surgical remission probably will prevent long-term survival after pulmonary metastasectomy, a surgeon has to take in account the phenomenon of unforeseeable, particularly contralateral presence of metastases. This has tremendous impact on the operative approach and surgical techniques. In the early studies deriving from the 1940s, diagnostics were X-ray pictures and conventional tomography, which remained the gold standard up to the beginning 1980s. CT scans became more important and currently are the gold standard for the diagnosis of pulmonary nodules. The problem of unforeseeable metastases both unilateral and contralateral is well known with the advent of conventional X-ray tomography. Putnam et al. (1983) have discussed this item broadly with the conclusion that more than 16 nodules suggest inoperability. Furthermore, the unforeseeable presence of bilateral metastases indicates a double-sided approach for which their recommendation is sternotomy, per Takita et al. (1977). Johnston (1983) reported on a number of unforeseen nodules in 53% of 46 patients operated for pulmonary metastases. In 61% of patients thought to have unilateral disease, contralateral nodules were found that proved to be metastatic.

Accuracy of CT scans has always been a matter of investigation and discussion. CT scans have not increased to good predictive value even with modern 16- to 64-line scanners. Su et al. (2004) saw a bilateral operation, either performed as sternotomy or as double-sided thoracotomy, as the procedure of choice. In 78% of cases, unforeseen contralateral nodules were detected. Picci et al. (2001) found a poor predictive value (53%) with the generation of CT scanners from the 1990s. The development of higher resolution scanners did not solve this problem. Kayton et al. (2006) report on a continuously poor correlation with a coefficient between .5 and .45 ($p<.001$) with an underestimation in 35% of patients. They therefore recommend bilateral exploring and avoiding minimally invasive techniques. The latter will be discussed below. In contrast, only a few studies recommend the unilateral operation, and only when no contralateral nodule is detected in CT scan (Younes et al. 2002). In our series, all patients without contraindication {previous operations, lung function severely damaged by AFM [Adriamycin (doxorubicin, Adria Laboratories, Columbus, OH), 5-fluorouracil and methotrexate] chemotherapy} were operated on bilaterally by sternotomy or sequential lateral thoracotomy within the same hospitalization or at least within 3 months. The unilateral approach was regarded sufficient when nodules did not prove to be metastases and a CT scan showed no contralateral manifestation. This showed strategic consistency with most reviewed studies.

12.7.4
A Place for Minimally Invasive Surgery (VATS)?

All surgically conducted studies agree that palpation of the whole lung or both lungs is necessary to identify all existing nodules because of poor predictive values of diagnostics. McCormack et al. (1996) reported a rate of 56% overseen metastases in patients with thoracoscopic resection preceding clearing thoracotomy. Kayton et al. (2006) agreed in their opinion that minimally invasive techniques should be avoided when complete surgical remission is intended. Studies evaluating the place of video-assisted thoracoscopic surgery (VATS) report high recurrence rates, which may arise from reduced radicality (Yim et al. 1995). A variation of the VATS procedure enabling palpation of the lung was reported by Mineo et al. (2001). A transxiphoidal incision is performed to manually palpate both lungs in one session. However, due to the size of VATS stapling devices, this approach will be limited to pleural and near pleural lesions.

12.8
Conclusions

All reviewed studies show that patients with lung metastases in osteosarcoma have no chance of long-term survival without thoracic surgery. Long-term survival is possible in any stage of metastatic relapse if surgery is performed, even after multiple redo operations.

It is obvious that complete surgical remission is the main prognostic factor for overall and event-free survival. The point in time when presenting metastases may play a certain role, but only shows a statistical tendency, is still unclear. Although the number and localization of metastases often do not show statistical relevance, the role of tumour burden also remains unclear.

Bilaterality of pulmonary metastases creates a demand for bilateral surgery. Even modern high-tech CT scans do not demonstrate complete reliability. Bilateral surgical exploration therefore is necessary to achieve complete surgical remission. Whether sternotomy favours sequential bilateral thoracotomy has yet to be investigated.

Minimally invasive approaches are not appropriate for pulmonary metastasectomy. Palpation of all existing lung tissue remains essential for complete surgical remission.

References

Antunes M, Bernardo J, Salete M, Prieto D, Eugenio L, Tavares P (1999) Excision of pulmonary metastases of osteogenic sarcoma of the limbs. Eur J Cardiothorac Surg 15:592–596

Bacci G, Briccoli A, Mercuri M, Ferrari S, Bertoni F, Gasbarrini A, Fabbri N, Cesari M, Forni C, Campanacci M (1998) Osteosarcoma of the extremities with synchronous lung metastases: long-term results in 4neoadjuvant chemotherapy. J Chemother 10:69–76

Bacci G, Longhi A, Versari M, Mercuri M, Briccoli A, Picci P (2006) Prognostic factors for osteosarcoma of the extremity treated with neoadjuvant chemotherapy: 15-year experience in 789 patients treated at a single institution. Cancer 106:1154–1161

Bentzen SM (2001) Prognostic factor studies in oncology: osteosarcoma as a clinical example. Int J Radiat Oncol Biol Phys 49:513–518

Bielack SS, Kempf-Bielack B, Delling G, Exner GU, Flege S, Helmke K, Kotz R, Salzer-Kuntschik M, Werner M, Winkelmann W, Zoubek A, Jurgens H, Winkler K (2002) Prognostic factors in high-grade osteosarcoma of the extremities or trunk: an analysis of 1,702 patients treated on neoadjuvant cooperative osteosarcoma study group protocols. J Clin Oncol 20:776–790

Boyer LA (1807) The lectures of Boyer upon diseases of the bone. Arr. by Richerand A, vol 1. John Callow Press, London

Branscheid D, Krysa S, Wollkopf G, Bulzebruck H, Probst G, Horn M, Schirren J, Vogt-Moykopf I (1992) Does ND-YAG laser extend the indications for resection of pulmonary metastases? Eur J Cardiothorac Surg 6:590–596

Briccoli A, Rocca M, Salone M, Bacci G, Ferrari S, Balladelli A, Mercuri M (2005) Resection of recurrent pulmonary metastases in patients with osteosarcoma. Cancer 104:1721–1725

Carter SR, Grimer RJ, Sneath RS, Matthews HR (1991) Results of thoracotomy in osteogenic sarcoma with pulmonary metastases. Thorax 46:727–731

Diemel KD, Branscheid D, Goretzki PE (2006) Techniken der Thoraxchirurgie: Lunge und Bronchien. In: Becker H, Encke A, Röher HD (eds) Viszeralchirurgie, 2nd edn. Urban and Fischer, München

Divis G (1927) Ein Beitrag zur operativen Behandlung der Lungengeschwülste. Acta Chir Scand 62:329–334

Edlich RF, Shea MA, Foker JE, Grondin C, Castaneda AR, Varco RL (1966) A review of 26 years' experience with pulmonary resection for metastatic cancer. Dis Chest 49:587–594

Edwards AT (1934) Malignant disease of the lung. J Thorac Surg 4:107–124

Eve FS (1883) Lectures on cystic tumors of the jaws and on the etiology, general characters and relations of tumours. Br Med J 1:241–243

Goorin AM, Delorey MJ, Lack EE, Gelber RD, Price K, Cassady JR, Levey R, Tapper D, Jaffe N, Link M, et al (1984) Prognostic significance of complete surgical resection of pulmonary metastases in patients with osteogenic sarcoma: analysis of 32 patients. J Clin Oncol 2:425–431

Goorin AM, Shuster JJ, Baker A, Horowitz ME, Meyer WH, Link MP (1991) Changing pattern of pulmonary metastases with adjuvant chemotherapy in patients with osteosarcoma: results from the multiinstitutional osteosarcoma study. J Clin Oncol 9:600–605

Gordon N, Koshkina NV, Jia SF, Khanna C, Mendoza A, Worth LL, Kleinerman ES (2007) Corruption of the Fas pathway delays the pulmonary clearance of murine osteosarcoma cells, enhances their metastatic potential, and reduces the effect of aerosol gemcitabine. Clin Cancer Res 13:4503–4510

Harting MT, Blakely ML, Jaffe N, Cox CS, Hayes-Jordan A, Benjamin RS, Raymond AK, Andrassy RJ, Lally KP (2006) Long-term survival after aggressive resection of pulmonary metastases among children and adolescents with osteosarcoma. J Pediatr Surg 41:194–199

Heitmiller RF, Marasco WJ, Hruban RH, Marsh BR (1993) Endobronchial metastasis. J Thorac Cardiovasc Surg 106:537–542

Huth JF, Eilber FR (1989) Patterns of recurrence after resection of osteosarcoma of the extremity. Strategies for treatment of metastases. Arch Surg 124:122–126

Johnston MR (1983) Median sternotomy for resection of pulmonary metastases. J Thorac Cardiovasc Surg 85:516–522

Kager L, Zoubek A, Potschger U, Kastner U, Flege S, Kempf-Bielack B, Branscheid D, Kotz R, Salzer-Kuntschik M, Winkelmann W, Jundt G, Kabisch H, Reichardt P, Jurgens H, Gadner H, Bielack SS (2003) Primary metastatic osteosarcoma: presentation and outcome of patients treated on neoadjuvant Cooperative Osteosarcoma Study Group protocols. J Clin Oncol 21:2011–2018

Kaste SC, Pratt CB, Cain AM, Jones-Wallace DJ, Rao BN (1999) Metastases detected at the time of diagnosis of primary pediatric extremity osteosarcoma at diagnosis: imaging features. Cancer 86:1602–1608

Kayton ML, Huvos AG, Casher J, Abramson SJ, Rosen NS, Wexler LH, Meyers P, LaQuaglia MP (2006) Computed tomographic scan of the chest underestimates the number of metastatic lesions in osteosarcoma. J Pediatr Surg 41:200–206

Kempf-Bielack B, Bielack SS, Jurgens H, Branscheid D, Berdel WE, Exner GU, Gobel U, Helmke K, Jundt G, Kabisch H, Kevric M, Klingebiel T, Kotz R, Maas R, Schwarz R, Semik M, Treuner J, Zoubek A, Winkler K (2005) Osteosarcoma relapse after combined modality therapy: an analysis of unselected patients in the Cooperative Osteosarcoma Study Group (COSS). J Clin Oncol 23:559–568

Khanna C, Prehn J, Yeung C, Caylor J, Tsokos M, Helman L (2000) An orthotopic model of murine osteosarcoma with clonally related variants differing in pulmonary metastatic potential. Clin Exp Metastasis 18:261–271

Krönlein RU (1884) Über Lungenchirurgie. Berl Klin Wochenschrift 21:129–32

Koshkina NV, Khanna C, Mendoza A, Guan H, DeLauter L, Kleinerman ES (2007) Fas-negative osteosarcoma tumor cells are selected during metastasis to the lungs: the role of the Fas pathway in the metastatic process of osteosarcoma. Mol Cancer Res 5:991–999

Macewen W (1886) Carcinoma in its pathological and aetiological aspects with remarks on the principles of its surgical treatment. Glasgow Med J 25:271–291

Mannix EP (1953) Resection of multiple pulmonary metastases fourteen years after amputation for osteochondrogenic sarcoma of tibia; apparent freedom from recurrence two years later. J Thorac Surg 26:544–549

Marcove RC, Martini N, Rosen G (1975) The treatment of pulmonary metastasis in osteogenic sarcoma. Clin Orthop Relat Res 111:65–70

Martini N, Huvos AG, Mike V, Marcove RC, Beattie EJ Jr (1971) Multiple pulmonary resections in the treatment of osteogenic sarcoma. Ann Thorac Surg 12:271–280

McCormack PM, Bains MS, Begg CB, Burt ME, Downey RJ, Panicek DM, Rusch VW, Zakowski M, Ginsberg RJ (1996) Role of video-assisted thoracic surgery in the treatment of pulmonary metastases: results of a prospective trial. Ann Thorac Surg 62:213–216

Meyer WH, Schell MJ, Kumar AP, Rao BN, Green AA, Champion J, Pratt CB (1987) Thoracotomy for pulmonary metastatic osteosarcoma. An analysis of prognostic indicators of survival. Cancer 59:374–379

Meyers PA, Heller G, Healey JH, Huvos A, Applewhite A, Sun M, LaQuaglia M (1993) Osteogenic sarcoma with clinically detectable metastasis at initial presentation. J Clin Oncol 11:449–453

Mineo TC, Ambrogi V, Paci M, Iavicoli N, Pompeo E, Nofroni I (2001) Transxiphoid bilateral palpation in video-assisted thoracoscopic lung metastasectomy. Arch Surg 136:783–788

Mogulkoc N, Goker E, Atasever A, Veral A, Ozkok S, Bishop PW (1999) Endobronchial metastasis from osteosarcoma of bone: treatment with intraluminal radiotherapy. Chest 116:1811–1814

Morrow CE, Vassilopoulos PP, Grage TB (1980) Surgical resection for metastatic neoplasms of the lung: experience at the University of Minnesota Hospitals. Cancer 45:2981–2985

Morton DL, Joseph WL, Ketcham AS, Geelhoed GW, Adkins PC (1973) Surgical resection and adjunctive immunotherapy for selected patients with multiple pulmonary metastases. Ann Surg 178:360–366

Parham FW (1898) Thoracic resection for tumours growing from the bony wall of the chest. Trans South Surg Assoc 11:223–363

Pastorino U, Buyse M, Friedel G, Ginsberg RJ, Girard P, Goldstraw P, Johnston M, McCormack P, Pass H, Putnam JB (1997) Long-term results of lung metastasectomy: prognostic analyses based on 5206 cases. The International Registry of Lung Metastases. J Thorac Cardiovasc Surg 113:37–49

Pevarski DJ, Drane WE, Scarborough MT (1998) The usefulness of bone scintigraphy with SPECT images for detection of pulmonary metastases from osteosarcoma. AJR Am J Roentgenol 170: 319–322

Pfannschmidt J, Klode J, Muley T, Hoffmann H, Dienemann H (2006) Pulmonary resection for metastatic osteosarcomas: a retrospective analysis of 21 patients. Thorac Cardiovasc Surg 54: 120–123

Picci P, Vanel D, Briccoli A, Talle K, Haakenaasen U, Malaguti C, Monti C, Ferrari C, Bacci G, Saeter G, Alvegard TA (2001) Computed tomography of pulmonary metastases from osteosarcoma: the less poor technique. A study of 51 patients with histological correlation. Ann Oncol 12:1601–1604

Putnam JB, Roth JA, Wesley MN, Johnston MR, Rosenberg SA (1983) Survival following aggressive resection of pulmonary metastases from osteogenic sarcoma: analysis of prognostic factors. Ann Thorac Surg 36:516–523

Quénu, Longuet (1898) Des tumeurs du squelette thoracique. Rév Chir 15:396

Récamier JCA (1829) Récherches sur le traitement du cancer. Paris

Rolle A, Pereszlenyi A, Koch R, Bis B, Baier B (2006) Laser resection technique and results of multiple lung metastasectomies using a new 1,318 nm Nd:YAG laser system. Lasers Surg Med 38:26–32

Saltzman DA, Snyder CL, Ferrell KL, Thompson RC, Leonard AS (1993) Aggressive metastasectomy for pulmonic sarcomatous metastases: a follow-up study. Am J Surg 166:543–547

Seydel (1909) Über Operabilität von Lungen und Pleuratumoren. Munch Med Wochenschr 59:452–459

Su WT, Chewning J, Abramson S, Rosen N, Gholizadeh M, Healey J, Meyers P, La Quaglia MP (2004) Surgical management and outcome of osteosarcoma patients with unilateral pulmonary metastases. J Pediatr Surg 39:418–423

Takita H, Merrin C, Didolkar MS, Douglass HO, Edgerton F (1977) The surgical management of multiple lung metastases. Ann Thorac Surg 24:359–364

Thomford NR, Woolner LB, Clagett OT (1965) The surgical treatment of metastatic tumors in the lungs. J Thorac Cardiovasc Surg 49:357–363

Thompson RC, Cheng EY, Clohisy DR, Perentesis J, Manivel C, Le CT (2002) Results of treatment for metastatic osteosarcoma with neoadjuvant chemotherapy and surgery. Clin Orthop Relat Res 397:240–247

Tofuku K, Yokouchi M, Murayama T, Minami S, Komiya S (2006) HAS3-related hyaluronan enhances biological activities necessary for metastasis of osteosarcoma cells. Int J Oncol 29: 175–183

Torek F (1930) Removal of metastatic carcinoma of the lung and mediastinum. Arch Surg 21: 1416–1424

Tsuchiya H, Kanazawa Y, Abdel-Wanis ME, Asada N, Abe S, Isu K, Sugita T, Tomita K (2002) Effect of timing of pulmonary metastases identification on prognosis of patients with osteosarcoma: the Japanese Musculoskeletal Oncology Group study. J Clin Oncol 20:3470–3477

Vogt-Moykopf I, Fritz T, Meyer G, Bulzerbruck H, Daskos G (1986) Bronchoplastic and angioplastic operation in bronchial carcinoma: long-term results of a retrospective analysis from 1973 to 1983. Int Surg 71:211–220

Walshe WH (1846) The nature and treatment of cancer. Taylor and Walton, London

Ward WG, Mikaelian K, Dorey F, Mirra JM, Sassoon A, Holmes EC, Eilber FR, Eckardt JJ (1994)

Pulmonary metastases of stage IIB extremity osteosarcoma and subsequent pulmonary metastases. J Clin Oncol 12:1849–1858

Weinlechner K (1882) Zur Kasuistik der Tumoren ander Brustwand und deren Behandlung. Wien Med Wochenschr 32:590–591; 624–628

Winkler K, Beron G, Schellong G, Stollmann B, Prindull G, Lasson U, Brandeis W, Henze G, Ritter J, Russe W, Stengel-Rutkowski L, Treuner J, Landbeck G (1982) Kooperative Osteosarkomstudie COSS-77: Ergebnisse nach über 4 Jahren. Klin Padiatr 194:251–256

Yim AP, Lin J, Chan AT, Li CK, Ho JK (1995) Video-assisted thoracoscopic wedge resections of pulmonary metastatic osteosarcoma: should it be performed? Aust N Z J Surg 65:737–739

Younes RN, Gross JL, Deheinzelin D (2002) Surgical resection of unilateral lung metastases: is bilateral thoracotomy necessary? World J Surg 26:1112–1116

Part III
Soft Tissue Sarcomas

Standardized Approach to the Treatment of Adult Soft Tissue Sarcoma of the Extremities

Per-Ulf Tunn, Christoph Kettelhack, and Hans Roland Dürr

Abstract Soft tissue sarcomas are very rare tumors. Available data are based on only a few prospective randomized trials. Most studies are retrospective, reviewing the results of single institutions. Furthermore, universally accepted treatment protocols for adult patients are lacking. Several prognostic factors have been identified, including grading, tumor size and development of metastatic disease; however, the relevance of other important aspects in the treatment of patients with soft tissue sarcomas remains unknown or subject to controversy. The main issues concern: which surgical margin width is safe from an oncological perspective? Does local recurrence influence survival? Can systemic chemotherapy improve prognosis? Is radiotherapy necessary in every case? Should it be applied pre-, post- or intraoperatively? What is the value of assessing the response after neoadjuvant therapy? These topics are examined in this review.

Per-Ulf Tunn (✉)
Department of Orthopaedic Oncology
Sarkomzentrum Berlin-Brandenburg
Helios Klinikum Berlin-Buch
Schwanebecker Chaussee 50
13125 Berlin, Germany
E-mail: per-ulf.tunn@helios-kliniken.de

Abbreviations

AJCC	American Joint Committee on Cancer
CNB	Core needle biopsy
CT	Computer tomography
EIA	Etoposide, ifofamide, adriamycin
EORTC	European Organisation for Research and Treatment of Cancer
FNA	Fine needle aspiration biopsy
Gy	Gray
ILP	Isolated limb perfusion
IORT	Intraoperative radiation therapy
MRI	Magnetic resonance imaging
MRS	Magnetic resonance spectroscopy
31P-MRS	^{31}Phosphorus-magnetic resonance spectroscopy
MSKCC	Memorial Sloan-Kettering Cancer Center
NCI	National Cancer Institute
PET	Positron emission tomography

18-FDG-PET	18-Fluorodeoxyglucose-positron emission tomography
RHT	Regional hyperthermia
RT	Radiotherapy
STS	Soft tissue sarcoma
SUV	Standard uptake value
TNF-α	Tumor necrosis factor-alpha
UICC	Union Internationale Contre Cancer

13.1
Introduction

Soft tissue sarcomas (STS) are rare, representing 1%–2% of all malignant neoplasms in adulthood. There are approximately 8,300 new cases in the United States annually, 1,800 in Great Britain and 2,200 in Germany. The sex distribution is almost equal with a slight dominance in males. The tumors are more common in the second half of life [17, 23, 34, 46, 62]. More than 50 subgroups can be distinguished immunohistologically [27, 28]; liposarcoma is the most frequent type, comprising approximately 20% of all soft tissue sarcomas.

At the time of primary diagnosis, about 30% of the patients have stage I disease (UICC 2003), a further 30% have stage II, 20% have stage III and 20% have stage IV disease [72]. In general, soft tissue sarcomas can be treated curatively with R0 resection in stages I–III. The surgical resection in combination with radiotherapy constitutes the basic treatment of localized high-grade sarcomas. Compartmental resections (for intracompartmental tumors) and wide resections (for extracompartmental tumors) are predominantly applied. Neoadjuvant concepts (e.g. radiotherapy, isolated limb perfusion and systemic chemotherapy with or without regional hyperthermia) should be considered for locally advanced tumors when achieving a primary R0 resection is uncertain. These modalities have the goal of local tumor remission, in order to provide more favourable conditions for the subsequent resection. Primary surgical therapy is performed in about 45% of patients with soft tissue sarcoma, up to 35% undergo neoadjuvant therapy with subsequent resection and approximately 20% receive palliative systemic therapy due to the presence of metastatic disease at first diagnosis. Taking into account the available multimodal treatment approaches, limb-preserving surgery is feasible in well over 80% of patients.

Several retrospective studies have shown that grading, tumor size, deep tumor location and the presence of metastasis are independent prognostic factors in multivariate analysis [12, 24, 44, 66, 73, 82]. Due to the rarity of soft tissue sarcomas there are only a few prospective randomized studies available, so that the relevance of many clinical issues remains unknown or subject to controversy. The most common topics are going to be addressed and analyzed in this review.

13.2
Biopsy Techniques

If a soft tissue sarcoma is suspected clinically and on imaging, histopathological confirmation of the diagnosis prior to definite treatment is the logical consequence. An exception to this rule pose superficially located tumors up to 3 cm in size that can be completely (R0) resected by primary surgery without functional deficits. Representative tumor tissue can be obtained by means of image-guided fine-needle aspiration biopsy (FNA), core needle biopsy (CNB) or incisional biopsy [30, 33, 58].

FNA is the least invasive method; an accurate diagnosis is feasible in 72% of cases [1]. The probability of a correct diagnosis rises to over 90% with CNB [1, 16], though these results could be obtained only in tumor centres and were only reproducible there. Employing this imaging-guided technique to confirm diagnosis is reasonable particularly in the case of large, very heterogeneous or retroperitoneal-located tumors.

Incisional biopsy provides several advantages. It yields the highest volume of tumor, and along with preserving tissue for the tumor bank (e.g. for molecular genetic diagnostics) it also enables intraoperative frozen section analysis. The disadvantage of incisional biopsy by definition is the invasiveness of the procedure.

Both open biopsy and minimally invasive methods must be carefully planned to obtain diagnosis without complicating subsequent tumor resection. In summary, the following recommendations for obtaining tissue can be made depending on the presence of primary tumor versus recurrence:

A. Histological confirmation of the primary tumor using either

- Ultrasound-/CT-/MRI-guided CNB, possibly insufficient regarding grading and typing
- Open incisional biopsy

B. Histological confirmation of local recurrence

- Ultrasound-/CT-/MRI-guided CNB or FNA biopsy, usually sufficient combined with a documented diagnosis of the primary tumor

The biopsy must be planned in co-operation with the surgical/orthopaedic oncologist so that the tumor is reached by the shortest route and definitive tumor resection is not impeded. Open biopsies in the limbs are performed with a longitudinal skin incision with no exceptions. Careful haemostasis and the placement of a wound drain are obligatory, in order to avoid ecchymosis resulting in the spread of tumor cells. The skin should be closed with an intracutaneous suture. When core biopsies are performed, a precise anatomical description or, even better, a marking of the biopsy tract on the skin is essential to ensure that the tract can later be included in the resected specimen during definitive tumor resection, which is occasionally delayed by neoadjuvant treatment [72].

13.3 Surgical Therapy in Soft Tissue Sarcoma: General Principles

Surgical therapy forms the basis of local tumor control of soft tissue sarcomas. The treatment strategy is essentially determined by the tumor stage and location. The defined aim is R0 resection with a good functional outcome. Ablative procedures can be justified only if all multimodal treatment options have been exhausted, and in these cases obtaining a second opinion is strongly advised. With the exception of superficially located tumors with a longitudinal diameter of up to 3 cm, where a primary wide resection is feasible without functional impairment, a valid histological confirmation prior to local surgical treatment is imperative [34, 46].

Regardless of the resection technique, the R0 situation must always be striven for in curative treatment modalities (Table 13.1). In order for this to be accomplished, the resection always incorporates the biopsy and drain tract. Compartmental resection or, more often, functional compartmental resection is applied for intracompartmental soft

Table 13.1 Definition of the R-classification for soft tissue sarcomas

R0	The surgical margins are macroscopically and microscopically negative for tumor cells
R1	A surgical margin is microscopically contaminated with tumor cells or the tumor was marginally resected along its pseudocapsule
R2	An intralesional tumor resection was performed

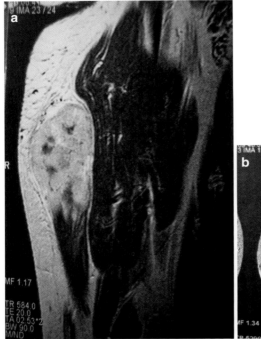
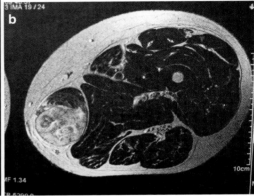

Fig. 13.1 a,b MRI of a dedifferentiated liposarcoma of the left thigh, localized within the gracilis muscle. Optimal surgical treatment consists of functional compartmental resection

tissue sarcomas. When performing a functional compartmental resection the affected muscle compartment is not removed from the insertion to the origin; allowing for a muscular safety margin, the muscle stumps can be preserved in case of smaller sarcomas, resulting in a better functional outcome. Compartmental resection, i.e. resection of a muscle or a muscle group from its origin to its insertion, is only necessary when the tumor contaminates the entire compartment.

The surgical treatment of choice for extra-compartmental-located soft tissue sarcomas is wide resection. R0 resections can usually be achieved by co-resecting a layer of healthy tissue (e.g. muscle fascia, periosteum, bone lamella, epineurium or vessel adventitia), occasionally with the aid of neoadjuvant treatment modalities.

So far there has been no evidence-based and clinically comprehensible definition of the term "wide resection". The question is not so much what is "wide" as what is "safe" from an oncologic perspective. For clinical practice, the R-classification is currently the most useful to facilitate comparison of surgical outcome, regardless of whether the tumor is located intra- or extracompartmentally. Marginal (along the tumor pseudocapsule) or even intralesional resections are oncologically inadequate and usually cannot be compensated for by additional treatment modalities [78].

Primary tumor resection in adults is the treatment of choice when distant metastases are undetectable and R0 resection with preservation of a functional limb is deemed feasible (Fig. 13.1). Should a primary R0 resection be impossible or achievable only by means of amputation, a neoadjuvant treatment (radiation therapy, systemic chemotherapy, isolated limb perfusion) ought to be recommended with the objective of local tumor remission and subsequent limb-sparing surgery (Fig. 13.2).

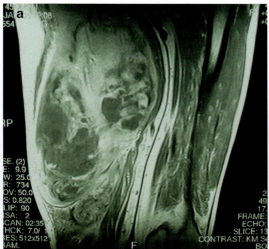
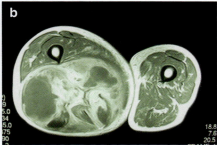

Fig. 13.2 a,b MRI of a locally advanced myxofibrosarcoma in the posterior compartment of the thigh. Due to the size and location of the tumor, neoadjuvant treatment is necessary prior to surgical resection

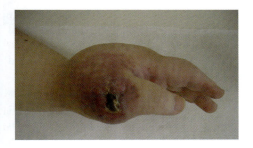

Fig. 13.3 Clinical presentation of a locally recurrent and exulcerated angiosarcoma of the left thumb. Amputation is the only surgical option available

An ablative procedure can be performed with curative or palliative intent. The former is the case when R0 resection cannot be achieved even when neoadjuvant treatment modalities are applied. The cause could be tumor infiltration of joints, several compartments, nerves, etc., leaving behind a non-functioning limb or limb segment after R0 resection (Fig. 13.3). Tumor ulceration, intractable pain, uncontrollable tumor bleeding, imminent sepsis or the goal of improving care and quality of life can justify amputation with palliative intent.

13.3.1
The Influence of Surgical Margins

Many textbooks still advocate the need to obtain a 2- to 3cm surgical margin width in all directions when resecting a soft tissue sarcoma. On the one hand this postulation has never been scientifically proved, while every orthopaedic and surgical oncologist actually performing such resections knows that this requirement would lead to an increase of ablative surgical procedures. Luckily, this is not true. The absolute metric width of the surgical margin is not as important as oncological safety. Is a safety margin of 1 cm inside a muscle, or a subcutaneous fat tissue layer of 2 cm comparable to an intact muscle fascia of less then 1 mm over a soft tissue sarcoma [15]? This question has yet to be definitely answered.

McKee et al. found better local recurrence-free survival rates with a safety distance of >10 mm compared to surgical margin widths of 0 mm and 1–9 mm in a cohort of 111 patients [47]. However, no significant difference regarding distant metastasis-free and overall survival could be shown between the patient groups. The authors concluded that a surgical margin of >10 mm was sufficient in terms of local control for patients with soft tissue sarcomas.

Gronchi et al. studied a series of 911 patients with soft tissue sarcomas and found that surgical margin status (R0 vs R1) was no independent prognostic factor ($p=0.338$) in multivariate analysis, compared to tumor size, grade, depth, histotype and the presence of local recurrence [23].

Contrary to that, Pisters et al. demonstrated in a prospectively collected database of 1,041 adult patients that microscopically positive surgical margins constitute an adverse prognostic factor [53]. Stojadinovic et al. produced similar results in a retrospective analysis of 2,084 patients [66], with an overall 5-year disease-specific survival rate of 83% for negative margins compared to 75% for positive margins ($p<0.001$). The local recurrence rate amounted to 15% for negative and 28% for positive margins. Furthermore, Baldini et al. showed in a series of 74 patients with primary soft tissue sarcoma of the extremities and trunk a 10-year local control rate of 87% for a negative surgical margin width of less than 1 cm, compared to 100% for a margin width of ≥1 cm, although one should take into account that more than half of the patients had grade I tumors [4].

A further issue concerns the prognostic influence of preoperative radiotherapy in regards to surgical margins. Sadoski et al. found in a series of 132 irradiated patients that the 5-year local control rate in patients presenting with primary tumors was 83% for positive margins and 97% for negative margins [63]. For margin widths equal to or less than 1 mm the rate amounted to 96%, compared to 97% for margin widths exceeding 1 mm. Tanabe et al. also came to the conclusion that local control following preoperative radiotherapy is significantly better with negative surgical margins ($p=0.005$), whereas overall survival is not influenced ($p=0.90$) [67].

In summary, there are no studies so far which can define an oncological safe surgical margin width; currently the R-classification is best suited to fulfil clinical needs in routine practice.

13.3.2
The Influence of an Unplanned Excision

Soft tissue sarcomas are often treated surgically having been mistaken by the treating physician for benign soft tissue tumors. In an analysis of a regional database in France, only 7% of the patients primarily treated for sarcoma were preoperatively evaluated by a multidisciplinary team [59]. Of the patients, 74% were resected without clear margins. Similar data were presented from an audit in the Trent region in the UK [21]. Only 15% of the patients were referred to a sarcoma specialist. The most common misdiagnoses included lipomas, fibromas and haematomas. Accordingly, an adequate primary diagnostic workup was lacking in most cases; patient and surgeon both were subsequently "surprised" by the result of the histopathological examination.

The surgical reports after an unplanned excision typically describe dissections or enucleations along the tumor capsule. As this is only a pseudocapsule along the margin of soft tissue sarcomas [78], tumor tissue is left behind in up to 65% of the cases (Table 13.2). As a result, secondary wide or compartmental resection, depending on the tumor location, is necessary after completion of staging. Several articles have also confirmed the logically expected relation between grading and the frequency of residual tumor.

Patients with secondary resection of a soft tissue sarcoma demonstrate similar or even improved local recurrence rates compared to patients with primary R0 resection [65]. A detailed analysis of local recurrence-free and overall survival was performed in a series of 1,092 patients of MSKCC, examining the impact of secondary resection after inadequate primary excision of a soft tissue sarcoma. Of the patients, 685 had been referred before any surgical treatment and subsequently underwent only one therapeutic operation at MSKCC (resection group), while 407 patients had been referred after undergoing excision without planned wide margins before referral and subsequently underwent a re-resection at MSKCC (re-resection group) [43]. The results are surprising and need to be put into the overall context, so as not to draw incorrect conclusions. The 5-year survival rate for the resection group was 70% versus 88% for the re-resection group. However, there were significantly more patients with T2b tumors in the first group. In multivariate analysis both grading ($p<0.0001$) and tumor size ($p<0.001$) proved to be decisive prognostic factors for disease-specific survival. After adjusting for factors predictive of outcome, such as grading, size, location and R classification, secondary resection after inadequate primary excision remained an independent positive predictor for survival ($p<0.005$). This observation applied for all AJCC stages. The authors could not provide a clear explanation for their findings, suggesting that they unwittingly selected a more favourable group; and yet their analysis could not confirm this.

Any interpretation of these results should take into account that the patients in the re-resection group were referred to a highly specialized center. The combination of wide secondary resection by an experienced team, adjuvant radiotherapy and occasionally chemotherapy led to a particularly favourable outcome. On no account may these observations support incomplete primary surgery without local imaging and histological confirmation for soft tissue tumors suspicious for malignancy. This approach can only be justified for small, superficially located tumors, resected with the intent of an excisional biopsy with adequate drainage and no contamination of surrounding layers of tissue. After an unplanned or inadequate resection of a soft tissue sarcoma, the previous operation field should be secondarily widely resected. Any seroma or haematoma cavities must remain closed.

Kepka et al. examined the results of radiation therapy alone in 72 patients, in whom re-resection after unplanned excision of a soft tissue sarcoma was not performed due to various causes [36]. The mean radiation dose given was 66 Gy. The 5-year local control rate amounted to 88%, although 10 cases of major radiotherapy complications were observed.

In conclusion, re-resection is the treatment of choice after prior unplanned excision. If this can only be achieved by means of an ablative

Table 13.2 Clinical outcome after re-resection due to an inadequate/unplanned excision of a soft tissue sarcoma

Author	No. of pat. (n)	Residual tumor (%)	R1-resection (%)	Rate of local recurrence (5 years) (%)
Fiore et al. 2006 [20]	318	24	-	18.7
Rougraff et al. 2005 [60]	106	65	-	11 (superficial tumors)
Goodland et al. 1996 [22]	95	59	17	-
Zornig et al. 1995 [84]	67	45	13	7
Davis et al. 1997 [11]	104	40	-	38
Noria et al. 1996 [50]	65	35	9	22
Lewis et al. 2000 [43]	407	39	9	14
Siebenrock et al. 2000 [65]	16	63	10	19
Zagars et al. 2003 [82]	295	46	12	15

procedure, neoadjuvant treatment protocols or radiation therapy alone could be applied.

13.3.3
The Influence of Local Recurrence

Whether a local recurrence after previous R0 resection of soft tissue sarcoma is an independent prognostic factor or merely another aspect of a highly malignant and locally aggressive tumor with no prognostic significance in multivariate analysis is subject to debate. There is a higher rate for local relapse within 2 years after completion of primary treatment; 65% of all local failures occur in this interval, while 90% occur within 4 years [17]. Expectedly, the local recurrence rates after R1 resection are significantly higher than those after R0 resection despite adjuvant treatment modalities; and have been correlated with a worse prognosis as well [23]. Lewis et al. also demonstrated in a retrospective study of 911 patients that local recurrence of high-grade soft tissue sarcoma was significantly associated both with a higher rate of distant metastasis ($p = 0.005$) and with an increase of disease-specific mortality ($p = 0.007$) [44].

Contrary to that, local relapse was not believed to influence overall survival in the 1980s [60]. In retrospect, the limited number of patients ($n = 27$) in this study was probably the main reason for the false conclusion. Subsequently, several larger studies analysed the prognostic impact of local recurrence on disease-specific survival. In 1997 Ueda et al. showed in a retrospective study that local relapse significantly worsens prognosis ($p = 0.006$) [73]. Another recent study of Gronchi et al. further validated the negative prognostic significance of local recurrence [24]. The authors showed that the 10-year disease-specific mortality rate amounted to 22% in the absence of local failure compared to up to 54% for patients with a local relapse. Should the surgical treatment of a local recurrence result in an R1 resection, the risk for a re-recurrence has been found to be significantly higher ($p = 0.004$), leading in turn to a further worsening of prognosis [49].

In conclusion, local recurrence is an independent negative prognostic factor, associated with a decrease in overall survival as a result of a higher risk of distant metastasis. The surgical treatment of a local recurrence should be based on the same principles that apply to the treatment of the primary tumor, although most cases are complicated by unfavourable local conditions, particularly when a local recurrence develops inside or around a radiation field, after isolated limb perfusion or following plastic reconstruction. Higher rates of local complications and a higher proportion of ablative procedures compared to the surgical treatment of the primary tumor should be expected in such cases [70].

13.4
Neoadjuvant and Adjuvant Treatment Modalities in Soft Tissue Sarcoma

Neoadjuvant therapy is a valuable option that should always be implemented in cases of locally advanced tumors. It aims at the devitalization of the tumor, in order to facilitate limb salvage with improved local tumor control. Tumor response is evaluated by histological examination after surgical resection.

Several neoadjuvant treatment modalities have been clinically validated; radiation therapy [10, 52, 57, 63, 79], isolated hyperthermic limb perfusion with TNF-α and melphalan [26, 42] and systemic chemotherapy with or without regional hyperthermia in the context of study protocols (e.g. EORTC protocols) for extremity soft tissue sarcomas and radiation therapy for retroperitoneal sarcomas and sarcomas of the trunk [31, 68]. On the other hand, published data on the surgical procedures and surgical treatment outcomes after neoadjuvant therapy are rather scarce; there are no persuasive data from randomized studies showing a benefit in terms of overall survival for patients treated with neoadjuvant therapy. Furthermore, whether the extent of the tumor resection can be adjusted to the response of the tumor has yet to be clarified. To complicate matters further, most multimodal treatment studies were only designed as phase II trials for locally advanced soft tissue sarcomas [13, 25, 39, 55].

13.4.1
The Role of Systemic Chemotherapy

Systemic chemotherapy has been established in the treatment of soft tissue sarcomas in children and adolescents, in the setting of therapy optimization studies [17, 48]. In adulthood, systemic chemotherapy of highly malignant soft tissue sarcomas remains a subject of clinical studies. So far there is no consensus on the patients, the stage (with the exception of stage IV) and the tumor entities that would primarily benefit from systemic chemotherapy. Randomized trials examining the effect of chemotherapy on STS have produced conflicting results. Several factors, for instance older patient age, significant comorbidities, etc., could provide a plausible explanation for this inconsistency. Despite all this, response rates around 30%–42% have been recorded [18, 19, 25, 39].

Data regarding neoadjuvant chemotherapy for adult soft tissue sarcoma are based on only a few prospective, randomized, multicenter trials. Most studies are retrospective, so that binding guidelines are lacking. The "MAID"-study [13], published in 2003, analysed 48 patients who received three cycles of neoadjuvant chemotherapy with mesna, adriamycin, ifosfamide and dacarbazine combined with 44 Gy of radiotherapy, followed by surgery. Another three cycles were administered postoperatively, while further 16 Gy were delivered to patients with positive surgical margins. Outcome was compared with the data of a historical control group of 48 patients, matched for tumor size, grade, age and era of treatment. Statistical analysis revealed an improved overall survival ($p=0.0003$) and disease-free survival ($p=0.0016$) for the patients who received neoadjuvant chemotherapy and radiotherapy, while the increase in 5-year actuarial local control rate wasn't significant. Since this study was neither prospective nor randomized, the results provide little help for clinical practice. Furthermore, one should not ignore the fact that 29% of the patients in the MAID group developed wound healing complications and 25% febrile neutropenia.

Issels et al. recently demonstrated in a multi-institutional trial of the EORTC (EORTC 62961/ESHO-RHT 95-study) a positive impact of regional hyperthermia (RHT) combined with neoadjuvant systemic chemotherapy consisting of etoposide, ifosfamide and adriamycin (EIA) in the treatment of high-risk soft tissue sarcomas in adults, compared to chemotherapy alone, for the first time in the context of a phase III trial [31, 32]. Recruited for this study between 1997 and 2007 were 341 patients; 169 were randomly assigned to receive systemic chemotherapy combined with regional hyperthermia (EIA+RHT), while 172 patients were treated with EIA alone, both prior to and after local aggressive treatment with surgery and radiotherapy. Analysis showed that, compared to chemotherapy alone, regional hyperthermia combined with chemotherapy leads to a statistically significant improvement in tumor response ($p=0.002$), disease-free survival ($p=0.003$) and local progression-free survival ($p=0.015$) in patients with locally advanced, high-grade STS.

In 1988 Chang et al. reported the results of applying adjuvant chemotherapy in patients with high-grade extremity soft tissue sarcomas, in the setting of a prospective, randomized study of the NCI [9]. The outcome of 36 patients who received adjuvant chemotherapy with adriamycin, cyclophosphamide and methotrexate was compared to that of 28 patients who were treated by surgery alone. There was no significant benefit in the 5-year overall survival ($p=0.124$), while the benefit in disease-free survival was only marginally significant ($p=0.037$). Similar were the findings of Bramwell et al. [6]. In a randomized study of 468 patients between 1977 and 1988, the authors showed that adjuvant chemotherapy with cyclophosphamide, vincristine, adriamycin and dacarbazine (CYVADIC) in adult patients with soft tissue sarcoma improved local recurrence-free survival ($p=0.004$), but not overall survival ($p=0.64$). A major limitation of this study is that a lot of the patients recruited had highly differentiated (G1) sarcomas.

In a meta-analysis of over 1,500 patients with soft tissue sarcomas, Tierney et al. also failed to demonstrate a convincing benefit from adjuvant systemic chemotherapy compared to the control group [69]. The difference in overall survival was not statistically significant between the two groups ($p=0.12$), although this study also showed an improved overall recurrence-free survival ($p=0.0001$) in the chemotherapy group. All in all, adjuvant chemotherapy appears to have no significantly positive effect, at least in terms of overall survival.

In summary, whether and which patients benefit from systemic chemotherapy with the aim of reducing the risk of local recurrence and distant metastasis is by no means proved. Administrating adjuvant systemic chemotherapy outside clinical studies cannot be justified.

13.4.2
The Role of Isolated Limb Perfusion

Isolated hyperthermic limb perfusion (ILP) with TNF-α and melphalan provides an excellent therapeutic option to obtain local control and avoid or delay limb amputation in patients with advanced, irresectable extremity soft tissue sarcoma. The technique of ILP allows 15 to 25 times higher regional drug concentrations in the tumor-bearing extremity, which is isolated from systemic circulation, than the ones reached after systemic administration.

ILP with TNF-α and melphalan is a well-established and safe method, if applied by experienced surgeons, but is not yet as widely practiced for extremity sarcomas as it could be. It has revolutionized the local management of locally advanced extremity STS, which should be equally effective whether the intent is curative or palliative, as local control improves quality of life. Tumor response rates after ILP are excellent, facilitating limb salvage in approximately 85% of patients [26, 42]; however, to date there are no data to support that ILP has any impact on overall survival.

13.4.3
The Role of Radiotherapy

Several studies have shown that radiotherapy (RT) in patients with high-grade STS has a positive effect on local recurrence-free survival, regardless of the timing (neoadjuvant or adjuvant) or the technique (external beam radiotherapy, intraoperative radiotherapy, brachytherapy), yet it does not influence overall survival [2, 12, 38, 52, 54, 57, 63, 79, 83]. Accordingly, radiotherapy appears to have no impact on metastasis.

A detailed analysis of data available on patients with STS reveals that, taking into consideration tumor location, size, surgical margin status, etc., there are no general rules regarding when to employ radiation therapy. For low-grade STS, data available show that RT combined with surgical treatment does not improve local tumor control, whereas in patients with high-grade STS, adjuvant radiotherapy plays an important role in multimodal treatment approaches, as validated by two large prospective trials. Pisters et al. demonstrated in 1996 that local tumor control after adjuvant brachytherapy of high-grade STS was significantly better compared to surgery alone (89% vs 66%, $p=0.0025$); no significant difference was observed in low-grade lesions ($p=0.49$) [54].

Yang et al. confirmed the results 2 years later for high-grade tumors and additionally showed an improved local control in low-grade sarcoma [79]. In a series of 91 patients with high-grade STS who underwent limb-sparing surgery and adjuvant systemic chemotherapy, 47 patients were randomized to additionally receive adjuvant external beam RT and 44 patients not to receive RT. Local recurrence-free survival was significantly higher in the radiotherapy group ($p=0.0028$), while no difference in overall survival between the two groups was shown ($p=0.71$). Of a further 50 patients with low-grade STS randomized in the same study to surgical treatment alone ($n=24$), or surgery and adjuvant radiotherapy ($n=26$), there was also a lower probability of local recurrence in patients who received RT ($p=0.016$), again without a difference in overall survival.

DeLaney et al. examined the efficacy of radiation therapy in a retrospective study of 154 soft tissue sarcoma patients with microscopically or grossly positive surgical margins, all of whom underwent RT with curative intent [12]. The authors reported a 5-year actuarial local control rate of 76% and found that local control was highest with extremity lesions, radiation dose greater than 64 Gy, microscopically (vs grossly) positive margins and superficial lesions. However, if a wide re-resection is feasible without functional deficits, it should not be replaced by radiotherapy alone.

It remains unclear whether every patient with a high-grade STS, taking into account surgical margin status, profits from adjuvant radiotherapy. Khanfir et al. showed in a retrospective study of 133 patients that adjuvant RT in multivariate analysis correlates with a statistically significant improvement of local tumor control only in patients with a surgical margin of less than 10 mm ($p=0.005$), and not in patients with a surgical margin of 10 mm or greater [38]. Similar results were published by Baldini et al. [4]. Furthermore, Pisters et al. recently demonstrated in a prospective trial that patients with T1 STS (high- and low-grade) and microscopically negative surgical margins may be spared adjuvant RT without a higher risk of local recurrence [56].

The value of neoadjuvant versus adjuvant radiotherapy in terms of local recurrence-free and overall survival was examined by O'Sullivan et al. in a prospective randomized study of 190 patients [52]. The local recurrence rate did not differ between the two groups ($p=0.7119$), while overall survival was slightly higher in the preoperative group ($p=0.0481$). More patients had wound complications after neoadjuvant RT compared to those in the adjuvant RT group (35% vs 17%, $p=0.01$). More patients in the adjuvant RT group developed subcutaneous fibrosis, joint stiffness and radiogenic oedema than in the neoadjuvant group (68% vs 36%, $p<0.0001$). Partially retrospective studies came to almost identical results as well [10, 57, 71, 79].

Zagars et al. demonstrated in a retrospective study of 517 patients, 271 of which received preoperative and 246 postoperative RT, that the local recurrence rate after preoperative RT was significantly lower ($p=0.005$) compared to postoperative RT [83], while disease-free survival was almost identical in both groups. Given that the adjuvant RT group included more patients with positive surgical margins and patients presenting with local recurrence, the authors showed in multivariate analysis that the apparent differences in local control found on univariate analysis were entirely explained by differences in the distribution of prognostic factors between the two treatment groups, and concluded that differences in disease outcome could not be attributed to the timing of RT.

In a further retrospective study, Zagars and Ballo evaluated the influence of neoadjuvant and adjuvant RT after inadequate surgical treatment of STS followed by re-resection in a specialist centre [81]. A mean dose of 50 Gy was preoperatively administered in 121 patients, while 159 patients received postoperative RT with a mean dose of 60 Gy. As expected, this study also found no difference in local recurrence-free ($p=0.378$) and overall survival ($p=0.129$) at 5, 10 and 15 years after treatment. Preoperative RT has the advantages of a lower dosage and a smaller radiation field due to the clearly defined tumor size.

The combined use of chemotherapy and radiotherapy has the potential to induce tumor shrinkage prior to surgery in large, high-grade soft tissue sarcomas, but, until now, this treatment option remains under investigation; results from prospective, randomized trials are awaited [13, 55]. In the case of anatomically determined narrow surgical margins, local tumor control can be improved by intraoperative radiation therapy (IORT), facilitating the preservation of functional structures [14, 51, 77]. The use of IORT has been shown to improve local tumor control by up to 40% [41]. The high costs involved at present are a serious limitation of the technique.

Kepka et al. evaluated the results of definitive radiotherapy for STS in a series of 121 patients with no acceptable surgical options [35]. The radiation dose ranged from 25 to 87.5 Gy, with a median of 64 Gy. The 5-year local control rate amounted to 45%, disease-free survival to 24% and overall survival to 35%. Delivering a dose of 63 Gy or higher was associated with a significant improvement in results, while a significant increase in complications occurred in patients who received doses of 68 Gy or more, providing a therapeutic window for these patients.

Late treatment-related complications following pre- or postoperative radiotherapy combined with limb-sparing surgery for extremity STS include pathological fractures, severe sclerosis and peripheral nerve damage [29, 45]. The risk of a radiation-induced second malignancy is currently estimated to be low and dose-dependent [40], but no solid data are available. Whether a combined radiochemotherapy further increases this risk is just as unclear.

13.4.4
Response Assessment After Neoadjuvant Treatment in Soft Tissue Sarcoma

Neoadjuvant treatment (systemic chemotherapy, radiation therapy, isolated hyperthermic limb perfusion) of localized extremity soft tissue sarcomas aims at preventing ablative surgical procedures, while systemic chemotherapy also attempts to decrease the risk of metastasis. Accordingly, non-invasive procedures are required to assess local tumor response, in order to provide an estimation of prognosis and optimize interdisciplinary decisions regarding the continuation of chemotherapy and defining when surgical resection should be performed [28, 76], so as, for instance, to be able to promptly terminate an unnecessary and expensive chemotherapy in the case of poor response, minimizing the risk of adverse effects. Until now tumor progression, stable disease, partial and complete remission after neoadjuvant treatment were defined according to changes in the size of the tumor, so that the MRI played an important role in the evaluation of tumor response to treatment. However, clinical experience has shown that tumor size alone is not a reliable parameter. Thus, MRI criteria of stable disease or tumor progression do not necessarily correlate with tumor response. For instance, extensive, liquefying necrosis could feign progression.

More promising appear to be imaging techniques which can evaluate the metabolic activity of a tumor (positron emission tomography— PET, magnetic resonance spectroscopy—MRS), or its vascularization pattern (angiography) before, during and after neoadjuvant therapy.

One possibility for a non-invasive assessment of tumor response is provided by magnetic resonance spectroscopy. MRS is able to detect the distribution of certain atoms in a tissue mass using frequency-selective pulses; ^{31}phosphorus-MRS (31P-MRS) has been most commonly employed for the evaluation of tumor response [37, 74]. In 2002, Kettelhack et al. demonstrated that 31P-MRS could predict histological response with a specificity of 94% in patients with locally advanced extremity STS who underwent ILP with TNF-α and melphalan [37].

PET is a nuclear imaging technique that uses radioactive tracers to provide crude spatial information about metabolic processes [3]. The list of available tracers is growing constantly; the substance most widely used is ^{18}F-labelled fluoro-2-deoxy-D-glucose ([^{18}F]-FDG). The European Organisation for Research and Treatment of Cancer (EORTC) has defined criteria regarding the assessment of tumor response after neoadjuvant treatment with PET imaging (Table 13.3) [68, 80]. Although available evidence-based data for soft tissue tumors are limited [8, 75], the first clinical results concerning the evaluation of tumor response are promising. Schuetze et al. demonstrated, for instance, in a study of 46 patients with high-grade soft tissue sarcomas treated with neoadjuvant chemotherapy, that patients with a baseline maximal tumor standard uptake value (SUV max) at or exceeding 6 and with a less than 40% decrease in FDG uptake were at high risk of systemic disease recurrence, estimated to be 90% at 4 years from the time of initial diagnosis. On the other hand, patients whose tumors had a 40% or greater decline in the SUV_{max} in response to chemotherapy were at a significantly lower risk of recurrent disease and death after complete resection and adjuvant radiotherapy [64].

Isolated hyperthermic limb perfusion (ILP) for locally advanced extremity soft tissue sarcoma offers an ideal model to examine the accuracy of non-invasive response assessment after a one-time cytostatic therapy. Been et al. recently described a statistically significant decrease (p=0.002) of mean SUV after ILP in a series of 10 patients [5]. However, the prognostic significance of this observation is still unknown. For the time being, the use of PET in multimodal treatment of soft tissue sarcoma is still experimental and should therefore be restricted to clinical studies.

Table 13.3 Measurement of tumor response using [^{18}F]-FDG [80]

Response criteria	[^{18}F]-FDG
Complete metabolic response (CMR)	Complete resolution of [^{18}F]-FDG uptake within the tumor volume, so that it is indistinguishable from surrounding normal tissue
Partial metabolic response (PMR)	≥15% reduction in tumor [^{18}F]-FDG SUV after one cycle of chemotherapy
	>25% reduction in tumor [^{18}F]-FDG SUV after more than one treatment cycle
	A reduction in the extent of the tumor [^{18}F]-FDG uptake is not a requirement for PMR
Stable metabolic disease (SMD)	Neither PMD nor PMR
Progressive metabolic disease (PMD)	>25% increase in tumor-SUV within the tumor region defined on the baseline scan
	Visible increase in the extent of [^{18}F]-FDG tumor uptake (>20% in the longest dimension)
	Appearance of new [^{18}F]-FDG uptake in metastatic lesions

Summary

Soft tissue sarcomas are rare tumors. The treatment of choice in localized, high-grade sarcomas consists of surgical resection and radiotherapy. Should surgical treatment be possible only by means of ablative procedures, neoadjuvant therapy options (ILP, radiation therapy, systemic chemotherapy with or without regional hyperthermia) are to be included in multimodal treatment concepts. At least one imaging modality is required before every tumor resection, in order to reduce unplanned resections. Local control can be effectively improved with ILP, chemotherapy with RHT or RT.

The most important independent prognostic factors are tumor size, grading, location, the presence of distant metastasis and local recurrence. Whether systemic chemotherapy improves overall prognosis in patients with localized disease remains the subject of clinical studies. It is, however, undoubtedly established in the treatment of stage IV disease.

A lot of questions have still not been sufficiently clarified. Is an incorrect biopsy a negative prognostic factor? When should radiotherapy be administered pre-, post- or intraoperatively? Which surgical margins are ideal and what is the impact of surgical margins on local tumor control and overall survival? Evidence-based answers are available for none of these questions. Nevertheless, prognosis of STS has improved in the last 20 years and limb-sparing surgery can be performed in a growing number of patients.

References

1. Akerman M, Ryd W, Skytting B (2003) Fine-needle aspiration of synovial sarcoma: criteria for diagnosis: retrospective reexamination of 37 cases, including ancillary diagnostics. A Scandinavian Sarcoma Group study. Diagn Cytopathol 28:232–238
2. Alektiar KM, Brennan MF, Singer S (2005) Influence of site on the therapeutic ratio of adjuvant radiotherapy in soft-tissue sarcoma of the extremity. Int J Radiat Oncol Biol Phys 63:202–208
3. Aoki J, Endo K, Watanabe H, Shinozaki T, Yanagawa T, Ahmed AR, Takagishi K (2003) FDG-PET for evaluating musculoskeletal tumors: a review. J Orthop Sci 8:435–441
4. Baldini EH, Goldberg J, Jenner C, Manola JB, Demetri GD, Fletcher CD, Singer S (1999) Long-term outcomes after function-sparing surgery without radiotherapy for soft tissue sarcoma of the extremities and trunk. J Clin Oncol 17: 3252–3259
5. Been LB, Suurmeijer AJ, Elsinga PH, Jager PL, van Ginkel RJ, Hoekstra HJ (2007) 18F-fluorodeoxythymidine PET for evaluating the response to hyperthermic isolated limb perfusion for locally advanced soft-tissue sarcomas. J Nucl Med 48:367–372
6. Bramwell V, Rouesse J, Steward W, Santoro A, Schraffordt-Koops H, Buesa J, Ruka W, Priario J, Wagener T, Burgers M (1994) Adjuvant CYVADIC chemotherapy for adult soft tissue sarcoma—reduced local recurrence but no improvement in survival: a study of the European Organization for Research and Treatment of Cancer Soft Tissue and Bone Sarcoma Group. J Clin Oncol 12:1137–1149
7. Brecht IB, Ferrari A, Int-Veen C, Schuck A, Mattke AC, Casanova M, Bisogno G, Carli M, Koscielniak E, Treuner J (2006) Grossly-resected synovial sarcoma treated by the German an Italian Pediatric Soft Tissue Sarcoma Cooperative Groups: discussion on the role of adjuvant therapies. Pediatr Blood Cancer 46:11–17
8. Bredella MA, Caputo GR, Steinbach LS (2002) Value of FDG positron emission tomography in conjunction with MR imaging for evaluating-therapy response in patients with musculoskel et al sarcomas. Am J Roentgenol 179:1145–1150
9. Chang AE, Kinsella T, Glatstein E, Baker AR, Sindelar WF, Lotze MT, Danforth DN Jr, Sugarbaker PH, Lack EE, Steinberg SM (1988) Adjuvant chemotherapy for patients with high-grade soft-tissue sarcomas of the extremity. J Clin Oncol 6:1491–1500
10. Cheng EY, Dusenbery KE, Winters MR, Thompson RC (1996) Soft tissue sarcomas: preoperative versus postoperative radiotherapy. J Surg Oncol 61:90–99
11. Davis A, Kandel RA, Wunder JS, Unger R, Meer J, O'Sullivan B, Catton CN, Bell RS (1997) The impact of residual disease on local

recurrence in patients treated by initial unplanned resection for soft tissue sarcoma of the extremity. J Surg Oncol 66:81–87
12. DeLaney TF, Kepka L, Goldberg SI, Hornicek FJ, Gebhardt MC, Yoon SS, Springfield DS, Raskin KA, Harmon DC, Kirsch DG, Mankin HJ, Rosenberg AE, Nielsen GP, Suit HD (2007) Radiation therapy for control of soft-tissue sarcomas resected with positive margins. Int J Radiat Oncol Biol Phys 67:1460–1469
13. DeLaney TF, Spiro IJ, Suit HD, Gebhardt MC, Hornicek FJ, Mankin HJ, Rosenberg AL, Rosenthal DI, Miryousefi F, Ancukiewicz M, Harmon DC (2003) Neoadjuvant chemotherapy and radiotherapy for large extremity soft-tissue sarcomas. Int J Radiat Oncol Biol Phys 56:1117–1127
14. De Paoli A, Bertola G, Boz G, Frustaci S, Massarut S, Innocente R, De Cicco M, Sartor G, Trovo MG, Rossi C (2003) Intraoperative radiation therapy for retroperitoneal soft tissue sarcoma. J Exp Clin Cancer Res 22:157–161
15. Dickinson IC, Whitwell DJ, Battistuta D, Thompson B, Strobel N, Duggal A, Steadman P (2006) Surgical margin and its influence on survival in soft tissue sarcoma. ANZ J Surg 76:104–109
16. Domanski HA, Akerman M, Carlen B, Engellau J, Gustafson P, Alvegard TA, Nilbert M, Rydholm A (2005) Core-needle biopsy performed by the cytopathologist: a technique to complement fine-needle aspiration of soft tissue and bone lesions. Cancer 105:229–239
17. Eilber FC, Brennan MF, Riedel E, Alektiar KM, Antonescu CR, Singer S (2005) Prognostic factors for survival in patients with locally recurrent extremity soft tissue sarcoma. Ann Surg Oncol 12:228–236
18. Eilber FC, Tap WD, Nelson SD, Eckardt JJ, Eilber FR (2006) Advances in chemotherapy for patients with extremity soft tissue sarcoma. Orthop Clin North Am 37:15–22
19. Fernberg JO, Hall KS (2004) Chemotherapy in soft tissue sarcoma. The Scandinavian Sarcoma Group experience. Acta Orthop Scand 75:77–86
20. Fiore M, Casali PG, Miceli R, Mariani L, Lozza L, Collini P, Olmi P, Mussi C, Gronchi A (2006) Prognostic effect of re-excision in adult soft tissue sarcoma of the extremity. Ann Surg Oncol 13:110–117
21. Glencross J, Balasubramanian SP, Bacon J, Robinson MH, Reed MW (2003) An audit of the management of soft tissue sarcoma within a health region in the UK. Eur J Surg Oncol 2003 29:670–675
22. Goodland JR, Fletcher CDM, Smith MA (1996) Surgical resection of primary soft tissue sarcoma. J Bone Joint Surg Br 78:658–661
23. Gronchi A, Casali PG, Mariani L, Miceli R, Fiore M, Lo Vullo S, Bertulli R, Collini P, Lozza L, Olmi P, Rosai J (2005) Status of surgical margins and prognosis in adult soft tissue sarcomas of the extremities: a series of patients treated at a single institution. J Clin Oncol 23:96–104
24. Gronchi A, Miceli R, Fiore M, Collini P, Lozza L, Grosso F, Mariani L, Casali PG (2007) Extremity soft tissue sarcoma: adding to the prognostic meaning of local failure. Ann Surg Oncol 14:1583–1590
25. Grobmeyer SR, Maki RG, Demetri GD, Mazumdar M, Riedel E, Brennen MF, Singer S (2004) Neo-adjuvant chemotherapy for primary high-grade extremity soft tissue sarcoma. Ann Oncol 15:1667–1672
26. Grunhagen DJ, de Wilt JH, Graveland WJ, Verhoef C, van Geel AN, Eggermont AM (2006) Outcome and prognostic factor analysis of 217 consecutive isolated limb perfusions with tumor necrosis factor alpha and melphalan for limb-threatening soft tissue sarcoma. Cancer 106:1776–1784
27. Guillou L, Coindre JM (1997) Prognostic factors in soft tissue sarcoma in the adult. Ann Pathol 17:375–377
28. Gustafson P, Akerman M, Alvegard TA, Coindre JM, Fletcher CD, Rydholm A, Willen H (2003) Prognostic information in soft tissue sarcoma using tumor size, vascular invasion and microscopic tumor necrosis-the SIN-system. Eur J Cancer 39:1568–1576
29. Holt GE, Griffin AM, Pintilie M, Wunder JS, Catton C, O`Sullivan B, Bell RS (2005) Fractures following radiotherapy and limb-salvage surgery for lower extremity soft-tissue sarcomas. A comparison of high dose and low dose radiotherapy. J Bone Joint Surg Am 87:315–319
30. Issakov J, Flusser G, Kollender Y, Merimsky O, Lifschitz-Mercer B, Meller I (2003) Computed tomography-guided core needle biopsy for bone and soft tissue tumors. Isr Med Assoc J 5:28–30
31. Issels RD (2006) High-risk soft tissue sarcoma: clinical trial and hyperthermia combined chemotherapy. Int J Hyperthermia 22:235–239
32. Issels RD, Lindner LH, Wust P, Hohenberger P, Jauch K, Daugaard S, Mansmann U,

Hiddemann W, Blay J, Verweij J (2007) Regional hyperthermia (RHT) improves response and survival when combined with systemic chemotherapy in the management of locally advanced, high grade soft tissue sarcomas of the extremities, the body wall and the abdomen: a phase III randomised prospective trial. EORTC 62961/ESHO-RHT 95 Intergroup Trial, ASCO
33. Jones C, Liu K, Hirschowitz S, Klipfel N, Layfield LJ (2002) Concordance of histopathologic and cytological grading in musculoskeletal sarcomas: can grades obtained from analysis of the fine-needle aspirates serve as the basis for therapeutic decisions? Cancer 96:83–91
34. Junginger T, Kettelhack C, Schönfelder M, Saeger HD, Rieske H, Krummenauer F, Hermanek P (2001) Therapeutic strategies in malignant soft tissue tumors. Results of the soft tissue tumor register study of Surgical Oncology Working Group. Chirurg 72:138–148
35. Kepka L, DeLaney TF, Suit HD, Goldberg SI (2005) Results of radiation therapy for unresected soft-tissue sarcomas. Int J Radiat Oncol Biol Phys 63:852–859
36. Kepka L, Suit HD, Goldberg SI, Rosenberg AE, Gebhardt MC, Hornicek FJ, DeLaney TF (2005) Results of radiation therapy performed after unplanned surgery (without re-excision) for soft tissue sarcomas. J Surg Oncol 92:39–45
37. Kettelhack C, Wickede M, Vogl T, Schneider U, Hohenberger P (2002) [31]Phosphorus-magnetic resonance spectroscopy to assess histologic tumor response noninvasively after isolated limb perfusion for soft tissue tumors. Cancer 94:1557–1564
38. Khanfir K, Alzieu L, Terrier P, Le Péchoux C, Bonvalot S, Vanel D, Le Cesne A (2003) Does adjuvant radiation therapy increase loco-regional control after optimal resection of soft-tissue sarcoma of the extremities? Eur J Cancer 39:1872–1880
39. Kraybill WG, Harris J, Spiro IJ, Ettinger DS, DeLaney TF, Blum RH, Lucas DR, Harmon DC, Letson GD, Eisenberg B (2006) Radiation Therapy Oncology Group Trial 9514. Phase II study of neoadjuvant chemotherapy and radiation therapy in the management of high-risk, high-grade, soft tissue sarcomas of the extremities and body wall: radiation Therapy Oncology Group Trial 9514. J Clin Oncol 24:619–625
40. Kuttesch JF Jr, Wexler LH, Marcus RB, Fairclough D, Weaver-McClure L, White M, Mao L, DeLaney TF, Pratt CB, Horowitz ME, Kun LE (1996) Second malignancies after Ewing's sarcoma: radiation dose-dependency of secondary sarcomas. J Clin Oncol 14:2818–2825
41. Lehnert T, Schwarzbach M, Willeke F, Treiber M, Hinz U, Wannenmacher MM, Herfarth C (2000) Intraoperative radiotherapy for primary and locally recurrent soft tissue sarcoma: morbidity and long term prognosis. Eur J Surg Oncol 26[Suppl A]:21–24
42. Lejeune FJ, Pujol N, Nienard D, Mosimann F, Raffoul W, Genton A (2000) Limb salvage by neoadjuvant isolated perfusion with TNF-alpha and melphalan for non resectable soft tissue sarcoma of the extremities. Eur J Surg Oncol 26:669–678
43. Lewis JJ, Leung D, Espat J, Woodruff JM, Brennan MF (2000) Effect of reresection in extremity soft tissue sarcoma. Ann Surg 231:655–663
44. Lewis JJ, Leung D, Heslin M, Woodruff JM, Brennan MF (1997) Association of local recurrence with subsequent survival in extremity soft tissue sarcoma. J Clin Oncol 15:646–652
45. Livi L, Santoni R, Paiar F, Bastiani G, Beltrami G, Caldora P, Capanna R, De Biase P, Detti B, Fondelli S, Meldolesi E, Pertici M, Polli C, Simontacchi G, Biti G (2006) Late treatment-related complications in 214 patients with extremity soft-tissue sarcoma treated by surgery and postoperative radiation therapy. Am J Surg 191:230–234
46. Mankin HJ, Hornicek FJ (2005) Diagnosis, classification, and management of soft tissue sarcomas. Cancer Control 12:5–21
47. McKee MD, Liu DF, Brooks JJ, Gibbs JF, Driscoll DL, Kraybill WG (2004) The prognostic significance of margin width for extremity and trunk sarcoma. J Surg Oncol 85:68–76
48. Modritz D, Ladenstein R, Pötschger U, Amman G, Dieckmann K, Horcher E, Urban C, Meister B, Schmitt K, Jones R, Kaulfersch W, Haas H, Moser R, Stöllinger O, Peham M, Gadner H, Koscielniak E, Treuner J (2005) Treatment for soft tissue sarcoma in childhood and adolescence. Austrian results within the CWS 96 study. Wien Klin Wochenschr 117:196–209
49. Moureau-Zabotto L, Thomas L, Bui BN, Chevreau C, Stockle E, Martel P, Bonneviale P, Marques B, Coindre JM, Kantor G, Matsuda T, Delannes M (2004) Management of soft tissue sarcomas (STS) in first isolated local recurrence: a retrospective study of 83 cases. Radiother Oncol 73:313–319

50. Noria S, Davis A, Kandel R, Levesque J, O'Sullivan B, Wunder J, Bell R (1996) Residual disease following unplanned excision of a soft tissue sarcoma of an extremity. J Bone Joint Surg Am 78:650–655
51. Oertel S, Treiber M, Zahlten-Hinguranage A, Eichin S, Roeder F, Funk A, Hensley FW, Timke C, Niethammer AG, Huber PE, Weitz J, Eble MJ, Buchler MW, Bernd L, Debus J, Krempien RC (2006) Intraoperative electron boost radiation followed by moderate doses of external beam radiotherapy in limb-sparing treatment of patients with extremity soft-tissue sarcoma. Int J Radiat Oncol Biol Phys 64:1416–1423
52. O'Sullivan B, Davis AM, Turcotte R, Bell R, Catton C, Chabot P, Wunder J, Kandel R, Goddard K, Sadura A, Pater J, Zee B (2002) Preoperative versus postoperative radiotherapy in soft-tissue sarcoma of the limbs: a randomised trial. Lancet 359:2235–2241
53. Pisters PW, Leung DH, Woodruff J, Shi W, Brennan MF (1996) Analysis of prognostic factors in 1.041 patients with localized soft tissue sarcomas of the extremities. J Clin Oncol 14:1679–1689
54. Pisters PW, Harrison LB, Leung DH, Woodruff JM, Casper ES, Brennan MF (1996) Long-term results of a prospective randomized trial of adjuvant brachytherapy in soft tissue sarcoma. J Clin Oncol 14:859–868
55. Pisters PW, Patel SR, Prieto VG, Thall PF, Lewis VO, Feig BW, Hunt KK, Yasko AW, Lin PP, Jacobson MG, Burgess MA, Pollock RE, Zagars GK, Benjamin RS, Ballo MT (2004) Phase I trial of preoperative doxorubicin-based concurrent chemoradiation and surgical resection for localized extremity and body wall soft tissue sarcomas. J Clin Oncol 22:3375–3380
56. Pisters PW, Pollock RE, Lewis VO, Yasko AW, Cormier JN, Respondek PM, Feig BW, Hunt KK, Linn PP, Zagars G, Wei C, Ballo MT (2007) Long-term results of prospective trial of surgery alone with selective use of radiation for patients with T1 extremity and trunk soft tissue sarcoma. Ann Surg 246:675–682
57. Pollack A, Zagars GK, Goswitz MS, Pollock RA, Feig BW, Pisters PW (1998) Preoperative vs postoperative radiotherapy in the treatment of soft tissue sarcomas: a matter of presentation. Int J Radiat Oncol Biol Phys 42:563–572
58. Ray-Coquard I, Ranchere-Vince D, Thiesse P, Ghesquieres H, Biron P, Sunyach MP, Rivoire M, Lancry L, Meeus P, Sebban C, Blay JY (2003) Evaluation of core needle biopsy as a substitute to open biopsy in the diagnosis of soft-tissue masses. Eur J Cancer 39:2021–2025
59. Ray-Coquard I, Thiesse P, Ranchère-Vince D, Chauvin F, Bobin JY, Sunyach MP, Carret JP, Mongodin B, Marec-Bérard P, Philip T, Blay JY (2004) Conformity to clinical practice guidelines, multidisciplinary management and outcome of treatment for soft tissue sarcomas. Ann Oncol 2004 15:307–315
60. Rosenberg SA, Tepper J, Glatstein E, Costa J, Baker A, Brennan M, DeMoss EV, Seipp C, Sindelar WF, Sugarbaker P, Wesley R (1982) The treatment of soft tissue sarcoma of the extremities: prospective randomized evaluations of (1) limb-sparing surgery plus radiation therapy compared with amputation and (2) the role of adjuvant chemotherapy. Ann Surg 196:305–315
61. Rougraff BT, Davis K, Cudahy T (2005) The impact of previous surgical manipulation of subcutaneous sarcoma on oncologic outcome. Clin Orthop Relat Res 438:85–91
62. Rydholm A, Berg NO, Gullberg B, Thorngren KG, Persson BM (1984) Epidemiology of soft-tissue sarcoma in the locomotor system. A retrospective population-based study of the inter-relationships between clinical and morphologic variables. Acta Pathol Microbiol Immunol Scand 92:363–374
63. Sadoski C, Suit HD, Rosenberg A, Mankin H, Efird J (1993) Preoperative radiation, surgical margins, and local control of extremity sarcomas of soft tissues. J Surg Oncol 52:223–230
64. Schuetze SM, Rubin BP, Vernon C, Hawkins DS, Bruckner JD, Conrad EU 3rd, Eary JF (2005) Use of positron emission tomography in localized extremity soft tissue sarcoma treated with neoadjuvant chemotherapy. Cancer 103:339–348
65. Siebenrock KA, Hertel R, Ganz R (2000) Unexpected resection of soft-tissue sarcoma. More mutilating surgery, higher local recurrence rates, and obscure prognosis as consequences of improper surgery. Arch Orthop Trauma Surg 120:65–69
66. Stojadinovic A, Leung DH, Hoos A, Jaques DP, Lewis JJ, Brennan MF (2002) Analysis of the prognostic significance of microscopic margins in 2.084 localized primary adult soft tissue sarcomas. Ann Surg 235:424–434
67. Tanabe KK, Pollock RE, Ellis LM, Murphy A, Sherman N, Romsdahl MM (1994) Influence of surgical margins on outcome in patients with

preoperatively irradiated extremity soft tissue sarcomas. Cancer 73:1652–1659
68. Therasse P, Arbuck SG, Eisenhauer EA, Wanders J, Kaplan RS, Rubinstein L, Verweij J, van Glabbeke M, van Oosterom AT, Christian MC, Gwyther SG (2006) New guidelines to evaluate the response to treatment in solid tumors. European Organization for Research and Treatment of Cancer, National Cancer Institute of the United States, National Cancer Institute of Canada. J Natl Cancer Inst 98:232–234
69. Tierney JF, Mosseri V, Stewart LA, Souhami RL, Parmar MK (1995) Adjuvant chemotherapy for soft-tissue sarcoma: review and meta-analysis of the published results of randomised clinical trials. Br J Cancer 72:469–475
70. Torres MA, Ballo MT, Butler CE, Feig BW, Cormier JN, Lewis VO, Pollock RE, Pisters PW, Zagars GK (2007) Management of locally recurrent soft-tissue sarcoma after prior surgery and radiation therapy. Int J Radiat Oncol Biol Phys 67:1124–1129
71. Tseng JF, Ballo MT, Langstein HN, Wayne JD, Cormier JN, Hunt KK, Feig BW, Yasko AW, Lewis VO, Lin PP, Cannon CP, Zagars GK, Pollock RE, Pisters PW (2006) The effect of preoperative radiotherapy and reconstructive surgery on wound complications after resection of extremity soft-tissue sarcomas. Ann Surg Oncol 13:1209–1215
72. Tunn PU, Gebauer B, Fritzmann J, Hunerbein M, Schlag PM (2004) Soft tissue sarcoma. Chirurg 75:1165–1173
73. Ueda T, Yoshikawa H, Mori S, Araki N, Myoui A, Kuratsu S, Uchida A (1997) Influence of local recurrence on the prognosis of soft-tissue sarcomas. J Bone Joint Surg Br 79:553–557
74. Vaidya SJ, Payne GS, Leach MO, Pinkerton CR (2003) Potential role of magnetic resonance spectroscopy in assessment of tumor response in childhood cancer. Eur J Cancer 39:728–735
75. Vernon CB, Eary JF, Rubin BP, Conrad EU 3rd, Schuetze S (2003) FDG PET imaging guided re-evaluation of histopathologic response in a patient with high-grade sarcoma. Skeletal Radiol 32:139–142
76. Weber WA, Wieder H (2006) Monitoring chemotherapy and radiotherapy of solid tumors. Eur J nucl Med Mol Imaging 33[Suppl 1]:27–37
77. Willett CG (2001) Intraoperative radiation therapy. Int J Clin Oncol 6:209–214
78. White LM, Wunder JS, Bell RS, O'Sullivan B, Catton C, Ferguson P, Blachstein M, Kandel RA (2005) Histological assessment of peritumoral edema in soft tissue sarcoma. Int J Radiat Oncol Biol Phys 61:1439–1445
79. Yang JC, Chang AE, Baker AR, Sindelar WF, Danforth DN, Topalian SL, DeLaney T, Glatstein E, Steinberg SM, Merino MJ, Rosenberg SA (1998) Randomized prospective study of the benefit of adjuvant radiation therapy in the treatment of soft tissue sarcomas of the extremity. J Clin Oncol 16:197–203
80. Young H, Baum R, Cremerius U, Herholz K, Hoekstra O, Lammertsma AA, Pruim J, Price P (1999) Measurement of clinical and subclinical tumor response using [18F]-fluorodeoxyglucose and positron emission tomography: review and 1999 EORTC recommendations. European Organization for Research and Treatment of Cancer (EORTC) PET Study Group. Eur J Cancer 35:1773–1782
81. Zagars GK, Ballo MT (2003) Sequencing radiotherapy for soft tissue sarcoma when re-resection is planned. Int J Radiat Oncol Biol Phys 56:21–27
82. Zagars GK, Ballo MT, Pisters PW, Pollock RE, Patel SR, Benjamin RS (2003) Surgical margins and reresection in the management of patients with soft tissue sarcoma using conservative surgery and radiation therapy. Cancer 97:2544–2553
83. Zagars GK, Ballo MT, Pisters PW, Pollock RE, Patel SR, Benjamin RS (2003) Preoperative vs postoperative radiation therapy for soft tissue sarcoma: a retrospective comparative evaluation of disease outcome. Int J Radiat Oncol Biol Phys 56:482–484
84. Zornig C, Peiper M, Schröder S (1995) Re-excision of soft tissue sarcoma after inadequate initial operation. Br J Surg 82:278–279

Evaluating Surgery Quality in Soft Tissue Sarcoma

14

Eberhard Stoeckle, Jean-Michel Coindre, Michèle Kind, Guy Kantor, and Binh N. Bui

Abstract To identify pertinent indicators for oncologic outcomes in assessing surgery in soft tissue sarcomas, only local recurrences are considered here. Functional outcomes and treatment morbidity, equally important end-points for evaluating surgery quality, are less frequently reported and are not taken into account in this review. Herein, we review recent publications reporting indicators of surgery quality in soft tissue sarcoma treatment. Local recurrence-free interval is the major end-point in evaluating the quality of surgery. Disease-free survival should not be used because the risk factors for metastases are different from those for local recurrence. Five-year local recurrence-free estimations for limb and trunk wall sarcoma should be below 20%, and best approach 10%. The risk of local recurrence depends on tumour biology (i.e. grade) and quality of surgery as defined by the quality of margins. Better than margin width as measured on the tumour specimen, margin quality determined consensually between surgeons and pathologists is the best indicator for local outcome. Quality of margin should be expressed according the UICC residual disease definitions (R0: *in sano*, R1: microscopic residual disease, R2: macroscopic residual disease). Other important indicators for surgery quality are treatment in specialised centres, a planned, organised surgery, and treatment within a multi-disciplinary team. Soft tissue sarcoma should also be treated in specialised centres. Surgery quality depends on obtained margins that are determined best by close collaboration between the surgeon and the pathologist.

14.1
Introduction

Treatment outcome in soft tissue sarcoma (STS) depends mainly on the quality of the surgery, the mainstay of sarcoma treatment. In contrast to bone sarcoma, STS show a great variety of presentations, including more than 50 histological subtypes, ubiquitous tumour locations and quite different behaviours according tumour biology (Fletcher et al. 2002). There are several consequences from this tumour

Eberhard Stoeckle (✉)
Department of Surgery
Institut Bergonie, Regional Cancer Centre
229 Cours de l'Argonne
33076 Bordeaux Cedex, France
E-mail: Stoeckle@bergonie.org

heterogeneity: (1) the quality of surgery may improve only with better knowledge of these tumours; (2) progress in knowledge is slow because of the rarity and heterogeneity of STS; and (3) different treatment approaches are indicated according the various tumour presentations. Adequate surgery should give a high tumour control and favourable functional outcome with minimal morbidity. These exigencies are often contradictory. In order to perform the surgery most appropriate for the patient's situation, the surgeon must be familiar with STS physiopathology and work with a team highly specialised in sarcoma treatment.

Local tumour control is the first end-point in evaluating quality of surgery of STS. The "price to pay", however, in terms of functional outcome and surgical complications, is a major consideration when planning an operation for STS. Other chapters in this collection already deal, at least partially, with these important issues (e.g. Chaps. 13 and 18), allowing us to focus this contribution on the oncological issue of tumour control.

In this review, which emphasises the local outcome part of surgery quality, we first define pertinent end-points for local outcome. Next, reported local recurrence rates are compiled and definitions of margins determined. Risk factors for local recurrence are analysed with the final objective of predicting resectability of STS in order to integrate surgery in multidisciplinary treatments.

14.2
What End-Points for Assessing Local Tumour Control?

An apparently easy question that is more difficult to be answered than supposed: what are the best end-points for assessing local tumour control? Historically, in the 1940s–1950s, more than two-thirds of patients operated on for an STS had recurrent disease (Bowden and Booher 1958; Mazanet and Antman 1991). At that time, general outcome was thought linked to the quality of surgery. Radical surgery, i.e. amputations, therefore became the standard treatment of limb STS, and local treatments gave raise to 47% local recurrences (Firth 1979).

These high local recurrence rates suggest that surgery at that time was dictated more by technical considerations than by knowledge of tumour extension. After Cade in the early 1950s (Cade 1950), it is Bowden and Booher who first described the modalities of loco-regional extensions of STS, comprising a tumour growing centrifugally limited by a pseudocapsule and evolving within an anatomic compartment (Bowden and Booher 1958). Understanding that the risk of local recurrence was linked to surgical margin more than to type of procedure, Simon and Enneking (1976) developed a conservative surgical approach by compartmentectomy, based on Bowden and Booher's description. By their approach, they showed that local recurrence could be reduced to 15%–20% (Simon and Enneking 1976; Enneking et al. 1981). These results were confirmed in other series with limb-sparing surgery either by surgery alone (Cantin et al. 1968; Shiu et al. 1975; Simon and Enneking 1976) or by a combination of surgery with radiotherapy (Lindberg et al. 1981). In 1984, a United States NIH consensus conference recommended conservative surgery as standard in STS (NIH 1985). The rate of amputations in STS in the United States dropped from 29.3% in 1988 to 9% in 1993 (Pollock et al. 1996). The evidence that amputations did not prevent patients from dieing from metastases helped to bring about this breakthrough. Moreover, a small, randomised trial comparing conservative treatment to amputation demonstrated that survival was not affected by the conservative approach (Rosenberg et al. 1982). However, because local recurrences were associated with distant recurrences, a causal relationship remained suspected, keeping unclear the impact of surgery respectively on local and general outcome. Therefore, most series reported surgical results by disease-free survival that takes into account both local and distant recurrences.

It took some 20 years more to recognise that prognostic factors for local and general outcomes were different (Bell et al. 1989; Coindre et al. 1996; Mandard et al. 1989; Markhede et al. 1982; Pisters et al. 1996; Ravaud et al. 1992; Rydholm et al. 1984; Saddegh et al. 1992) and that surgical margins or local recurrences had no influence (Dickinson et al. 2006; Gerrand et al. 2003; Gustafson et al. 1991; Rööser et al. 1990; Trovik et al. 2000; Vraa et al. 2001), or if so, only in specific locations (i.e. retroperitoneal and head and neck locations) or with certain subtypes of STS (Gronchi et al. 2005; LeVay et al. 1993; Stojadinovic et al. 2002a; Zagars et al. 2003). Separating metastatic recurrence from outcome, local recurrence therefore remains the best end-point expressing the quality of surgery in STS. To be valid, it should be given in actuarial local recurrence-free estimates, in order to erase differences in local recurrence figures due to differences in follow-up. This is best illustrated by a series of 171 patients treated at the Royal Marsden Hospital in London. In their initial article, Pitcher et al. reported a local recurrence rate of 9% (15/171) isolated and 14% (24/171) crude after a follow-up of 20 months (Pitcher et al. 1994). In a second report it became 20.6% (35/171) after 5.3 years of follow-up, giving an actuarial local recurrence-free rate of 26% (Pitcher et al. 2000).

Besides the establishment of conservative surgery, another breakthrough in sarcoma treatment was the definition of grading systems for prognosis. Among them, the French Federation of Cancer Centres (FNCLCC) system (Trojani et al. 1984) emerged as the most reproducible and reliable (Coindre et al. 1986; Guillou et al. 1997). It is based on factors independent from histopathology (differentiation, necrosis, and mitoses), hence leaving histology as a complementary prognostic factor (Coindre et al. 2001). Together with size, grade is the best prognosticator for metastases and survival, most representative of the biological aggressiveness of STS (Coindre et al. 1996; Guillou et al. 1997).

To the same degree that grade determines the risk of metastases, surgical margins predict local recurrence. Obtaining clear margins should be the goal of every surgical approach in STS. This objective depends on tumour biology and presentation, but also on skill and the surgeon's experience with STS. Paradoxically, despite these consensual observations and early experience with descriptions of tumour margins (Simon and Enneking 1976; Enneking et al. 1981), no universally accepted system for margin determination has been established yet. In this review we will analyse the different systems of margin determination. For this purpose, we will constrain the present work to limb and trunk wall sarcoma, the most frequent (60% of STS) and the best described of the sarcoma. Head and neck sarcoma, with its specific anatomic constraints and outcomes, need a different approach (Kotilingam et al. 2006; LeVay et al. 1993; Stojadinovic et al. 2002b; Zagars et al. 2003) that is not dealt with here, as does retroperitoneal sarcoma, which is explored in another chapter (see Chap. 17).

14.3
Local Recurrence Rates

For this overview, we have compiled several patient series, stratified according treatment by surgery alone or by surgery combined with radiotherapy. The result gives an indication of local outcome within broader collected patient information, perhaps representing a better picture of the reality than results exclusively from very specialised treatment centres. Crude local recurrence rates (actuarial estimations lacking in previous publications) are 21%, 22% and 16% in series with exclusive surgery, surgery plus partial radiotherapy and surgery plus systematic radiotherapy, respectively (Tables 14.1, 14.2 and 14.3). In more recent series, actuarial 5-year local recurrence-free intervals range from 10% to 18% (Eilber et al. 2003; Gerrand et al. 2003; Stoeckle et al. 2006; Stojadinovic et al. 2002b; Zagars et al. 2003). There has been some concern regarding the relatively unchanged survival data from the Memorial Sloan-Kettering Cancer Center (MSKCC) in patients treated during the period 1982 to 2001, with disease-specific survival progressing insignificantly from 78% to 84% (Weitz et al. 2003). When looking further back to series from the same institution dating from the 1930's, only little progress has been seen in local outcome (as depicted in Table 14.4). That may mean that the most productive efforts affecting tumour control have already been made in this specialised institution, and there may be little hope of further progress by surgery alone. In our own experience at Institut Bergonié, the rate of local recurrence has dropped from 24% to 13% between the 1970s and the 1990s (Ravaud et al. 1992; Stoeckle et al. 2006). Within the French Sarcoma Group (FSG-GETO), a multicentric group, local recurrences dropped from 32% to 21% at the same time (Coindre et al. 1996; Stoeckle et al. 2007). It can be postulated that the 10% local recurrence rate constitutes a difficult-to-pass barrier when using limb-sparing treatment, even in specialised centres. Contrarily, outside specialised centres, frequent inadequate

Table 14.1 Primary STS. Local recurrences by surgery alone

Authors	Total patients	Recurrences (n)	Percentage (range)
9 References[a]	1,721	363	21 (7–30)%

[a]References: Cantin et al. 1968; Shiu et al. 1975; Simon and Enneking 1976; Enneking et al. 1981; Markhede et al. 1982; Karakousis et al. 1986; Rydholm et al. 1991; Gaynor et al. 1992; Trovik et al. 2000
Amputations: 0%–35%

Table 14.2 Primary STS. Local recurrences by surgery and partial radiotherapy

Authors	Total patients	No. of recurrences	Percentage (range)
13 References[a]	5,591	1,217	22 (10–41)%

[a]Ruka et al. 1989; Ravaud et al. 1992; Azzarelli 1993; LeVay et al. 1993; Gustafson 1994; Keus et al. 1994; Coindre et al. 1996; Peiper et al. 1997; Bauer et al. 2001; Stefanovski et al. 2002; Eilber et al. 2003; McKee et al. 2004; Dickinson et al. 2006
Radiotherapy: 18%–78%

Table 14.3 Primary STS. Local recurrences by surgery and systematic radiotherapy

Authors	Total patients	No. of recurrences(n)	Percentage (range)
10 References[a]	2,185	341	16 (12–46) %

[a]Lindberg et al. 1981; Wood et al. 1984; Mandard et al. 1989; Avizonis et al. 1990; Stotter et al. 1990; Langlois et al. 1991; Herbert et al. 1993; Sadoski et al. 1993; Zagars et al. 2003; Khanfir et al. 2003

initial approaches are responsible for deeply altered local control rates and reduced survival (Bauer et al. 2001; Clasby et al. 1997; Gustafson et al. 1994; Ray-Coquard et al. 2004; Rydholm 1998; Siebenrock et al. 2000; Trovik et al. 2000). This is a clear signal that STS should be treated in specialised centres.

14.4
Margins and Their Impact on Local Control

14.4.1
Margin Determination and Local Outcome

Recent publications reporting tumour margins and their influence on local outcome are compiled in Table 14.5. In most reports, the impor-

Table 14.4 Local outcomes at MSKCC over time

Author	Period	Location	No. at presentation	Amputation (%)	F-up	N	5-y LR Crude(%)	5-y LR Actuarial (%)
Cantin et al. 1968	1935–1959	L+T	653 (A) 324 (P)	NP	>5 y	187 74	29% 23%	–
Shiu et al. 1975	1949–1968	Lower L	297 (A) 161 (P)	47	>5 y	19	18% 12%	–
Gaynor et al. 1992	1968–1978	L	403 (A)	33	8.7 y	119	30%	–
Stojadinovic et al. 2002	1982–2000	L	1156 (P)	8	50 m	181	16%	18%

A, all, primary and recurrent; F-up, follow-up; L, limb; LR, local recurrence; m, months; MSKCC, Memorial Sloan-Kettering Cancer Center, New York; NP, not provided; P, primary; T, trunk wall; y, years

tance of margin is determined at pathological examination of the specimen of excision. Margin width is determined mainly by the distance from the tumour edge to the periphery of the specimen. The definition of margin quality is therefore given according distances with lower cut-off values ranging from 0 mm (LeVay et al. 1993; McKee et al. 2004; Stefanovski et al. 2002) to upper cut-offs at 4 cm (LeVay et al. 1993), most limits being at 1 mm (Dickinson et al. 2006; Gronchi et al. 2005; Koea et al. 2003; Stojadinovic et al. 2002a). In a majority, margin quality is expressed as either negative or positive. Some have conserved the Enneking system (i.e. intralesional, marginal, wide) secondarily translated in adequate and inadequate excisions (Trovik et al. 2000). Others add realisation of radiotherapy to margin width in order to define adequacy of margins (Keus et al. 1994). In close margins, Gerrand et al. (2001) introduce tumour type and the notion of planned surgery, giving, by combining these criteria, a highly predictive feature of the local recurrence risk. Uncertain margins are also given (Zagars et al. 2003), or close margins of less than 1 cm (LeVay et al. et al. 1993; McKee et al. 2004), leading to three categories of margins (negative—close or uncertain—positive). Dickinson et al. (2006) have categorised nine varieties of margins, going from radical and wide (>20 mm) to wide contaminated, passing over ill-defined margins. Globally, in all studies with two categories of margins, a twofold difference in local recurrences between them is found (Gronchi et al. 2005; Koea et al. 2003; Stefanovski et al. 2002; Stojadinovic et al. 2002b; Trovik et al. 2000). Results are more variable when three or more categories are defined (Dickinson et al. 2006; Keus et al. 1994; LeVay et al. 1993; McKee et al. 2004; Zagars et al. 2003).

In the French Sarcoma Group (FSG-GETO) system, reporting quality of surgery employs the UICC definition of residual disease (R) (Sobin and Wittekind 2002) that defines three categories: R0=*in sano*, R1=(possible) microscopic residual disease, R2=macroscopic residual disease. In the FSG-GETO procedure, the residual disease definition is obtained after combining (through a "thesis, antithesis, and synthesis" procedure) surgical findings and pathological analysis. In order to reduce subjectivity of surgical findings ("always wide excision"), a checklist for surgery reporting has been established (Stoeckle 1997; Stoeckle et al. 2005),

Table 14.5 Resection margins and local recurrences in primary soft tissue sarcoma

Reference; center	Location	No. of pts	Median follow-up (months)	Determination of margin	Quality of resection: Result	Quality of resection: Frequencies	5-year LR: According margin	5-year LR: Global
LeVay et al. 1994 PMH	All	321	80	NP	Wide 1–4 cm Close <1 cm Positive 0 mm	NP	7% 17%	22%
Keus et al. 1994; NCI/ALH	Limb+ girdles	143	114	Pathol. margin 2 cm/ XRT	Wide Narrow XRT Incompl. XRT	18% 45% 37%	19% 8% 16%	17%
Trovik et al. 2000; SSG	Limb+ trunk	559	89	Pathol. margin Enneking	Adequate Inadequate	75% 25%	15%[b] 32%[b]	NP
Stefanovski et al. 2002; CRO	All	395; (L+T: 273)	35	Pathol. margin at edge	Negative Positive	68% 32%	20% 35%	26%
Stojadinovic et al. 2002b; MSKCC	Limb	1,156	50	Pathol. margin at edge	Negative Positive	81% 19%	18%[a] 35%[a]	18%
Koea et al. 2003; MSKCC	Limb strict	911	35	Pathol. margin 1 mm	Negative Positive	83% 17%	13% 22%	14% crude
Eilber et al. 2003; UCLA	Limb	607	88	Pathol. margin at edge	Negative Positive	98% 2%	NS NS	10%
Zagars et al. 2003; MDA	All	1,225 (L+T: 601)	114	Pathol. margin at edge	Negative Uncertain Positive	66% 19% 15%	12%[b] 26%[b] 38%[b]	17%
McKee et al. 2004; RPCI/ SUNY	Limb+ trunk	111	80	Pathol. margin in mm	>10 mm 1–9 mm 0 mm	47% 41% 12%	16% 42% 42%	26% crude; 29/111

Gronchi et al. 2005; INSCT	Limb+ Girdles	642	Pathol. margin 1 mm	Negative Positive	87% 13%	12% 26%	14%
Dickinson et al. 2006; WMC	NP	324	107	Pathol margin 1 mm[c]	>/=1 mm <1 mm	67% 33%	2- to 3.7-fold	~10% crude; (27/279)
Stoeckle et al. 2006; IB	Limb+ trunk wall	200	32	Surg/pathol. consensus UICC	R0 R1	74% 26%	7% 30%	13%

CRO, Centro di Riferimento Oncologico, Aviano, Italy; IB, Institut Bergonié, Bordeaux, France; INSCT, Istituto Nazionale per lo Studio e la Cura dei Tumori, Milano, Italy; L, limb; LR, local recurrence; MDA, M.D. Anderson Cancer Center, Houston, Texas; MSKCC, Memorial Sloan Kettering Cancer Center, New York; NCI/ALH, The Netherlands Cancer Institute, Antoni van Leeuwenhoek Hospital, Amsterdam, NL; NP, not provided; NS, not significant; PMH, Princess Margaret Hospital, Toronto, Canada; pts, patients; T, trunk; RPCI/SUNY, Roswell Park Cancer Institute/State University of New York, Buffalo, NY; SSG, Scandinavian Sarcoma Group; UCLA, University of California, Los Angeles; WMC, The West Medical Centre, Brisbane, Australia; XRT, radiotherapy
[a] Concerning 2,084 STS of all anatomic sites
[b] Estimated from survival curves
[c] Nine categories of margins overall

including notions such as "tumour seen during dissection?" underlining a close dissection, and "tumour rupture?", which figures unfavourably for outcome (Tanabe et al. 1994). The shrinkage of the tumour specimen, especially the retraction of the muscle initially covering the tumour, giving way to the tumour surface, can falsely be interpreted as a contaminated margin. Therefore, pathological reporting has also been stressed with an important recommendation for the pathologist to describe the tumour, but not to draw a conclusion about surgery quality (Ghnassia et al. 1998). Finally, quality of surgery is determined collegially, by analysing the different descriptions during regular group meetings. Important issues in this three-category system centre around the first two categories, R0 and R1, for which treatment adaptation is discussed; the R2 categories require no discussion. In a prospective evaluation of this system at Institut Bergonié, a fourfold difference in local outcomes between the two resection types, R0 and R1, was found (Stoeckle et al. 2006).

The Japanese Orthopaedic Association has set out a system of reporting margins that combines margin width in centimetres (up to 4 cm) and margin quality, comprising a conversion of margin quality (strong or thin) into thickness in centimetres. This somewhat complex system, conceived both for bone and STS, is probably more suitable for bone sarcoma where margin width is easier to measure because of the stable anatomic rapports (Kawaguchi et al. 2004).

14.4.2
Co-factors Influencing Margin Quality

14.4.2.1
Surgery Planning

Unplanned surgery is probably the most important risk factor in obtaining unclear margins. At re-excision, about 50% of specimens contain residual tumour (Chap. 13).

14.4.2.2
Tumour Capsule

In their initial report, Simon and Enneking (1976) described a zone of compressed tissue formed by stretched muscle around the tumour surface, pushed by the centrifugal spread of the tumour. At the periphery of these stretched muscles they observed a reactive zone, able to harbour satellite tumour nodules especially in high-grade tumours. They used the term of "pseudocapsule" for this reactive zone, underlying the fact that dissection within this plane, called shelling-out, leaves microscopic residues and favours recurrence (Enneking et al. 1981).

The presence of microsatellites in high-grade tumours constituted the rationale for Enneking's staging system, based on the compartmental location of the tumour and its grade. They then measured surgery quality according the distance of the surgical plane to the pseudocapsule. However, this term is confusing because the authors situated the pseudocapsule within the reactive zone. In current experience, especially after unplanned excision, the observed surgical plane is frequently closer to the tumour surface, with no compressed muscle or reactive zone surrounding it. However, when re-excision is performed, in half of the cases no residual tumour is found. This observation means that (1) microsatellite tumours are not systematically within the reactive zone, (2) a real, very fine capsule at the tumour surface may exist, (3) there are different meanings for marginal surgery and shelling-out, the last could be directly at the tumour surface, and (4) there are tumours without a real delimitation at their periphery. Ill-limited tumour growth is seen in epithelioid sarcoma, dermatofibrosarcoma protuberans, angiosarcoma, most high-grade malignant fibrous histiocytoma (MFH) and undifferentiated sarcoma. These tumours can extend close to, or more rarely involve (Ferguson et al. 2006), neurovascular bundles, bone and skin, an extension corresponding to the T3-stage of the 1978 UICC classification, abandoned in 1997. These and other high-grade tumours can also show multifocal growth, comprising satellite nodules in the reactive zone (frequent) or skip metastases in the compartment (rare). This extensive growth occurs in about 1/3 of cases (Stoeckle et al. 2006).

Infiltrative and multinodular patterns have been described as early as 1968 by Cantin et al. (1968) and have been confirmed by others (LeVay et al. 1993; Manoso et al. 2006; Sastre-Garau et al. 1997; Shiu et al. 1975). Extensive tumour growth not only constitutes an independent risk factor for unclear margins, but also for metastatic-free survival (Coindre et al. 2001). Therefore, contrary to the statement of Simon and Enneking (1976), pseudoencapsulation is not a constant characteristic of STS and a description of surgery quality based on the notion of pseudocapsule only can be inappropriate. More recent systems, based on observations of whole-tumour sections, distinguish between "pushing" and infiltrating tumours. Combined with vascular invasion and necrosis, these peripheral growth patterns have been shown to be highly predictive for metastases and local recurrence (Engellau et al. 2005). Infiltrating peripheral tumour growth can be predicted by MRI (Fernebro et al. 2006), helping to predict resectability. In an earlier study from FSG-GETO, Sastre-Garau et al. demonstrated that the co-existence of tumour necrosis, deep location (i.e. intra-abdominal) and the ancient T3 involvement pattern were highly predictive of poor resectability (Sastre-Garau et al. 1997).

14.4.2.3
Tumour Size

A huge tumour size may prevent the surgeon from obtaining wide resection margins. In contrast with the schematic representation by Enneking et al. (1981) of a tumour in the thigh, showing a 2-mm tumour in a 30-mm thigh (equivalent to a 1.2 cm tumour in a 18 cm thigh), STS in this location can easily measure 10 cm in diameter (Stoeckle et al. 2006; Grimer 2006). Azzarelli et al. demonstrated that this size made it nearly impossible to obtain 2 cm margins in all directions (Azzarelli 1993). McKee et al. showed that margins exceeding 1 cm were obtained in only 47% of their patients (McKee et al. 2004). Dickinson et al. obtained margins exceeding 5 mm in only 54% of cases (Dickinson et al. 2006). It is therefore somewhat illusory to claim a margin of up to 4 cm qualified as adequate, as is recommended by the Japanese Orthopaedic Association (Kawaguchi et al. 2004). In order to preserve important functional structures (sciatic, median nerves), a close dissection can be adequate, when it is prior planned and adapted to tumour type and low grade (Gerrand et al. 2001) as well as type of extension (Lin et al. 2007). Furthermore, prior planning allows for the delivery of pre-operative treatments such as radiotherapy (Sadoski et al. 1993), chemotherapy (Cany et al. 1992), radiochemotherapy (Eilber et al. 2003), isolated limb perfusion (Eggermont et al. 1996; Bonvalot et al. 2005) and intra-operative treatments such as intraoperative radiotherapy (Oertel et al. 2006) or brachytherapy (Llacer et al. 2006).

14.4.2.4 Tumour Grade

As stated, high-grade tumours are more likely to be ill-limited and to harbour microsatellite tumours at their periphery. High grade is an important risk factor for unclear margins and therefore for local recurrence (Table 14.6).

14.4.3 Impact of Margin and Other Factors on Local Recurrence

Independent prognostic variables for local outcome by multivariate analysis are compiled in Table 14.6. Interestingly, despite different

Table 14.6 Independent prognostic factors for local recurrence

Reference	Location	Margin (HR)	Grade (HR)	Other significant variables
LeVay et al. 1993	L+G+H&N	S (NP)	S (NP)	Age, direct extension
Keus et al. 1994	L+G	S (NP)	S (NP)	-
Trovik et al. 2000	L+T	S (2.9)	S (3.0)	-
Gerrand et al. 2001	L	S (3.2)	NA	-
Stefanovski et al. 2002	All	S (1.8)	S (2.8)	Stage
Stojadinovic et al. 2002b	L	S (2.4)	S (1.7)	Size, histology, location
Koea et al. 2003	L	S (2.0)	NS	Age, histology
Eilber et al. 2003	L	NS[a]	S (2.6)	Age, histology
Zagars et al. 2003	All	S (2.5)	S (1.5)	Age, histology, location, size, recurrence
McKee et al. 2004	L+G+T	S (NP)	NS	Size
Gronchi et al. 2005	L+G	S (1.9)	NS	-
Stoeckle et al. 2006	L+G+T	S (4.3)	S (3.9)	-
Frequencies	12	11	8	Age 4, histology 4, size 3, location 2

G, girdles; H&N, head and neck; HR, hazard ratio; L, limb; NP, not provided; NS, not significant; T, trunk wall; S, significant
[a]Only 2% positive margins

techniques employed to determine it, surgical margin is systematically found as an independent prognostic factor for local outcome. The only negative study comprises a series with 98% margin-negative patients, making it difficult to compare with the 2% of margin-positive patients (Eilber et al. 2003). Hazard ratios (HR) when reported, range between 1.8 and 3.2; it is 4.3 in the prospective study of Institut Bergonié (Stoeckle et al. 2006). Grade, determined according several systems, is found as the second most frequent independent risk factor for local recurrence in eight studies. The other variables, including age, size, histopathology, and location, are more accessorily reported. These results underline the predominant influence on local control of both surgery quality (margin) and tumour biology (grade).

14.5
Long-Term Follow-Up with Actuarial Estimates in Homogeneous Patient Groups

About 70%–80% of local recurrences occur within 3 years. Short-term follow-up misses late recurrences that could be linked to particular tumour biology. Gronchi et al. (2005) did not find a difference in local outcome between margin-negative and -positive patients at early follow-up, a difference that became significant only after longer follow-up. As shown also by Stojadinovic et al. (2002a), systemic risks prevail early but local risks become more important later. Local recurrence-free intervals should be used to report local outcome, allowing better comparisons between reports and between the same patient groups over time (see the experience of the Royal Marsden Hospital; Pitcher et al. 1994 and 2000). Data about recurrence should concern homogeneous groups. It is well known that the risk of a second recurrence is enhanced after a first one. Because prognosis is quite different between primary and recurrent STS, reporting results should be limited to either primary or recurrent STS, without mixing them together.

14.6
Recapitulation: Criteria for Evaluating Surgery Quality with STS

– Surgery has to be planned.
– Treatment should be performed in specialised centres.
– Surgery has to be embedded in multidisciplinary treatment.
– The extent of resection should be adapted to tumour presentation and grade.
– Margins should be determined collaboratively between the surgeon and the pathologist.
– Quality of margins (negative vs positive, R0 vs R1) is more precise in predicting outcome than quantity (in mm).
– The end-point for surgery quality is local recurrence (LR), not disease-free survival.
– LR data should be given by actuarial methods (local recurrence-free estimation).
– The greater the difference in LR between margin negative and margin positive, the better the system for margin determination is.
– LR rates for limb and trunk wall STS should not exceed 20% at 5 years with the objective of approaching 10% in future series.

References

Avizonis VN, Sause WT, Menlove RL (1990) Utility of surgical margins in the radiotherapeutic management of soft tissue sarcomas. J Surg Oncol 45:85–90
Azzarelli A (1993) Surgery in soft tissue sarcomas. Eur J Cancer 29A:618–623

Bauer H, Trovik C, Alvegard T, Berlin Ö, Erlanson M, Gustafson P, et al (2001) Monitoring referral and treatment in soft tissue sarcoma. Study based on 1,851 patients from the Scandinavian Sarcoma Group register. Acta Orthop Scand 72:150–159

Bell RS, O'Sullivan B, Liu FF, Powell J, Langer F, Fornasier VL, et al (1989) The surgical margin in soft tissue sarcoma. J Bone Joint Surg 71:370–375

Bonvalot S, Laplanche A, Lejeune F, Stoeckle E, Le Pechoux C, Vanel D, et al (2005) Limb salvage with isolated perfusion for soft tissue sarcoma: could less TNF-alpha be better? Ann Oncol 16:1061–1068

Bowden L, Booher RJ (1958) The principle and techniques of resection of soft parts of sarcoma. Surgery 44:963–977

Cade S (1950) Soft tissue tumours, their natural history and treatment. Proc R Soc Med 44:19–36

Cantin J, Mc Neer GP, Clin FC, Booher RJ (1968) The problem of local recurrence after treatment of soft tissue sarcoma. Ann Surg 168:47–53

Cany L, Bui NB, Stöckle E, Coindre JM, Kantor G, ravaud A (1992) Chimiothérapie d'induction et traitement combiné conservateur des sarcomes des tissus mous de l'adulte. Bull Cancer 79:1077–1085

Clasby R, Tilling K, Smith MA, Fletcher CD (1997) Variable management of soft tissue sarcoma: regional audit with implications for specialist care. Br J Surg 84:1692–1696

Coindre JM, Trojani M, Contesso G, David M, Rouessé J, Bui NB, et al (1986) Reproducibility of a histopathologic grading system for adult soft tissue sarcoma. Cancer 58:306–309

Coindre JM, Terrier P, Bui NB, Bonichon F, Collin F, Le Doussal V, et al (1996) Prognostic factors in adult patients with locally controlled soft tissue sarcoma. A study on 546 patients from the French Federation of Cancer Centers Sarcoma Group. J Clin Oncol 14:869–877

Coindre JM, Terrier P, Guillou L, Le Doussal V, Collin F, Ranchère D, et al (2001) Predictive value of grade for metastasis development in the main histologic types of adult soft tissue sarcomas. A study of 1240 patients from the French Federation of Cancer Centers Sarcoma Group. Cancer 91:1919–1926

Dickinson IC, Whitwell DJ, Battistuta D, Thompson B, Strobel N, Duggal A, Steadman P (2006) Surgical margin and its influence on survival in soft tissue sarcoma. ANZ J Surg 76:104–109

Eggermont AM, Schraffordt KH, Klausner JM, Kroon BB, Schlag PM, Lienard D, et al (1996) Isolated limb perfusion with tumor necrosis factor and melphalan for limb salvage in 186 patients with locally advanced soft-tissue sarcomas. The cumulative multicenter European experience. Ann Surg 224:756–764

Eilber FC, Rosen G, Nelson SD, Selch M, Dorey F, Eckardt J, Eilber FR (2003) High-grade extremity soft tissue sarcomas. Factors predictive of local recurrence and its effect on morbidity. Ann Surg 2:218–226

Engellau J, Bendahl PO, Persson A, Domanski H, Akerman M, Gustafson P, et al (2005) Improved prognostication in soft tissue sarcoma: independent information from vascular invasion, necrosis, growth pattern, and immunostaining using whole-tumor sections and tissue microarrays. Hum Pathol 36:994–1002

Enneking WF, Spanier SS, Malawer MM (1981) The effect of the anatomic setting on the results of surgical procedures for soft parts sarcoma of the thigh. Cancer 47:1005–1022

Ferguson PC, Griffin AM, O'Sullivan B, Catton CN, Davis AM, Murji A, et al (2006) Bone invasion in extremity soft-tissue sarcoma. Impact on disease outcomes. Cancer 106:2692–2700

Fernebro J, Wiklund M, Jonsson K, Bendahl PO, Rydholm A, Nilbert M, Engellau J (2006) Focus on the tumour periphery in MRI evaluation of soft tissue sarcoma: infiltrative growth signifies poor prognosis. Sarcoma 21:1–5

Firth LA (1979) The relative roles of surgery and radiotherapy in the management of soft tissue sarcomas of adults. Clin Radiol 30:155–159

Fletcher CDM, Unni KK, Mertens F (eds) (2002) Pathology and genetics of tumours of soft tissue and bone. World Health Organization classification of tumours, vol 5. IARC Press, Lyon

Gaynor JJ, Tan CC, Casper ES, Collin CF, Friedrich C, Shiu M, et al (1992) Refinement of clinicopathologic staging for localized soft tissue sarcoma of the extremity: a study of 423 adults. J Clin Oncol 10:1317–1329

Gerrand CH, Wunder JS, Kandel RA, O'Sullivan B, Catton CN, Bell RS, et al (2001) Classification of positive margins after resection of soft-tissue sarcoma of the limb predicts the risk of local recurrence. J Bone Joint Surg 83:1149–1155

Gerrand CH, Bell RS, Wunder JS, Kandel RA, O'Sullivan B, Catton CN, et al (2003) The influence of anatomic location on outcome in patients with soft tissue sarcoma of the extremity. Cancer 97:485–492

Ghnassia JP, Vilain MO, Coindre JM, Bertrand G, Château MC, Collin F, et al (1998) Recommendations pour la prise en charge anatomo-pathologique des sarcomes des tissus mous de l'adulte. Ann Pathol 18:505–511

Grimer R (2006) Size matters for sarcomas. Ann R Coll Surg Engl 88:519–524

Gronchi A, Casali PG, Mariani L, Miceli R, Fiore M, Lo Vullo S, et al (2005) Status of surgical margins and prognosis in adult soft tissue sarcomas of the extremities: a series of patients treated at a single institution. J Clin Oncol 23:96–104

Guillou L, Coindre JM, Bonichon F, Bui NB, Terrier P, Collin F, et al (1997) Comparative study of the National Cancer Institute and French Federation of Cancer Centers Sarcoma Group grading systems in a population of 410 adult patients with oft tissue sarcoma. J Clin Oncol 15:350–362

Gustafson P (1994) Soft tissue sarcoma. Epidemiology and prognosis in 508 patients. Acta Orthop Scand 65[Suppl 259]:1–31

Gustafson P, Rööser B, Rydholm A (1991) Is local recurrence of minor importance for metastases in soft tissue sarcoma? Cancer 67:2083–2086

Gustafson P, Dreinhofer K, Rydholm K (1994) Soft tissue sarcoma should be treated at a tumor center. A comparison of quality of surgery in 375 patients. Acta Orthop Scand 65:47–50

Herbert SH, Corn BW, Solin LJ, Lanciano RM, Schultz DJ, McKenna WG, Coia LR (1993) Limb-preserving treatment for soft tissue sarcomas of the extremities. The significance of surgical margins. Cancer 72:1230–1238

Karakousis CP, Emrich LJ, Rao U, Krishnamsetty RM (1986) Feasibility of limb salvage and survival in soft tissue sarcomas. Cancer 57:484–491

Kawaguchi N, Ahmed AR, Matsumoto S, Manabe J, Matsushita Y (2004) The concept of curative margin in surgery for bone and soft tissue sarcoma. Clin Orthop 419:165–172

Keus RB, Rutgers EJ, Ho GH, Gortzak E, Albus-Lutter CE, Hart AA (1994) Limb-sparing therapy of extremity soft tissue sarcomas: treatment outcome and long-term functional results. Eur J Cancer 30A:1459–1463

Khanfir K, Alzieu L, Terrier P, Le Pechoux C, Bonvalot S, Vanel D, et al (2003) Does adjuvant radiation therapy increase loco-regional control after optimal resection of soft-tissue sarcoma of the extremities? Eur J Cancer 39:1872–1880

Koea JB, Leung D, Lewis JJ, Brennan MF (2003) Histopathologic type: an independent prognostic factor in primary soft tissue sarcoma of the extremity? Ann Surg Oncol 10:432–440

Kotilingam D, Lev DC, Lazar AJ, Pollock RE (2006) Staging soft tissue sarcoma: evolution and change. CA Cancer J Clin Oncol 56:282–291

Langlois D, Bey P, Luporsi E, Hoffstetter S, Marchal C, Malissard L, et al (1991) Radiothérapie des sarcomes des parties molles: place et résultats. Bull Cancer Radiother 78:39–49

LeVay J, O'Sullivan B, Catton C, Bell R, Fornasier V, Cummings B, et al (1993) Outcome and prognostic factors in soft tissue sarcoma in the adult. Int J Radiat Oncol Biol Phys 27:1091–1099

Lin PP, Pino ED, Normand AN, Deavers MT, Cannon CP, Ballo MT, et al (2007) Periostal margin in soft-tissue sarcoma. Cancer 109:598–602

Lindberg RD, Martin RG, Romsdahl MM, Morton DL (1981) Conservative surgery and postoperative radiotherapy in 300 adults with soft tissue sarcomas. Cancer 47:2391–2397

Llacer C, Delannes M, Minsat M, Stoeckle E, Votron L, Martel P, et al (2006) Low-dose intraoperative brachytherapy in soft tissue sarcomas involving neurovascular structure. Radiother Oncol 78:10–16

Mandard AM, Petiot JF, Marnay J, Mandard JC, Chasle J, de Ranieri E, et al (1989) Prognostic factors in soft tissue sarcomas. A multivariate analysis of 109 cases. Cancer 63:1437–1451

Manoso MW, Pratt J, Healey JH, Boland PJ, Athanasian EA (2006) Infiltrative MRI pattern and incomplete initial surgery compromise local control of myxofibrosarcoma. Clin Orthop Relat Res 450:89–94

Markhede G, Angervall L, Stener B (1982) A multivariate analysis of the prognosis after surgical treatment of malignant soft tissue sarcomas. Cancer 49:1721–1733

Mazanet R, Antman K (1991) Sarcomas of soft tissues and bone. Cancer 68:463–473

McKee MD, Liu DF, Brooks JJ, Gibbs JF, Driscoll DL, Kraybill WG (2004) The prognostic significance of margin width for extremity and trunk sarcoma. J Surg Oncol 85:68–76

NIH (1985) Proceedings of the NIH Consensus Development Conference limb-sparing treatment of adult soft-tissue and osteogenic sarcomas. Bethesda, Md. December 3–5, 1984. Cancer Treat Symp 3:1–167

Oertel S, Treiber M, Zahlten-Hingurange A, Eichin S, Roeder F, Funk A, et al (2006) Intraoperative electron boost radiation followed by moderate doses of external beam radiotherapy in limb-sparing treatment of patients with extremity soft-tissue sarcoma. Int J Radiat Oncol Biol Phys 64:1416–1423

Peiper M, Zurakowski D, Zornig C (1997) Survival in primary soft tissue sarcoma of the extremities and trunk. Langenbecks Arch Chir 382:203–208

Pisters PWT, Leung DH, Woodruff J, Shi W, Brennan MF (1996) Analysis of prognostic factors in 1041 patients with localized soft tissue tumours of the extremities. J Clin Oncol 14:1679–1689

Pitcher ME, Fish S, Thomas JM (1994) Management of soft tissue sarcoma. Br J Surg 81:1136–1139

Pitcher ME, Ramanathan RC, Fish S, A'Hern R, Thomas JM (2000) Outcome of treatment for limb and limb girdle sarcomas at the Royal Marsden Hospital. Eur J Surg Oncol 26:548–551

Pollock RE, Karnell LH, Menck HR, Winchester DP (1996) The National Cancer Data base report on soft tissue sarcoma. Cancer 78:2247–2257

Ravaud A, Bui NB, Coindre JM, Lagarde P, Tramond P, Bonichon F, et al (1992) Prognostic variables for the selection of patients with operable soft tissue sarcomas to be considered in adjuvant chemotherapy trials. Br J Cancer 66:961–969

Ray-Coquard I, Thiesse P, Ranchère-Vince D, Chauvin F, Bobin JY, Sunyach MP, et al (2004) Conformity to clinical practice guidelines, multidisciplinary management and outcome of treatment for soft tissue sarcomas. Ann Oncol 15:307–315

Rööser B, Gustafson P, Rydholm A (1990) Is there no influence of local control on the rate of metastases in high-grade soft tissue sarcoma? Cancer 65:1727–1729

Rosenberg SA, Tepper J, Glatstein E, Costa J, Baker A, Brennan M, et al (1982) The treatment of soft-tissue sarcomas of the extremities. Prospective randomized evaluations of (1) limb-sparing surgery plus radiation therapy compared with amputation and (2) the role of adjuvant chemotherapy. Ann Surg 196:305–314

Ruka W, Emrich LJ, Driscoll DL, Karakousis CP (1989) Clinical factors and treatment parameters affecting prognosis in adult high-grade soft tissue sarcomas: a retrospective review of 267 cases. Eur J Surg Oncol 15:411–423

Rydholm A (1998) Improving the management of soft tissue sarcoma: diagnosis and treatment should be given in specialised centres. BMJ 317:93–94

Rydholm A, Berg NO, Gullberg BO, Persson BM, Thomeren KG (1984) Prognosis for soft-tissue sarcoma in the locomotor system. A retrospective population-based follow-up study of 237 patients. Acta Pathol Microbiol Immunol Scand 92:375–386

Rydholm A, Gustafson P, Rööser B, Willen H, Akerman M, Herrlin K (1991) Limb-sparing surgery without radiotherapy based on anatomic location of soft tissue sarcoma. J Clin Oncol 9:1757–1765

Saddegh MK, Lindholm J, Lundberg A, Nilsonne U, Kreicbergs A (1992) Staging of soft tissue sarcomas. Prognostic analysis of clinical and pathological features. J Bone Joint Surg 74:495–500

Sadoski C, Suit HD, Rosenberg A, Mankin H, Efird J (1993) Preoperative radiation, surgical margins, and local control of extremity sarcomas of soft tissues. J Surg Oncol 52:223–230

Sastre-Garau X, Coindre JM, Leroyer A, Terrier P, Ollivier L, Stoeckle E, et al (1997) Predictive factors for complete removal in soft tissue sarcomas: a retrospective analysis in a series of 592 cases. J Surg Oncol 65:175–182

Shiu MH, Castro EB, Hajdu SI, Fortner JG (1975) Surgical treatment of 297 soft tissue sarcomas of the lower extremity. Ann Surg 182:597–602

Siebenrock KA, Hertel R, Ganz R (2000) Unexpected resection of soft-tissue sarcoma. More mutilating surgery, higher local recurrence rates, and obscure prognosis as consequences of improper surgery. Arch Orthop Trauma Surg 120:65–69

Simon MA, Enneking WF (1976) The management of soft tissue sarcomas of the extremities. J Bone Joint Surg 58-A:317–327

Sobin LH, Wittekind C (2002) Tumours of bone and soft tissues. TNM Classification of malignant tumours. Wiley-Liss, New York

Stefanovski P, Bidoli E, de Paoli A, Buonadonna A, Boz G, Libra M, Morassut S, Rossi C, Carbone A, Frustaci S (2002) Prognostic factors in soft tissue sarcomas: a study of 395 patients. Eur J Surg Oncol 28:153–164

Stoeckle E (1997) Nouvelles techniques chirurgicales des sarcomes des tissus mous. Cancer Radiother 1:453–456

Stoeckle E, Coindre JM, Kantor G, Thomas L, Avril A, Lagarde P, et al (2005) Quality of surgery in soft tissue sarcoma: a single centre experience with the French Sarcoma Group (FSG) surgical system. Cancer Ther 3:31–39

Stoeckle E, Gardet H, Coindre JM, Kantor G, Bonichon F, Milbéo Y, Thomas L, Avril A, Bui BN (2006) Prospective evaluation of quality of surgery in soft tissue sarcoma. Eur J Surg Oncol 32:1242–1248

Stoeckle E, Coindre JM, Thomas L, Bui M, Kantor G, Kind M, Bui BN (2007) Chirurgie des sarcomes des tissues mous des membres et de la paroi du tronc. Oncologie 9:107–113

Stojadinovic A, Leung DH, Allen P, Lewis JJ, Jaques DP, Brennan MF (2002a) Primary adult soft tissue sarcoma: time-dependent influence of prognostic variables. J Clin Oncol 20:4344–4352

Stojadinovic A, Leung DH, Hoos A, Jaques DP, Lewis JJ, Brennan MF (2002b) Analysis of the prognostic significance of microscopic margin in

2,084 localized primary adult soft tissue sarcomas. Ann Surg 235:424–434

Stotter AT, A'Hern RP, Fisher C, Mott AF, Fallowfield ME, Westbury G (1990) The influence of local recurrence of extremity soft tissue sarcoma on metastases and survival. Cancer 65:1119–1129

Tanabe KK, Pollock RE, Ellis LM, Murphy A, Sherman N, Romsdahl MM (1994) Influence of surgical margins on outcome in patients with preoperatively irradiated extremity soft tissue sarcomas. Cancer 73:1652–1659

Trojani M, Contesso G, Coindre JM, Rouëssé J, Bui NB, de Mascarel A, et al (1984) Soft-tissue sarcoma of adults: study of pathological prognostic variables and definition of a histopathological grading system. Int J Cancer 1984 33:37–42

Trovik CS, Bauer HC, Alvegard TA, Anderson H, Blomqvist C, Berlin Ö, et al (2000) Surgical margins, local recurrence and metastasis in soft tissue sarcomas: 559 surgically-treated patients from the Scandinavian Sarcoma Group Register. Eur J Cancer 36:710–716

Vraa S, Keller J, Nielsen OS, Jurik AG, Jensen OM (2001) Soft-tissue sarcoma of the thigh: surgical margin influences local recurrence but not survival in 152 patients. Acta Orthop Scand 72:72–77

Weitz J, Antonescu CR, Brennan MF (2003) Localized extremity soft tissue sarcoma: improved knowledge with unchanged survival over time. J Clin Oncol 21:2719–2725

Wood WC, Suit HD, Mankin HJ, Cohen AM, Proppe K (1984) Radiation and conservative surgery in the treatment of soft tissue sarcoma. Am J Surg 147:537–541

Zagars GK, Ballo MT, Pisters PW, Pollock RE, Patel SR, Benjamin RS, Evans HL (2003) Prognostic factors for patients with localized soft-tissue sarcoma treated with conservation surgery and radiation therapy. An analysis of 1225 patients. Cancer 97:2530–2543

Peripheral Nerve Considerations in the Management of Extremity Soft Tissue Sarcomas

15

Peter C. Ferguson, Anna A. Kulidjian, Kevin B. Jones, Benjamin M. Deheshi, and Jay S. Wunder

Abstract Evaluation of peripheral nerves, both clinically and with imaging, is critical in the evaluation of patients with extremity soft tissue sarcomas. If an essential peripheral nerve is felt to be adjacent to a soft tissue sarcoma but not circumferentially surrounded, it can usually be salvaged using the technique of epineural dissection in the setting of adjuvant radiation. If, however, a critical nerve is circumferentially involved with tumor, it must be sacrificed for the sake of local control. Various reconstruction techniques are available in this situation, including nerve grafting, distal nerve transfer, and tendon transfer, with each technique having specific indications. Regardless of the technique, it is important to inform the patient that normal extremity function is not likely to be achieved. The issue of nerve involvement therefore becomes a critical factor in determining the possibility of limb salvage in borderline cases. For the situation in which postoperative function is already expected to be compromised due to vascular, bone, or extensive soft tissue resection, nerve resection may be the ultimate deciding factor in recommending amputation rather than limb salvage.

Peter C. Ferguson (✉)
University Musculoskeletal Oncology Unit
Mount Sinai Hospital
476G-600 University Avenue
Toronto, ON M5G 1X5
Canada
E-mail: pferguson@mtsinai.on.ca

15.1
Introduction

The increasingly narrow and specifically refined definitions of safe margins have been critical to the transition from amputation to limb salvage as the standard surgical technique for soft tissue sarcomas (STS) of the extremity. The 2-cm cuff of uninvolved tissue completely enclosing an excised sarcoma, which historically defined a wide margin, is a theoretical goal that is often mutually exclusive with the objective of functional limb salvage. Extremity anatomy simply provides too many spatial constraints on such margins for deep tumors of large sizes. Some of the most obvious anatomic constraints to the 2-cm definition of wide margins include the peripheral nerves, whose preservation is essential to maintain the function and comfort of more distal aspects of the limb to be salvaged (Davis et al. 2000).

As conventional radiotherapy techniques have demonstrated efficacy in improving local control of STS, the definition of a safe surgical margin has narrowed on many fronts. Perhaps the last of these fronts to advance have been those directed toward peripheral nerves. In the recent past, involvement of a major peripheral nerve such as the sciatic nerve was considered an absolute indication for amputation. Our understanding has improved in recent years of both the functional results of limb salvage in the setting of nerve resection, and, with the use of adjuvant or neoadjuvant radiotherapy, the potential for safe but very close margins on and around nerves. Such advances in the management of peripheral nerve involvement specifically have expanded the indication for limb salvage and have made amputations a much less common necessity.

Although loss of any peripheral nerve, whether mixed or purely sensory, may cause some degree of symptoms in the affected extremity, for the purposes of this chapter any reference to peripheral nerves implies major mixed motor and sensory nerves, in particular the sciatic, femoral, tibial, and peroneal nerves in the lower extremity, and axillary, musculocutaneous, median, radial, and ulnar in the upper extremity. Sacrifice of any of these peripheral nerves has been shown to be associated with significant functional impairment; their preservation, if oncologically safe, is therefore of critical importance.

15.2
Diagnosis of Peripheral Nerve Involvement

15.2.1
History and Physical Examination

It is unusual for peripheral nerves to be frankly invaded by STS. More commonly the nerve is encircled by adjacent tumor over a variable circumference. Despite this, patients are often asymptomatic and it may be difficult to clearly ascertain, on history and physical examination, whether or not a peripheral nerve is involved by a sarcoma. There are, however, some features of the history and physical examination that may provide clues to the possibility of peripheral nerve involvement by an extremity STS. Sarcomas, even when quite large, typically are not painful. Pain in the setting of an STS may imply direct nerve involvement, among other possible causes (Fig. 15.1). Furthermore, in patients who recollect the pain preceding a noticeable mass, tumors may occasionally arise from the peripheral nerves themselves. Burning pain, radicular pain in an anatomic peripheral nerve distribution, paraesthesias, and weakness all suggest either peripheral nerve involvement with tumor or compression of a peripheral nerve within a fascial compartment. The duration of symptoms can be important in predicting the possibility for nerve recovery after tumor resection. If a patient presents with longstanding nerve palsy then it is unlikely that a salvaged nerve

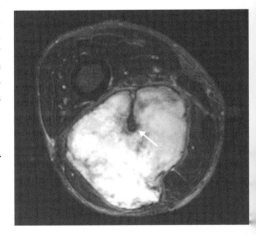

Fig. 15.1 This patient presented with a foot drop as well as paresthesiae and dysesthesiae both plantarly and dorsally on his foot. Imaging confirmed involvement of both the peroneal and tibial branches of his sciatic nerve by this high-grade sarcoma (*arrow* pointing to the sciatic nerve)

will function postoperatively. Although it is important to ascertain whether these symptoms exist, their absence does not necessarily preclude nerve involvement.

Physical examination of any sarcoma patient must include a detailed peripheral nerve examination in the affected extremity. This is especially crucial in patients with symptoms that suggest peripheral nerve involvement. A carefully documented sensory and motor examination is essential. A positive Tinel's sign with percussion may indicate a sarcoma arising from a peripheral nerve. Atrophy often signifies longstanding nerve dysfunction and can have ramifications for functional recovery after resection of the tumor. Proximity to other critical structures in the extremity must also be documented. Altered peripheral pulses or evidence of significant swelling in the extremity may indicate co-existent vascular involvement, and, together with peripheral nerve involvement, may preclude an attempt at limb salvage. Involvement of adjacent bone can be assessed by attempting to move the sarcoma over the surface of the bone—if it is mobile then there is usually a safe periosteal margin and the bone need not be resected. If the tumor is fixed to bone then it may need to be resected and again, combined with nerve resection, may imply severe functional limitations in the salvaged limb, making amputation a more likely alternative. Examination of the skin overlying the lesion is essential in planning soft tissue coverage. If it is anticipated that a peripheral nerve can be salvaged yet will be exposed due to significant skin resection, then flap reconstruction must be planned.

15.2.2
Imaging

Although medical history and physical examination are essential in patient assessment, the development of cross-sectional imaging, in particular high-resolution magnetic resonance imaging (MRI) scans, has greatly facilitated the management of extremity STS. By allowing for better appreciation of the anatomic extent of tumors and proximity to critical structures such as peripheral nerves, these technological advances have been essential to the establishment of limb salvage surgery as the standard management of extremity STS, and in particular they have set the stage for surgical techniques designed to salvage peripheral nerves.

Review of the preoperative MRI may demonstrate that important peripheral nerves are completely free of the sarcoma, with a clear fatty plane between nerve and tumor on T1 weighted images. In these situations the surgeon can anticipate that the peripheral nerve can be easily dissected free of the tumor with a negative margin. Quite often, however, the MRI fails to demonstrate a fatty plane between the tumor and a critical peripheral nerve, and the nerve may be partially surrounded by the tumor (Fig. 15.2). However, provided there is a portion of the nerve's circumference that is not surrounded by tumor, it can often be preserved using the technique of epineural dissection, which will be described. If a critical nerve is completely encased in tumor then nerve preservation would entail cutting through the tumor and obtaining a

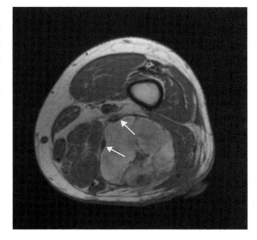

Fig. 15.2 MRI showing peroneal and tibial nerve on the surface of the tumor (*arrows* pointing to the nerves)

grossly positive margin, a procedure that would be ill-advised due to the very high risk of local recurrence. In this rare situation nerve resection becomes a necessity.

15.2.3
Other Diagnostic Considerations

Despite the advances in high-resolution MRI, peripheral nerves that lie on the tumor surface may occasionally be difficult to differentiate from those encased by it. In the situation in which it is difficult to assess nerve involvement on imaging, the decision on nerve salvage must be made intraoperatively. Therefore any patient in whom it cannot be determined on imaging whether nerve salvage is possible must be informed preoperatively that nerve sacrifice and nerve salvage are both potential outcomes of surgery. The patient should understand as clearly as possible the functional deficits to be expected from each technique and the limitations associated with nerve-deficient limbs.

Although other investigations of peripheral nerves, such as nerve conduction studies and electromyography, may be of use in documenting any preoperative nerve palsy, their utility is usually limited in the preoperative setting. These tests are usually reserved for documenting recovery of nerve palsies postoperatively, and may be useful in providing evidence of success of nerve reconstruction techniques.

15.3
Management of Peripheral Nerve Involvement

15.3.1
General Approach

In any patient in whom a sarcoma is adjacent to a peripheral nerve, surgery alone with preservation of the nerve will give inadequate margins, leading to a significant risk of local recurrence. In most of these instances the sarcomas are deep and also close to bone and critical blood vessels. In order to permit limb salvage with an acceptable risk of local recurrence, radiotherapy, in either the preoperative or postoperative period, will be essential. Preservation of the nerve can then ensue during surgical resection. If, however, imaging suggests that a major peripheral nerve will require resection due to circumferential involvement, then it is incumbent on the surgeon to ascertain whether functional limb salvage can still take place. As a general rule, if one peripheral nerve requires excision while other critical structures can be preserved, then limb salvage in association with radiotherapy should take place, as functional limitations are likely to be less than with amputation. If however, multiple nerves or a single nerve and other critical structures require resection, the surgeon must carefully consider whether the function of the salvaged limb would be superior to amputation and prosthetic fitting.

15.3.2
Epineural Dissection

Nerve resection, while no longer an absolute indication for amputation, nonetheless bears serious morbidity that is preferably avoided. Motor nerve resection has been shown to have significant detrimental effect on patient-reported functional outcome measures in a group of patients having undergone resection of extremity sarcomas (Davis et al. 1999, 2000). Defining the limits of a safely avoidable nerve resection is therefore pivotal.

In ascertaining risk of local recurrence after STS resection, it is now accepted that close surgical margins can safely be categorized as equivalent to "wide"—even in the sub-centimeter zone—when neoadjuvant or adjuvant radiation therapy is also used. Theoretically in keeping with the radical compartment resections described by William Enneking as treatment for sarcomas (Simon et al. 1979), such close margins engendered no additional risk of local recurrence in a large series of patients with carefully defined margins (Gerrand et al. 2001). In this study, a "planned positive" margin, adjacent to a fixed critical anatomic structure such as blood vessel, nerve, or bone, was associated with a local recurrence rate equivalent to that of a negative margin when radiotherapy was utilized as part of the treatment paradigm. This evidence, when applied to thoughts of proximate peripheral nerves, suggests that epineurium can serve as an adequate margin, with respect to protection against local recurrence.

The most directly enlightening outcomes specifically addressing peripheral nerves in this regard come from a retrospective review of a prospective cohort of patients (Clarkson et al. 2005). This article compared 43 patients undergoing epineural dissection of the sciatic nerve during STS resection in the thigh with 44 patients bearing tumors of similar size and grade, but located distantly from the sciatic nerve in the thigh. The technique of epineural dissection was utilized when the tumor encompassed the sciatic nerve on less than 270° of its circumference. Radiotherapy, usually neoadjuvant, was routinely employed. The epineural dissection group had only 3 local and 18 systemic relapses, compared to 1 local and 17 systemic relapses in the control group. These were not significantly different, statistically. These epineural dissection patients also had appreciably better functional outcomes when compared to a smaller cohort of patients undergoing sciatic nerve resection.

This series of patients offers adequate evidence of the safety of the technique, when embarked upon thoughtfully and carefully. The decision to proceed with epineural dissection can only be finally made intraoperatively, after dissecting out the involved nerve proximal and distal to the sarcoma.

15.3.2.1
Epineural Dissection Surgical Technique

Epineural dissection, a special technique, is utilized when a peripheral nerve is found to be adjacent to the surface of a sarcoma, usually without a clear plane on preoperative MRI. If the locations of critical peripheral nerves are not clear on preoperative cross-sectional imaging, intraoperative examination of the nerves is essential (Fig. 15.3). If a nerve appears to be passing directly into the tumor, then any attempt

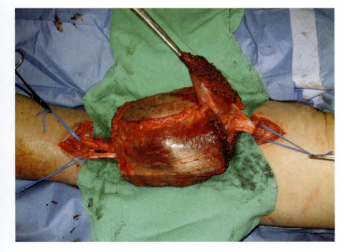

Fig. 15.3 Intraoperative photograph of the nerve completely encased by tumor, thus precluding salvage

at nerve salvage must be abandoned and it must be sacrificed (Fig. 15.4a, b). If the nerve is found to be on the surface of the tumor, with a portion of the nerve visible and not surrounded by tumor then epineural dissection may take place. Although it is debatable, for practical reasons at least 90° of the circumference of the nerve should be visible to attempt salvage. Anything less often makes nerve extrication from the tumor prohibitively difficult.

The surgical technique consists of dissection of all margins of the sarcoma except for the nerve that is in direct proximity to the tumor. The nerve is then isolated proximal and distal to the tumor such that the last remaining host structure attached to the tumor is the nerve itself (Fig. 15.5). The nerve at this point usually remains attached to the inflammatory tissue peripheral to the sarcoma, but not completely encased. This distinction is the critical final step in the decision to

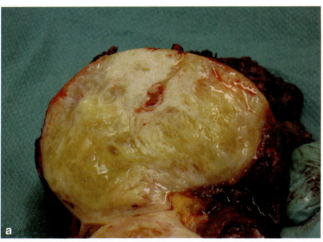
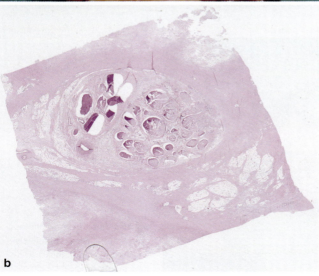

Fig. 15.4 a, b Photographs from the same patient with gross and microscopic pathologic confirmation of the sciatic nerve completely encased in tumor, precluding safe resection

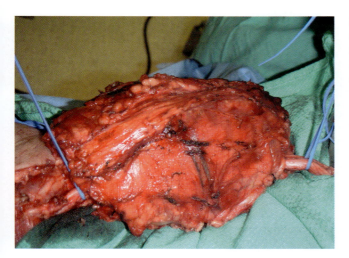

Fig. 15.5 Wide margin dissection of the tumor with the nerve isolated proximally and distally but abutting the tumor on the surface

salvage a nerve by epineural dissection. The relationship between tumor and nerve may be incompletely resolved on the preoperative imaging or may have even changed in the interval between the time of imaging and the surgical date. If a surgical plane directly to at least one uninvolved epineural surface of the nerve is not identifiable, the decision to sacrifice the nerve should be made. If, alternatively, the nerve itself is clearly visible and an uninvolved surface of the epineurium available, then the decision can be made to proceed with epineural dissection. Mobility of the nerve over the tumor within its epineurium is often an encouraging sign that safe dissection may take place, but a nerve that is firmly adherent to the tumor can still be salvaged with this technique.

Fresh drapes or towels are used to surround the tumor, placing them between the tumor and the wound (Fig. 15.6). If possible the tumor with its attached nerve may be placed over a basin. This setup protects the wound from potential tumor contamination in case the tumor is inadvertently entered during the epineural dissection. If this happens and the nerve becomes grossly contaminated with tumor, the nerve is sacrificed and the tumor specimen is passed off the surgical table in its isolating drapes or basin and with the offending instrument.

Sharp dissection using a fresh scalpel blade is used to split the epineurium longitudinally on the surface of the nerve (Fig. 15.7). The epineurium is reflected back to the surface of the tumor, keeping the nutrient vessels attached and reflected with it. The nerve fascicles then are lifted directly out of their epineural sheath. Any nerve fibers that enter into the gross substance of the tumor are sacrificed (Figs. 15.8 and 15.9). At our institution, standard wound irrigation is used after the removal of the tumor. Although some centers advocate use of distilled water or alcohol as the irrigation solution (Matsumoto et al. 2002), few data are available to support this practice and it has the potential to delay wound healing.

15.3.3
Nerve Resection Without Reconstruction

As has been detailed, nerve resection can be planned based on preoperative MRI with evidence of nerve encasement by the extremity STS. However, it is essential to confirm at the time of surgical resection that the nerve is indeed encased;

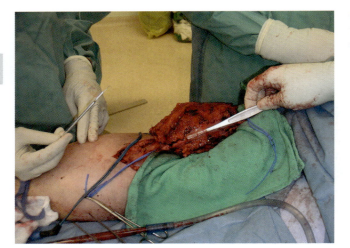

Fig. 15.6 Tumor isolated from the wound by towels, allowing the nerves to be inspected

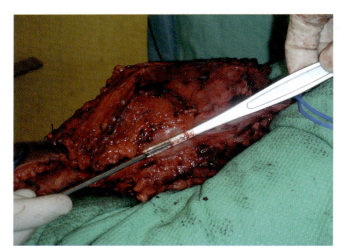

Fig. 15.7 Sharp epineural dissection

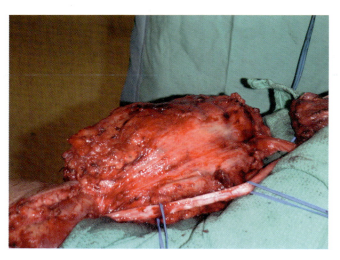

Fig. 15.8 Nerve dissected free of tumor with planned close surgical margins

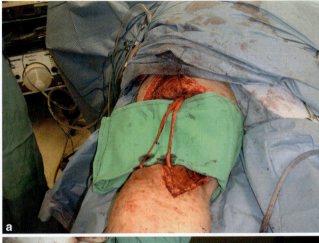
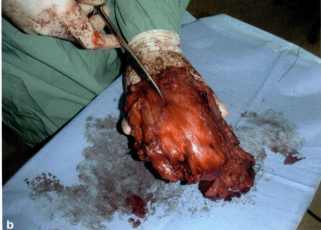

Fig. 15.9 a, b Intraoperative photographs with dissected nerves and the tumor with the surgeon pointing to the area where the nerve was dissected off

indeed; occasionally a nerve that appears to be non-salvageable on imaging will be noted intraoperatively to have an uninvolved surface to permit entry to the epineural sheath and epineural dissection for nerve salvage. If, however, maintenance of the nerve in question would require gross contamination by cutting directly through the tumor, then the nerve must be resected for the sake of local control.

It is essential for the surgeon to have a preoperative plan to deal with an expected nerve resection. The technique of management of a nerve defect depends on the expected functional deficit associated without reconstruction and the anticipated success of the reconstruction technique. In the upper extremity, resection of the median, radial, or ulnar nerves is often associated with severe functional limitations and significant impact on daily activities. Furthermore, techniques of reconstruction to overcome these functional deficits are fairly reliable. For this reason, upper extremity nerve resections are often associated with an attempted reconstructive procedure. Conversely, in the lower extremity, where bracing can frequently compensate for motor deficits and where sensory deficits, while potentially risky, do not incur devastating functional outcomes, different considerations are needed.

While resection of the femoral nerve has received no direct discussion in the literature, its sensory innervation is relatively expendable, so long as painful neuromas can be avoided at the resection site. The motor deficit left after resection of the femoral nerve is most importantly the loss of knee extension by the quadriceps. While receiving little attention in the literature, this is considered to be a well-tolerated deficit. The thigh is the most common originating site of STS in the extremities, and resection of major portions of the quadriceps is common during the process of limb salvage for extremity STS. Many patients manage a back-knee gait, with compensatory knee hyperextension. Others can maintain erect posture with a dynamic or locking brace for the knee.

The sciatic nerve presents an entirely different challenge. While the motor deficits are easily braced even with static orthoses and the sensory losses bear only minor functional impairments, these sensory deficits are thought to carry a risk of skin problems and Charcot arthropathy. The related, but importantly distinct, plight of the insensate diabetic foot probably fueled the reluctance with which sarcoma surgeons initially embraced the thought of limb salvage in the setting of sciatic nerve resection. Whether or not the difference is based on the absence of macro- and microvasculopathy—or whether there is some other physiological discrepancy between the denervated foot of a post-resection sarcoma patient and the insensate foot of a patient with diabetes mellitus—is not clear. What does seem to be clear is that a major difference exists and that patients who have an insensate foot due to sciatic nerve resection seem to be much less prone to long-term sequelae of this deficit than patients with diabetes mellitus.

The first two reports of sciatic nerve resection in the setting of limb salvage for STS were reported in 1984 (Nambisan et al. 1984) and 1991 (Young et al. 1991), both for tumors directly involving the nerve. O'Connor then discussed the theoretical functional advantage over high transfemoral amputation or hip disarticulation of a biological prosthesis in the form of a braced ankle and foot after sciatic nerve resection in the thigh (O'Connor 1998). The first functional outcome data came from a Toronto study documenting the plight of 10 patients undergoing resection of the sciatic nerve in the thigh. These cases were reported along with 10 other patients from other centers by Fuchs et al. (2001). One patient was noted to have ended up in amputation from plantar skin complications 6 years after sciatic nerve resection. Toronto Extremity Salvage Scores ranged from acceptable to excellent, averaging 73.5. Two other series followed the next year, detailing the outcomes from another 21 patients in total (Bickels et al. 2002; Brooks et al. 2002). All three reports concurred that all patients subjectively preferred the salvaged limb with an insensate foot to the possibility of an amputation.

Naturally, if sciatic nerve resection no longer remains an absolute indication for amputation, resection of its terminal branches are also generally preferable to amputation. More has been written about tibial and specifically peroneal nerve resections due to the frequency with which the need for these is encountered in the anatomically constrained popliteal space and leg. With or without reconstruction, resection of these is compatible with a very functional limb when appropriate bracing and skin precautions are utilized (Kim and Kline 1996; Ozaki et al. 1997; Shiu et al. 1986).

15.3.4
Nerve Resection and Reconstruction

When peripheral nerves are completely encased in sarcomas, removal of the involved segment of the nerve en bloc with the tumor is the only currently advisable strategy. In the past, this was often considered an indication for amputation. Even when a single peripheral nerve must be resected, if safe margins are otherwise surgically tenable in the extremity, limb salvage is still generally undertaken. The decision to proceed with nerve reconstruction or functional restoration, topics that will be discussed here, generally applies to upper extremity resections involving the median, ulnar, or radial nerve. The specific technique of reconstruction or functional restoration to be utilized depends on many factors, including patient age, the length of nerve resected, the specific nerve resected, the status of the soft tissues elsewhere in the extremity, the use of radiotherapy, and the presence of a pre-existing longstanding nerve palsy.

Modern advances in peripheral nerve surgery proffer great promise for future application in the setting of limb salvage. However, for the present, specific techniques can rarely be employed. Commercially available nerve conduits are currently only recommended for gaps of less than 2 cm. Most sarcomas that fully encompass nerves, generating the indication for nerve resection, are much larger than 2 cm. This unfortunate fact of nature renders such exciting technological advances powerless to help in the reconstruction of most peripheral nerve defects after sarcoma resection.

Similarly, autogenous nerve grafting—using the sural or other relatively expendable peripheral nerves—is less predictable with longer gaps (Kallio and Vastamaki 1993; Kalomiri et al. 1994; Meek et al. 2005; Stellini 1982). This challenge alone usually cancels the utility of grafting in the setting of major nerve reconstructions after sarcoma resections, but equally troublesome are the contraindications to grafting of large wounds, skin loss and muscle loss, most of which are also present following resection of a sarcoma large enough to fully encompass a major peripheral nerve.

Two other central difficulties with both grafting and nerve conduit reconstructions are the advanced age of many patients with STS and the proximal locations where the sarcomas are typically found. The mixed motor and sensory function of grafted nerves at this anatomic level makes successful recovery unpredictable and unreliable at best. Even direct repair of simple nerve lacerations in the brachium is successful in only about three-fourths of children and half of adults (Bolitho et al. 1999).

Although graft reconstruction of the sciatic nerve has been described after resection of STS, we do not recommend it given that functional recovery of sensation is the exception rather than the rule following such procedures (Lee et al. 1993; Melendez et al. 2001).

It seems apparent that nerve reconstruction, usually in the form of interposition grafting using the sural nerve, can only be counted on to reliably overcome functional deficits if certain specific criteria are met. Small deficits in young patients, ideally at a distal level in the upper extremity where the affected nerve is purely motor in nature, with otherwise healthy soft tissue, provides the ideal setting for nerve grafting. Nerve grafting in this situation often results in an excellent functional recovery. Unfortunately, it is indeed a rare sarcoma resection that meets all these criteria.

15.3.5
Distal Functional Restoration: Tendon Transfers

When major peripheral nerves are resected along with an extremity STS, and when the criteria for nerve reconstruction are not met, as is often the case, functional restoration of the nerve's distal motor functions is often quite possible. The gross motor deficit left after resection of any single major peripheral nerve in the upper extremity can be readily compensated for by transfer of adjacent muscles and tendons innervated by other unaffected nerves. Detailed descriptions of many techniques involved in the complex art of shoulder girdle, arm, and forearm tendon transfers are not well suited to this text, but many such options exist.

For radial nerve resection in the brachium a number of variations of the classic tendon transfer described originally by Robert Jones are possible. The pronator teres is transferred to the extensor carpi radialis brevis with or without inclusion of the extensor carpi radialis longus; either flexor carpi radialis or flexor carpi ulnaris is transferred to the finger extensors; and palmaris longus, flexor digitorum superficialis, or flexor carpi radialis is transferred into the thumb extensor. For median nerve resection in the brachium, extensor carpi radialis longus or the ulnar profundus tendons can be transferred into the index and long finger profundus tendons; flexor pollicis longus can be powered by the brachioradialis; both of these will depend heavily on the tenodesis effect, due to otherwise insufficient length of excursion. Flexor digitorum profundus from the long finger can be transferred to the ulnar profundus tendons if needed for strength after brachial resections of the ulnar nerve, but the loss of the intrinsics is more difficult to overcome, often requiring tenodesis or arthrodesis for maximal functional restoration (Giddens 2002).

While motor deficits other than the intrinsics are readily corrected for a single nerve, loss of any two of the radial, ulnar, and median nerves adds the additional challenges of scarce availability of innervated muscles available for transfer. Nevertheless, between fusion of some mobile elements and balanced transfers of available muscles, a limb more functional than an upper extremity prosthesis can occasionally be achieved.

Although it may be possible to restore motor function to a large extent with tendon transfers, sensory deficits persist. The functional value of a sensate distal upper extremity cannot be overemphasized and compensation for sensory deficits from resection of upper extremity peripheral nerves can often be more difficult to achieve than for motor deficits. A limb with neither ulnar nor median nerve function may therefore represent a relative indication for amputation.

15.3.6
Distal Functional Restoration: Distal Nerve Transfers

Some techniques other than tendon transfers also show some promise for reconstruction of both sensory and motor deficits left after peripheral nerve resection. Specialized microvascular surgeons and neurosurgeons in a number of tertiary medical centers are utilizing distal nerve transfers. This technique involves transferring redundant terminal branches of unaffected nerves into muscles rendered denervated by the STS resection. Furthermore, sensory fascicles can also be transferred to terminal sensory branches of the resected nerve. In this way both motor and sensory function can be restored. While documents of success do not abound in the literature, the technique is certainly gaining in popularity (O. Ozkan et al. 2002). One of the only widely available reports documents 15 of 25 patients' hands undergoing distal sensory nerve transfers as regaining two-point discrimination of less than 10 mm (T. Ozkan et al. 2001). This technique may hold great promise as not only does it restore both motor and sensory deficits, it does so with fewer constraints and limitations than nerve grafting.

15.3.7
Amputation

Wrought with an often overemphatic sense of surgical failure, amputation has become taboo to mention among many specialists in limb-salvage circles, but it remains the best course of therapy for some patients, even today. While absolute indications for amputation due to involvement of major peripheral nerves in STS are exceedingly rare, relative indications yet exist. Some combinations of non-reconstructible deficits will leave a patient with more challenges than function or satisfaction in a salvaged extremity. Specifically of note, complete resection of both the median and ulnar nerves needs to be considered very judiciously in the upper extremity, given the severe sensory loss that is expected. Similarly, combined resection of extensor innervation to both the knee and hip due to combined sciatic and femoral nerve resection will result in a very difficult functional situation for a patient.

Further, the undertaking of limb salvage is a laborious and time-consuming prospect for patients, especially at its extremes when major nerves will be resected requiring intensive rehabilitation and often distal reconstructions in the upper extremity. Such ventures are not the best course for every patient in whom they are technically feasible. Full disclosure of the risk and expected course of such treatment regimens must accompany a frank discussion of the patient's goals and desires prior to embarking on complex limb salvage. While excellent results are achievable, they will only be achieved when goals and expectations of the surgeon and patient are well aligned.

15.4 Conclusions

The peripheral nerves remain one of the last frontiers of limb salvage surgery for sarcomas. Bone resection can be overcome by reconstruction and vascular resection can be managed by bypass grafting, both with minimal functional limitations. Peripheral nerve resection, however, is associated with significant functional impairment and an often prolonged period of recovery after attempted reconstruction. Nonetheless, much has been learned in the last decade with regard to both the safety of planned close margins after adjuvant radiation and epineural dissection and the functional benefits of extremity salvage even with nerve resection contrasted to amputation. While research into the regeneration and reprogramming of peripheral nerves will hopefully render these techniques eventually obsolete,

for the present, a number of good options exist to manage sarcomas in close proximity to or directly involving peripheral nerves.

References

Bickels J, Wittig JC, Kollender Y, Kellar-Graney K, Malawer MM, Meller I (2002) Sciatic nerve resection: is that truly an indication for amputation? Clin Orthop Relat Res 399:201–204

Bolitho DG, Boustred M, Hudson DA, Hodgetts K (1999) Primary epineural repair of the ulnar nerve in children. J Hand Surg [Am] 24:16–20

Brooks AD, Gold JS, Graham D, Boland P, Lewis JJ, Brennan MF, Healey JH (2002) Resection of the sciatic, peroneal, or tibial nerves: assessment of functional status. Ann Surg Oncol 9:41–47

Clarkson PW, Griffin AM, Catton CN, O'Sullivan B, Ferguson PC, Wunder JS, Bell RS (2005) Epineural dissection is a safe technique that facilitates limb salvage surgery. Clin Orthop Relat Res 438:92–96

Davis AM, Bell RS, Badley EM, Yoshida K, Williams JI (1999) Evaluating functional outcome in patients with lower extremity sarcoma. Clin Orthop Relat Res 358:90–100

Davis AM, Sennik S, Griffin AM, Wunder JS, O'Sullivan B, Catton CN, Bell RS (2000) Predictors of functional outcomes following limb salvage surgery for lower-extremity soft tissue sarcoma. J Surg Oncol 73:206–211

Fuchs B, Davis AM, Wunder JS, Bell RS, Masri BA, Isler M, Turcotte R, Rock MG (2001) Sciatic nerve resection in the thigh: a functional evaluation. Clin Orthop Relat Res 382:34–41

Gerrand CH, Wunder JS, Kandel RA, O'Sullivan B, Catton CN, Bell RS, Griffin AM, Davis AM (2001) Classification of positive margins after resection of soft-tissue sarcoma of the limb predicts the risk of local recurrence. J Bone Joint Surg Br 83:1149–1155

Giddens G (2002) Nerve injuries. In: Bulstrode C, et al (eds) Oxford textbook of orthopedics and trauma, 3. Oxford University Press, New York, p 1848–1859

Kallio PK, Vastamaki M (1993) An analysis of the results of late reconstruction of 132 median nerves. J Hand Surg [Br] 18:97–105

Kalomiri DE, Soucacos PN, Beris AE (1994) Nerve grafting in peripheral nerve microsurgery of the upper extremity. Microsurgery 15:506–511

Kim DH, Kline DG (1996) Management and results of peroneal nerve lesions. Neurosurgery 39:312–319

Lee GW, Mackinnon SE, Brandt K, Bell RS (1993) A technique for nerve reconstruction following resection of soft-tissue sarcoma. J Reconstr Microsurg 9:139–144

Matsumoto S, Kawaguchi N, Manabe J, Matsushita Y (2002) "In situ preparation": new surgical procedure indicated for soft-tissue sarcoma of a lower limb in close proximity to major neurovascular structures. Int J Clin Oncol 7:51–56

Meek MF, Coert JH, Robinson PH (2005) Poor results after nerve grafting in the upper extremity: quo vadis? Microsurgery 25:396–402

Melendez M, Brandt K, Evans GR (2001) Sciatic nerve reconstruction: limb preservation after sarcoma resection. Ann Plast Surg 46:375–381

Nambisan RN, Rao U, Moore R, Karakousis CP (1984) Malignant soft tissue tumors of nerve sheath origin. J Surg Oncol 25:268–272

O'Connor MI (1998) Surgical management of malignant soft-tissue tumors. In: Simon MA, Springfield D (eds) Surgery for bone and soft-tissue tumors. Lipincott-Raven, Philadelphia, p 555–565

Ozaki T, Hillmann A, Lindner N, Winkelmann W (1997) Surgical treatment of bone sarcomas of the fibula. Analysis of 19 cases. Arch Orthop Trauma Surg 116:475–479

Ozkan O, Safak T, Vargel I, Demirci M, Erdem S, Erk Y (2002) Reinnervation of denervated muscle in a split-nerve transfer model. Ann Plast Surg 49:532–540

Ozkan T, Ozer K, Gulgonen A (2001) Restoration of sensibility in irreparable ulnar and median nerve lesions with use of sensory nerve transfer: long-term follow-up of 20 cases. J Hand Surg [Am] 26:44–51

Shiu MH, Collin C, Hilaris BS, Nori D, Manolatos S, Anderson LL, Hajdu SI, Lane JM, Hopfan S, Brennan MF (1986) Limb preservation and tumor control in the treatment of popliteal and antecubital soft tissue sarcomas. Cancer 57:1632–1639

Simon MA, Spanier SS, Enneking WF (1979) Management of adult soft-tissue sarcomas of the extremities. Surg Annu 11:363–402

Stellini L (1982) Interfascicular autologous grafts in the repair of peripheral nerves: eight years experience. Br J Plast Surg 35:478–482

Young JN, Friedman AH, Harrelson JM, Rossitch E Jr, Alston S, Rozear M (1991) Hemangiopericytoma of the sciatic nerve. Case report. J Neurosurg 74:512–515

16 Isolated Limb Perfusion with TNF-α and Melphalan in Locally Advanced Soft Tissue Sarcomas of the Extremities

Dirk J. Grünhagen, Johannes H.W. de Wilt, Albertus N. Van Geel, Cornelis Verhoef, and Alexander M.M. Eggermont

Abstract Limb-sparing surgery has become all the more important in soft tissue sarcoma (STS) of the extremities since we learned that amputation does not improve survival of these patients. In bulky tumours, however, preoperative strategies to reduce tumour size are then required. Isolated limb perfusion (ILP) with tumour necrosis factor (TNF) has been developed as a biochemotherapeutic therapy to act both on the tumour-associated vasculature and on the tumour itself. It has shown to be a very potent treatment modality, as in early reports response rates were around 80%. Limb salvage could then be achieved in a quite similar percentage. Many confirmatory studies have been performed since, with consistent results even in patients with multiple tumours, after extensive radiotherapy or with metastatic disease, all at the cost of very limited toxicity. This chapter gives an overview of the ILP studies performed in patients with soft tissue limb sarcoma, discusses the mechanism of TNF-mediated vasculotoxic effects on tumour vasculature, and places TNF-based ILP in the multimodality treatment of these patients with extensive STS of the extremities.

16.1 Introduction

The management of large extremity soft tissue sarcoma (STS) is as demanding as it is a challenge. Although the propensity of the tumour to develop systemic metastases is the primary cause of the high disease-specific mortality rate (up to 50%), the extremity tumours are often large at time of presentation, causing a local management problem (Cormier and Pollock 2004). Extensive and mutilating surgery (with or without radiotherapy) is often required, which

Alexander M.M. Eggermont (✉)
Department of Surgical Oncology
Erasmus MC
Daniel den Hoed Cancer Center
P.O. Box 5201
3008 AE Rotterdam
The Netherlands
E-mail: a.m.m.eggermont@erasmusmc.nl

can cause severe disability of the limb, while in some 10% of cases amputation may be inevitable. On the other hand, limb salvage has become all the more important in the light of evidence that amputations do not improve survival rates in patients with large (>5 cm) deep-seated high-grade sarcomas. Several studies have shown that marginal excisions with a high risk for local recurrence do not influence survival significantly (Gaynor et al. 1992; Gustafson et al. 1991; Potter et al. 1986; Stotter 1992). However, as STS in the extremity is often large at time of diagnosis, and radiotherapy mandatory after marginal excision, this treatment combination might mutilate and compromise limb function considerably. Preoperative therapies to improve limb salvage rates have been propagated. Preoperative radiotherapy alone or in combination with intra-arterial or intravenous chemotherapy has been reported to improve resectability rates of extremity soft tissue sarcomas (Eilber et al. 1980, 1984; Suit et al. 1981). Amputation may also be avoided and local control improved by combining a marginal resection in combination with brachytherapy to the tumour bed (Shiu et al. 1991). Isolated limb perfusion is another strategy to deal with locally advanced soft tissue sarcomas which can be applied also in case of multifocal primary or multiple sarcoma recurrences in limbs, thereby expanding the patient population that can be successfully treated.

16.2
Isolated Limb Perfusion

The technique of isolated limb perfusion (ILP) was pioneered by Creech and Krementz at Tulane University in New Orleans (Creech et al. 1958) and first applied in a patient with extensive melanoma metastases on the lower limb. The principal idea was that direct administration of a chemotherapeutic agent to the area to be treated by intra-arterial infusion would result in the maximum effect. However, venous return should be blocked to prevent the agents from entering the systemic circulation. This method of ILP was thus developed to be able to achieve regional concentrations of chemotherapeutic agents that are 15 to 25 times higher than can be reached with systemic administration, but without the systemic side-effects (Benckhuijsen et al. 1988).

A perfusion circuit is achieved by cannulating the major artery and vein of a limb and connecting these catheters to a pump oxygenator, thus

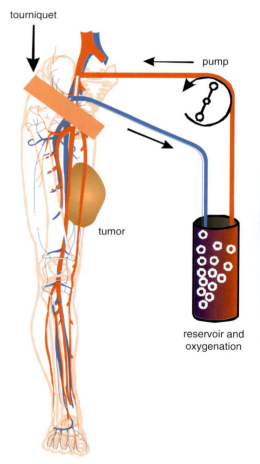

Fig. 16.1 Isolated limb perfusion circuit

creating extracorporeal circulation (Fig. 16.1). Further isolation of the limb from the corporeal circulation is guaranteed by the use of a tourniquet just proximal to the catheter tips. This revolutionary technique enables a locoregional therapy approach to tumours located in the extremity that fail other treatment options. Since the report of its effect in the treatment of melanoma in mice (Luck 1956), and because of the favourable local toxicity profile of the drug, melphalan (l-phenylalanine mustard) is used as the standard chemotherapeutic agent in the ILP setting. Melphalan is commonly used in doses of 10 mg/l perfused tissue for a leg and 13 mg/l for an arm (Thompson and Gianoutsos 1992). As cancer cells had been known to be selectively susceptible to high temperatures, hyperthermia was introduced in the ILP setting (Cavaliere et al. 1967). The now most commonly used technique of mild hyperthermia for ILP was described shortly hereafter (Stehlin 1969).

16.3
The Rationale for Using Tumour Necrosis Factor-α in ILP

A new era in the treatment of extremity cancer began in 1988, when the cytokine tumour necrosis factor-α (TNF) was introduced in ILP as both tumour cells and the tumour vasculature became targets for therapy (Lienard et al. 1992a). TNF was isolated as an endogenous factor, especially active in inflammation, with necrotizing ability on tumour cells (Carswell et al. 1975). Later studies revealed that TNF has a dual mechanism of action: high-dose TNF has an early direct cytotoxic impact to tumour cells (Sugarman et al. 1985), but more importantly the late TNF effect on the so-called tumour-associated vasculature induces a change in tumour morphology (Watanabe et al. 1988).

The addition of high-dose TNF to the perfusate results in a 4- to 6-fold increased uptake by the tumour of the cytostatic drug. For melphalan and for doxorubicin it was demonstrated that this uptake was tumour specific and no increased uptake was noted in the normal tissues, thus emphasizing the relative selectivity of TNF on the tumour-associated vasculature (de Wilt et al. 2000b; van der Veen et al. 2000). Moreover, it has been demonstrated that in hypervascularized tumours, synergistic effect between TNF and the chemotherapeutic agent is better compared to hypovascularized tumours (van Etten et al. 2003a). Whether a TNF-mediated drop in interstitial pressure (Kristensen et al. 1996) in the tumour plays a role in this mechanism remains speculative.

Tumour angiogenesis leads to tumour-associated vasculature that is different from normal vasculature mainly in the structure of the endothelium. The hypothesized mechanism of the selective destructive effects of TNF-ILP on tumour-associated vessels is loss of integrity of this altered endothelium by disrupting VE-cadherin complexes and reducing the activation of αVβ3 integrins (Menon et al. 2006; Ruegg et al. 1998). This leads to hyperpermeability of tumour vessels so that erythrocytes and other blood cells can extravasate to cause massive haemorrhagic necrosis. Moreover, direct cytotoxicity of TNF on endothelial cells leads to apoptosis of the endothelial cells, which contributes itself to increased permeability of the vessels (van Horssen et al. 2006). This destruction of the tumour-associated vasculature has been illustrated by means of pre- and post-perfusion angiographies (Eggermont et al. 1996b; Fig. 16.2) and in sarcoma patients' magnetic resonance spectrometry studies, in which it was clearly shown that the metabolic shutdown of the tumour is virtually complete within 16 h after the perfusion (Sijens et al. 1995). These observations confirm that TNF has its major effect on larger tumours with well-developed vasculature in contrast to small tumours which lack of developed capillary bed. TNF may exert its effect mainly through the neovasculature of the tumour, which is more abundant in large tumours.

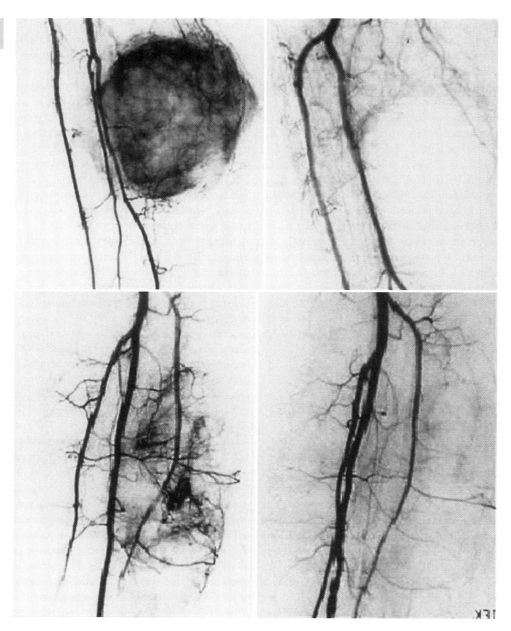

Fig. 16.2 Pre- and post-perfusion angiographies showing the TNF effect on tumour-associated vasculature

The application of TNF in the ILP setting was further studied in the preclinical setting. It turned out that for effective ILP a minimum duration of ILP of 30 min is required. The perfusion temperature should be above 38°C for maximum effect, but should not exceed 42°C in order to avoid unacceptable toxicity to the normal tissue (de Wilt et al. 1999). Hypoxia, although enhancing the effect of melphalan activity and TNF activity alone, did not further enhance the synergistic effect of the combination of TNF and melphalan (de Wilt et al. 1999). These studies form the basis of the clinical application of TNF-based ILP (TM-ILP) in both melanoma and sarcoma patients.

16.4
TNF-Based Isolated Limb Perfusion for STS

In contrast to the efficacy of melphalan-based ILP in patients with multiple in-transit melanoma metastases, results with ILP with melphalan, doxorubicin and a variety of other drugs for large soft tissue sarcomas were disappointing. After studies in the 1970s and 1980s with poor response rates, ILP for advanced SIS was largely abandoned (Klaase et al. 1989; Krementz et al. 1977; Muchmore et al. 1985; Pommier et al. 1988; Rossi et al. 1994), and this was supported by a study from the MD Anderson Cancer Center that found no objective response, but massive toxicity after ILP with doxorubicin alone (Feig et al. 2004).

Thanks to the pioneering work of Lejeune and Lienard this situation changed dramatically with the application of high-dose TNF in the ILP setting (Lienard et al. 1992a). TNF-based ILP has been established as a highly effective new method of induction biochemotherapy in extremity soft tissue sarcomas, with a 20%–30% complete remission (CR) rate and about a 50% partial remission (PR) rate (Eggermont et al. 1996a, b, 1999; Gutman et al. 1997; Hill et al. 1993; Santinami et al. 1996). On the basis of results in a multicentre programme in Europe, TNF was approved and registered in Europe for the sarcoma-indication in 1998 (Eggermont et al. 1999). The European TNF/ILP assessment group evaluated 246 patients with irresectable STS enrolled for 10 years in 4 studies. All cases were reviewed by an independent review committee and compared with conventionally treated patients (often by amputation) of a population-based Scandinavian STS database. In this patient population with locally very advanced disease, major responses were seen in 56.5%–82.6% of the patients, thus making resection of the sarcoma possible. Limb salvage was achieved in 74%–87% in these 4 studies and in 71% of the 196 patients who had been classified by the independent review committees as cases that normally could only have been managed by amputation (87%) or by functionally debilitating resection plus radiotherapy (13%). Comparison with the survival curves based on a matched control study with cases from the Scandinavian Soft Tissue Sarcoma Databank showed that TNF had no negative effect on survival ($p=0.96$). It was concluded that the application of TNF in combination with melphalan in the setting of isolated limb perfusion represents a new and successful option in the management of irresectable locally advanced extremity soft tissue sarcomas (Eggermont et al. 1999; Table 16.1).

This approval by the European Medicine Evaluation Agency of TNF in the treatment of STS in the ILP setting led to single-centre series that confirmed the efficacy of this procedure. Lejeune et al. (2000) reported a 17% CR and 64% PR rate in 22 STS patients treated for limb-threatening STS tumours, and achieved limb salvage in 77% of the patients. A similar limb-salvage rate of 84% and excellent functional results were reported from the Berlin team regarding their experience in a series of 55 patients (Hohenberger et al. 2001). The Amsterdam group reported somewhat less favourable results in their experience in 49 patients (overall response rate 63%). The limb salvage rate of 57% was felt to reflect the selection patients with particularly unfavourable characteristics (Noorda et al. 2003). We reported the large single-centre study of the Rotterdam group on STS patients, in which we found an overall response rate of 75% and were able to achieve limb salvage in 87% of the patients (Grünhagen et al. 2006b). Recent reports from groups in Milan and Groningen show very similar results (Pennacchioli et al. 2007; van Ginkel et al. 2007). All in all, these studies on the overall STS population show that overall response on TM-ILP varies between 63%

and 96% and a limb salvage that ranges from 58% to 94% (Table 16.1).

A point of discussion that has been studied in overall populations is whether high doses of TNF (3–4 mg) are necessary or whether lower doses (1 mg) suffice. An early clinical report by Hill and co-workers suggested that low doses of TNF (up to 1 mg) were sufficient, as in 9 patients with soft tissue tumours 9 complete responses were observed (Hill et al. 1993). The small study sample, the concomitant use of high doses of corticosteroids and the fact that a different type of TNF was used did not allow for definitive conclusions. After the Italian studies on ILP with low-dose TNF in combination with doxorubicin (Rossi et al. 1999; Rossi et al. 2005), the French group reported recently on their experience in 72 patients. In a randomized phase II trial, utilizing various doses of TNF ranging from 0.5 mg to 4 mg, they observed a 35% CR rate and an overall limb-salvage rate of 84%. No significant differences between the various TNF dosage groups were observed (Bonvalot et al. 2005). Our own experience on low-dose ILP for STS confirms these data (Grunhagen et al. 2005b), although we know from our laboratory data that at a very low TNF dose, all effect is lost (de Wilt et al. 1999; Table 1).

16.5
Results with TNFPlus Doxorubicin

Very similar results have been obtained by Italian perfusion groups with the drug doxorubicin in combination with TNF. Interestingly similar response and limb salvage rates are achieved while using lower doses of only 1 mg TNF instead of the usual doses of 2–4 mg in combination with melphalan (Rossi et al. 1999; Rossi et al. 2005; Table 16.1). The perfusions were performed at much higher temperatures (40–41°C), which is associated with higher locoregional toxicity. Grade IV locoregional toxicity was reported in 25% as opposed to only 5% in the large multicentre TNF plus melphalan series (Eggermont et al. 1996b, 1999). We found that with melphalan ILPs, grade IV toxicity was clearly related to tissue temperatures of above 39°C when melphalan was administered (Vrouenraets et al. 2001). Therefore, the last 8 years we have only allowed tissue temperatures to rise to 39°C after melphalan has been added to the perfusion circuit and have hardly seen any cases with grade IV toxicity since, without a drop in response rates (Eggermont et al. 1999; Grunhagen et al. 2006b). Most likely, the higher regional toxicity in the Italian experience with doxorubicin is primarily related to the hyperthermia, although doxorubicin may be responsible in part.

16.6
Toxicity of a TNF-Based ILP

Toxicity after an ILP procedure can be divided into local toxicity to the limb and systemic toxicity due to leakage from TNF to the systemic circulation. Wieberdink et al., already in the pre-TNF era, developed an ILP-specific scoring system for local toxicity. In this, grade 1 means no reaction; grade 2, slight erythema or oedema; grade 3, considerable erythema or oedema with some blistering, slightly disturbed motility permissible; grade 4, extensive epidermolysis or obvious damage to the deep tissues, causing definite functional disturbance, and threatening or manifest compartmental syndrome; and grade 5 means a reaction that may necessitate amputation (Wieberdink et al. 1982). In our experience in Rotterdam on 217 TNF-based ILPs for STS, no treatment-related amputation had to be performed, and Wieberdink grade 3 and 4 toxicity occurred in only 21% and 2% of cases, respectively (Grunhagen et al. 2006b). Whether TNF increases local toxicity compared to a melpha-

Table 16.1 Study reports of TNF-based ILP for irresectable soft tissue sarcomas

Drugs	No. of pts	CR	PR	NC/PD	Limb salvage	Reference
TNF+melphalan[a]	9	100%[b]	0%	0%	64%	Hill et al. 1993
TNF+IFN+melphalan	55	18%[b]	64%[b]	18%[b]	84%	Eggermont et al. 1996b
		36%[c]	51%[c]	13%[c]		
TNF+melphalan	10	70%[b]	20%[b]	10%[b]	89%	Santinami et al. 1996
TNF±IFN+melphalan	186	18%[b]	57%[b]	25%[b]	82%	Eggermont et al. 1996a
		29%[c]	53%[c]	18%[c]		
TNF±IFN+melphalan	35	37%[c]	54%[c]	9%[c]	85%	Gutman et al. 1997
TNF±IFN+melphalan	246	28%[d]	48%[d]	24%[d]	76%	Eggermont et al. 1999
	196	17%[d]	48%[d]	35%[d]	71%[e]	
TNF+Doxorubicin	20	26%[f]	64%[f]	10%[f]	85%	Rossi et al. 1999
TNF±IFN+melphalan	22	18%[c]	64%[c]	82%[c]	77%	Lejeune et al. 2000
TNF±IFN+melphalan	55	NS	NS	NS	84%	Hohenberger et al. 2001
TNF±IFN+melphalan	49	8%[c]	55%[c]	37%[c]	58%	Noorda et al. 2003
TNF±IFN+melphalan	217	18%[b]	51%[b]	31%[b]	75%	Grünhagen et al. 2006b
		26%[c]	49%[c]	25%[c]		
TNF±IFN+melphalan	73	25%[b]	69%[b]	6%[b]	61%[g]	van Ginkel et al. 2007
TNF + melphalan[h,a]	72	49%	17%	34%	84%	Bonvalot et al. 2005
		35%	22%	43%		
TNF+Doxorubicin[a]	21	5%[b]	57%[b]	38%[b]	71%	Rossi et al. 2005
		55%[f]	35%[f]	10%[f]		
TNF+Doxorubicin/melphalan[a]	51	41%[b]	55%[b]	4%[b]	82%	Pennacchioli et al. 2007
TNF±IFN+melphalan[a]	48	38%[c]	31%[c]	29%[c]	85%	Grünhagen et al. 2005b

CR, complete response; IFN, interferon-γ; NC, no change; No. of Pts, number of patients; NS, not stated; PD, progressive disease; PR, partial response; TNF, tumour necrosis factor
[a] Low dose (<4 mg for leg-ILP, <3 mg for arm-ILP)
[b] Objective clinical response rate by WHO criteria
[c] CR is clinical CR or 100% necrosis; PR is clinical PR or >50%–99% necrosis
[d] CR only recognized by EMEA (European Medicine Evaluation Agency) when histopathology showed 100% necrosis
[e] Independent committee recognized 196 patients as pure amputation candidates
[f] No clinical response data; CR: histopathological >90% necrosis; PR: radiological and/or histopathological >50% necrosis
[g] Overall 10 years' limb salvage rate
[h] Different scoring system: upper panel: CR/PR: loss of vasculature on ultrasound/MRI; lower panel CR: >90% necrosis on histopathology

lan-only ILP is still under debate. Initial reports in melanoma patients explicitly state that no increased local toxicity was observed in a triple drug (TNF, melphalan, IFN) regimen (Lienard et al. 1992a, b). However, in a TNF dose-escalation study with TNF doses up to 6 mg, Fraker et al. report that local toxicity was significantly related to the TNF dose (Fraker et al. 1996). The authors speculate that the reason for this observation is the increased uptake of melphalan in the tissue, as experimental ILPs with TNF only did not reveal local toxicity at all. Melphalan dose (total dose, peak concentration, concentration at equilibrium and area under curve) is a major determinant of acute local toxicity (Klaase et al. 1994; Thompson et al. 1996). The one study specifically addressing the local toxicity of TM-ILP, again of course in melanoma patients, showed a significant increase of local toxicity with TNF compared to melphalan-only ILPs (Vrouenraets et al. 2001). The confounding factor here, however, was that the patients in that study participating in the TNF-ILP protocol were, due to trial prescriptions, exposed to higher temperatures during melphalan circulation. This difference might partly explain the observed difference in toxicity. Minimizing local toxicity is essential, as it has been shown to be directly correlated with the incidence of long-term morbidity (tissue fibrosis, muscle atrophy and limb malfunction; Vrouenraets et al. 1995). At present, TM-ILP is performed under mild hyperthermic conditions with gradual administration of melphalan instead of a bolus injection causing no difference in acute local toxicity or in long-term morbidity between TM-ILP and melphalan-only perfusions (Noorda et al. 2004).

Systemic toxicity is directly correlated with leakage of the chemotherapeutics to the systemic circulation (Eggermont et al. 1996a; Stam et al. 2000; Swaak et al. 1993; Thom et al. 1995). In the present situation of leakage-free ILPs, the systemic toxicity is mostly limited to fever in the first 24 h postoperatively, which can be easily avoided by the immediate postoperative application of indomethacin and/or paracetamol. Furthermore, the patients commonly show a period of 6–10 h of a slightly elevated circulation due to a drop in peripheral resistance, which is compensated for by a mild tachycardia and a small drop in blood pressure. Essential in the management of this circulatory change is a policy of ample hydration of the patient during ILP and for the first 12–24 h after ILP. This policy assures adequate diuresis in all patients in order to keep the period of high-circulating TNF levels post-ILP as short as possible (Stam et al. 2000). Standard use of vasopressors is not recommended. A further reduction of systemic toxicity by reducing the TNF dose could not be demonstrated (Grünhagen et al. 2005b).

As ILP is only part of a treatment strategy in patients with STS, including post-ILP resection and postoperative radiotherapy when resection is marginal, recent interest has risen in the vascular toxicity of this treatment triad. Although it has been shown that a TNF-ILP has little effect on normal tissue vasculature (opposed to tumour associated vasculature) (van Horssen et al. 2006), the arteriotomy site can be subject to thrombosis directly postoperative. Moreover, the combination of ILP and radiotherapy can lead to periarterial fibrosis. Recent reports from the Groningen group indicate that this can lead to delayed amputation (up to 10 years post-ILP) due to critical leg ischaemia (Hoven-Gondrie et al. 2007; van Ginkel et al. 2007). However, it is unclear what the attributive toxic effect of ILP was in these cases. In light of this discussion, the question whether to use standard postoperative radiotherapy after a resection of a STS post-ILP remains unanswered. This issue has been studied only in a retrospective manner, and whereas a recent report states that radiotherapy reduces the risk of local recurrence (Thijssens et al. 2006), our analyses of the Rotterdam database could not support such a beneficial effect (Grünhagen et al. 2006b). Future studies might provide more information on the role of radiotherapy in ILP.

16.7
Special Patient Categories

16.7.1
Patients with Overt Metastatic Disease

Patients with overt metastatic disease and a limb-threatening tumour constitute a special category where tumour control can be relatively easily achieved, and thereby an amputation avoided, by a palliative TNF-based ILP. A 77% response rate with an 89% limb-salvage rate was reported in 9 such cases (Olieman et al. 1998), and we observed in 37 cases an 84% response rate and a 97% limb-salvage rate (Grunhagen et al. 2006a). This demonstrates that TNF-based ILP is an attractive option to improve quality of life in these patients in the final phase of their lives.

16.7.2
Patients with Multiple Tumours in the Extremity

Patients with multifocal primary tumours, such as Kaposi's sarcomas (Lev-Chelouche et al. 1999b), multiple lymphangio-sarcomas (Steward–Treves syndrome; Lans et al. 2002), or with multiple primary tumours of various histologies or multiple recurrences after prior surgery (Lev-Chelouche et al. 1999a) all present very difficult problems where TNF-based ILP is the ideal alternative to amputation. Remarkably good results have been reported. In Rotterdam, we observed after 16 ILPs in 10 patients with Steward–Treves Syndrome an 87% response rate, and an 80% limb-salvage rate. In our overall experience with patients with multiple tumours we observed after 64 ILPs a 77% response rate, and a limb-salvage rate of 82% (Grunhagen et al. 2005a). These results indicate that TNF-based ILP is very effective for patients with multiple tumours.

16.7.3
Patients with Recurrent Tumours in an Irradiated Field

A Rotterdam report on 29 ILPs in 26 such patients showed that in contrast to the belief that recurrent tumours in an irradiated field are unlikely to respond, a response rate of 70% and a limb-salvage rate of 65% could be achieved (Lans et al. 2005), indicating that in this very difficult patient category a TNF-based ILP is also an attractive treatment option.

16.7.4
Elderly Patients (>75 Years Old)

A very important message is given by the report on the Rotterdam experience with 50 TNF-based ILPs in patients older than 75 years with limb-threatening tumours. Results were very favourable in the 34 perfusions for limb-threatening sarcomas, with a 38% CR and a 38% PR rate, achieving limb salvage in 76% of the patients as well as in 16 perfusions for bulky melanoma in-transit metastases, resulting in a 75% CR and 25% PR rate. The procedure was proved safe in the elderly with the high reward of limb salvage, which is of overriding importance in this age group, where amputations tend to lead to loss of independence (van Etten et al. 2003b).

16.7.5
TNF-Based ILP Activity in Other Histologies

Since the tumour vasculature is the target of TNF and of the TNF plus chemotherapy combination it can be expected that this treatment is effective against a wide variety of tumour types as long as there is a well-developed vascular stromal component to the tumour. This is indeed the case. Apart from activity in some 20 different histological types of soft tissue sarcoma and activity in melanoma, the efficacy of TNF plus melphalan ILP has also been demonstrated in various skin tumours (Olieman et al. 1999) and bony sarcomas (Bickels et al. 1999). Even in patients with desmoid tumours/aggressive fibromatosis, who often present with recurrent disease that is difficult to treat surgically with or without radiotherapy, TM-ILP proves effective. Lev-Chelouche et al. and our own study both report on very similar results in 6 and 12 such cases. Response rates were 83% and 75%, respectively, and the limb-salvage rate was 100% in both reports, demonstrating the utility of the procedure (Grunhagen et al. 2005; Lev-Chelouche et al. 1999c).

16.8
Future Perspectives

To create further insight in the mechanisms underlying the positive results obtained with ILP in humans, we developed in rats extremity perfusion models in which various vasoactive drugs have been and are being studied. Nitric oxide (NO) is an important molecule in the maintenance of both vascular tone and the integrity of the vascular wall and is highly produced in experimental and human tumours. Inhibition of NO synthase during ILP resulted in hypoxia and an enhancement of TNF early vascular effects in the tumour. The anti-tumour effect of this TNF plus l-NAME/LNA (NO synthase inhibitors) is normally only observed when hypoxia or melphalan are added to TNF (de Wilt et al. 2000a). Other vasoactive drugs, such as histamine and IL-2, have been shown to have a clear synergy with melphalan in our tumour models (Brunstein et al. 2004; Hoving et al. 2005). These findings show the importance of agents that can change the pathophysiology of tumour vasculature and rheological conditions and thereby can improve drug uptake in tumours. Moreover, this underlines the importance of investigating how to modulate tumour physiology and the potential that this approach has to improve efficacy of various standard agents, even in systemic chemotherapy (Seynhaeve et al. 2007).

16.9
Conclusions

Isolated limb perfusion methodology provides us with an excellent tool in the clinic to obtain local control and avoid amputations of limbs in patients with limb-threatening tumours. This has been largely achieved by the success of the anti-vascular TNF-based biochemotherapy in this setting. TNF-based ILPs are now performed in some 30 cancer centres in Europe with referral programmes for limb salvage. TNF-based anti-vascular therapy of cancer is here to stay and its potential needs to be studied further (ten Hagen et al. 2001). Other drugs will follow and we may well learn through this model how to use them systemically more effectively as well.

References

Benckhuijsen C, Kroon BB, van Geel AN, Wieberdink J (1988) Regional perfusion treatment with melphalan for melanoma in a limb: an evaluation of drug kinetics. Eur J Surg Oncol 14:157–163

Bickels J, Manusama ER, Gutman M, Eggermont AM, Kollender Y, Abu-Abid S, Van Geel AN, Lev-Shlush D, Klausner JM, Meller I (1999) Isolated limb perfusion with tumour necrosis factor-alpha and melphalan for unresectable bone sarcomas of the lower extremity. Eur J Surg Oncol 25:509–514

Bonvalot S, Laplanche A, Lejeune F, Stoeckle E, Le Pechoux C, Vanel D, Terrier P, Lumbroso J, Ricard M, Antoni G, Cavalcanti A, Robert C, Lassau N, Blay JY, Le Cesne A (2005) Limb salvage with isolated perfusion for soft tissue sarcoma: could less TNF-alpha be better? Ann Oncol 16:1061–1068

Brunstein F, Hoving S, Seynhaeve AL, van Tiel ST, Guetens G, de Bruijn EA, Eggermont AM, ten Hagen TL (2004) Synergistic antitumor activity of histamine plus melphalan in isolated limb perfusion: preclinical studies. J Natl Cancer Inst 96:1603–1610

Carswell EA, Old LJ, Kassel RL, Green S, Fiore N, Williamson B (1975) An endotoxin-induced serum factor that causes necrosis of tumors. Proc Natl Acad Sci U S A 72:3666–3670

Cavaliere R, Ciocatto EC, Giovanella BC, Heidelberger C, Johnson RO, Margottini M, Mondovi B, Moricca G, Rossi-Fanelli A (1967) Selective heat sensitivity of cancer cells. Biochemical and clinical studies. Cancer 20:1351–1381

Cormier JN, Pollock RE (2004) Soft tissue sarcomas. CA Cancer J Clin 54:94–109

Creech O Jr, Krementz ET, Ryan RF, Winblad JN (1958) Chemotherapy of cancer: regional perfusion utilizing an extracorporeal circuit. Ann Surg 148:616–632

de Wilt JH, Manusama ER, van Tiel ST, van Ijken MG, ten Hagen TL, Eggermont AM (1999) Prerequisites for effective isolated limb perfusion using tumour necrosis factor alpha and melphalan in rats. Br J Cancer 80:161–166

de Wilt JH, Manusama ER, van Etten B, van Tiel ST, Jorna AS, Seynhaeve AL, ten Hagen TL, Eggermont AM (2000a) Nitric oxide synthase inhibition results in synergistic anti-tumour activity with melphalan and tumour necrosis factor alpha-based isolated limb perfusions. Br J Cancer 83:1176–1182

de Wilt JH, ten Hagen TL, de Boeck G, van Tiel ST, de Bruijn EA, Eggermont AM (2000b) Tumour necrosis factor alpha increases melphalan concentration in tumour tissue after isolated limb perfusion. Br J Cancer 82:1000–1003

Eggermont AM, Schraffordt Koops H, Klausner JM, Kroon BB, Schlag PM, Lienard D, van Geel AN, Hoekstra HJ, Meller I, Nieweg OE, Kettelhack C, Ben-Ari G, Pector JC, Lejeune FJ (1996a) Isolated limb perfusion with tumor necrosis factor and melphAalan for limb salvage in 186 patients with locally advanced soft tissue extremity sarcomas. The cumulative multicenter European experience. Ann Surg 224:756–764

Eggermont AM, Schraffordt Koops H, Lienard D, Kroon BB, van Geel AN, Hoekstra HJ, Lejeune FJ (1996b) Isolated limb perfusion with high-dose tumor necrosis factor-alpha in combination with interferon-gamma and melphalan for nonresectable extremity soft tissue sarcomas: a multicenter trial. J Clin Oncol 14:2653–2665

Eggermont AMM, Schraffordt Koops H, Klausner JM, Schlag PM, Lienard D, Kroon BBR, Gustafson P, Steinmann G, Clarke J, Lejeune F (1999) Limb salvage by isolated limb perfusion (ILP) with TNF and melphalan in patients with locally advanced soft tissue sarcomas: outcome of 270 ILPs in 246 patients. Proc Am Soc Clin Oncol 18:2067

Eilber FR, Mirra JJ, Grant TT, Weisenburger T, Morton DL (1980) Is amputation necessary for sarcomas? A seven-year experience with limb salvage. Ann Surg 192:431–438

Eilber FR, Morton DL, Eckardt J, Grant T, Weisenburger T (1984) Limb salvage for skeletal and soft tissue sarcomas. Multidisciplinary preoperative therapy. Cancer 53:2579–2584

Feig BW, Ross MI, Hunt KK (2004) A prospective evaluation of isolated limb perfusion with doxorubicin in patients with unresectable extremity sarcomas. Ann Surg Oncol 1[suppl S80]:Abstr 98

Fraker DL, Alexander HR, Andrich M, Rosenberg SA (1996) Treatment of patients with melanoma of the extremity using hyperthermic isolated limb perfusion with melphalan, tumor necrosis factor, and interferon gamma: results of a tumor necrosis factor dose-escalation study. J Clin Oncol 14:479–489

Gaynor JJ, Tan CC, Casper ES, Collin CF, Friedrich C, Shiu M, Hajdu SI, Brennan MF (1992) Refinement of clinicopathologic staging for localized soft tissue sarcoma of the extremity: a study of 423 adults. J Clin Oncol 10:1317–1329

Grunhagen DJ, Brunstein F, Graveland WJ, van Geel AN, de Wilt JH, Eggermont AM (2005a) Isolated limb perfusion with tumor necrosis factor and melphalan prevents amputation in patients with multiple sarcomas in arm or leg. Ann Surg Oncol 12:473–479

Grunhagen DJ, de Wilt JH, van Geel AN, Graveland WJ, Verhoef C, Eggermont AM (2005b) TNF dose reduction in isolated limb perfusion. Eur J Surg Oncol 31:1011–1019

Grunhagen DJ, de Wilt JH, Verhoef C, van Geel AN, Eggermont AM (2005c) TNF-based isolated limb perfusion in unresectable extremity desmoid tumours. Eur J Surg Oncol 31:912–916

Grunhagen DJ, de Wilt JH, Graveland WJ, van Geel AN, Eggermont AM (2006a) The palliative value of tumor necrosis factor alpha-based isolated limb perfusion in patients with metastatic sarcoma and melanoma. Cancer 106:156–162

Grünhagen DJ, de Wilt JH, Graveland WJ, Verhoef C, van Geel AN, Eggermont AM (2006b) Outcome and prognostic factor analysis of 217 consecutive isolated limb perfusions with tumor necrosis factor-alpha and melphalan for limb-threatening soft tissue sarcoma. Cancer 106:1776–1784

Gustafson P, Rooser B, Rydholm A (1991) Is local recurrence of minor importance for metastases in soft tissue sarcoma? Cancer 67:2083–2086

Gutman M, Inbar M, Lev-Shlush D, Abu-Abid S, Mozes M, Chaitchik S, Meller I, Klausner JM (1997) High dose tumor necrosis factor-alpha and melphalan administered via isolated limb perfusion for advanced limb soft tissue sarcoma results in a >90% response rate and limb preservation. Cancer 79:1129–1137

Hill S, Fawcett WJ, Sheldon J, Soni N, Williams T, Thomas JM (1993) Low-dose tumour necrosis factor alpha and melphalan in hyperthermic isolated limb perfusion. Br J Surg 80:995–997

Hohenberger P, Kettelhack C, Hermann A, Schlag PM (2001) Functional outcome after preoperative isolated limb perfusion with rhTNFalpha/melphalan for high-grade extremity sarcoma. Eur J Cancer 37:S34–S35

Hoven-Gondrie ML, Thijssens KM, Van den Dungen JJ, Loonstra J, van Ginkel RJ, Hoekstra HJ (2007) Long-term locoregional vascular morbidity after isolated limb perfusion and external-beam radiotherapy for soft tissue sarcoma of the extremity. Ann Surg Oncol 14:2105–2112

Hoving S, Brunstein F, aan de Wiel-Ambagtsheer G, van Tiel ST, de Boeck G, de Bruijn EA, Eggermont AM, ten Hagen TL (2005) Synergistic antitumor response of interleukin 2 with melphalan in isolated limb perfusion in soft tissue sarcoma-bearing rats. Cancer Res 65:4300–4308

Klaase JM, Kroon BB, Benckhuijsen C, van Geel AN, Albus-Lutter CE, Wieberdink J (1989) Results of regional isolation perfusion with cytostatics in patients with soft tissue tumors of the extremities. Cancer 64:616–621

Klaase JM, Kroon BB, van Geel BN, Eggermont AM, Franklin HR, Hart GA (1994) Patient- and treatment-related factors associated with acute regional toxicity after isolated perfusion for melanoma of the extremities. Am J Surg 167:618–620

Krementz ET, Carter RD, Sutherland CM, Hutton I (1977) Chemotherapy of sarcomas of the limbs by regional perfusion. Ann Surg 185:555–564

Kristensen CA, Nozue M, Boucher Y, Jain RK (1996) Reduction of interstitial fluid pressure after TNF-alpha treatment of three human melanoma xenografts. Br J Cancer 74:533–536

Lans TE, de Wilt JH, van Geel AN, Eggermont AM (2002) Isolated limb perfusion with tumor necrosis factor and melphalan for nonresectable Stewart-Treves lymphangiosarcoma. Ann Surg Oncol 9:1004–1009

Lans TE, Grunhagen DJ, de Wilt JH, van Geel AN, Eggermont AM (2005) Isolated limb perfusions with tumor necrosis factor and melphalan for locally recurrent soft tissue sarcoma in previously irradiated limbs. Ann Surg Oncol 12:406–411

Lejeune FJ, Pujol N, Lienard D, Mosimann F, Raffoul W, Genton A, Guillou L, Landry M, Chassot PG, Chiolero R, Bischof-Delaloye A, Leyvraz S, Mirimanoff RO, Bejkos D, Leyvraz PF (2000) Limb salvage by neoadjuvant isolated perfusion with TNFalpha and melphalan for non-resectable soft tissue sarcoma of the extremities. Eur J Surg Oncol 26:669–678

Lev-Chelouche D, Abu-Abeid S, Kollander Y, Meller I, Isakov J, Merimsky O, Klausner JM, Gutman M (1999a) Multifocal soft tissue sarcoma: limb salvage following hyperthermic isolated limb perfusion with high-dose tumor necrosis factor and melphalan. J Surg Oncol 70:185–189

Lev-Chelouche D, Abu-Abeid S, Merimsky O, Isakov J, Kollander Y, Meller I, Klausner JM, Gutman M (1999b) Isolated limb perfusion with high-dose tumor necrosis factor alpha and melphalan for Kaposi sarcoma. Arch Surg 134:177–180

Lev-Chelouche D, Abu-Abeid S, Nakache R, Issakov J, Kollander Y, Merimsky O, Meller I, Klausner JM, Gutman M (1999c) Limb desmoid tumors: a possible role for isolated limb perfusion with tumor necrosis factor-alpha and melphalan. Surgery 126:963–967

Lienard D, Ewalenko P, Delmotte JJ, Renard N, Lejeune FJ (1992a) High-dose recombinant tumor necrosis factor alpha in combination with interferon gamma and melphalan in isolation perfusion of the limbs for melanoma and sarcoma. J Clin Oncol 10:52–60

Lienard D, Lejeune FJ, Ewalenko P (1992b) In transit metastases of malignant melanoma treated by high dose rTNF alpha in combination with interferon-gamma and melphalan in isolation perfusion. World J Surg 16:234–240

Luck JM (1956) Action of p-[di(2-chloroethyl)]-amino-l-phenylalanine on Harding-Passey mouse melanoma. Science 123:984–985

Menon C, Ghartey A, Canter R, Feldman M, Fraker DL (2006) Tumor necrosis factor-alpha damages tumor blood vessel integrity by targeting VE-cadherin. Ann Surg 244:781–791

Muchmore JH, Carter RD, Krementz ET (1985) Regional perfusion for malignant melanoma and soft tissue sarcoma: a review. Cancer Invest 3:129–143

Noorda EM, Vrouenraets BC, Nieweg OE, van Coevorden F, van Slooten GW, Kroon BB (2003) Isolated limb perfusion with tumor necrosis factor-alpha and melphalan for patients with unresectable soft tissue sarcoma of the extremities. Cancer 98:1483–1490

Noorda EM, Vrouenraets BC, Nieweg OE, van Geel BN, Eggermont AM, Kroon BB (2004) Isolated limb perfusion for unresectable melanoma of the extremities. Arch Surg 139:1237–1242

Olieman AF, van Ginkel RJ, Molenaar WM, Schraffordt Koops H, Hoekstra HJ (1998) Hyperthermic isolated limb perfusion with tumour necrosis factor-alpha and melphalan as palliative limb-saving treatment in patients with locally advanced soft-tissue sarcomas of the extremities with regional or distant metastases. Is it worthwhile? Arch Orthop Trauma Surg 118:70–74

Olieman AF, Lienard D, Eggermont AM, Kroon BB, Lejeune FJ, Hoekstra HJ, Koops HS (1999) Hyperthermic isolated limb perfusion with tumor necrosis factor alpha, interferon gamma, and melphalan for locally advanced nonmelanoma skin tumors of the extremities: a multicenter study. Arch Surg 134:303–307

Pennacchioli E, Deraco M, Mariani L, Fiore M, Mussi C, Collini P, Olmi P, Casali PG, Santinami M, Gronchi A (2007) Advanced extremity soft tissue sarcoma: prognostic effect of isolated limb perfusion in a series of 88 patients treated at a single institution. Ann Surg Oncol 14:553–559

Pommier RF, Moseley HS, Cohen J, Huang CS, Townsend R, Fletcher WS (1988) Pharmacokinetics, toxicity, and short-term results of cisplatin hyperthermic isolated limb perfusion for soft-tissue sarcoma and melanoma of the extremities. Am J Surg 155:667–671

Potter DA, Kinsella T, Glatstein E, Wesley R, White DE, Seipp CA, Chang AE, Lack EE, Costa J, Rosenberg SA (1986) High-grade soft tissue sarcomas of the extremities. Cancer 58:190–205

Rossi CR, Vecchiato A, Foletto M, Nitti D, Ninfo V, Fornasiero A, Sotti G, Tregnaghi A, Melanotte P, Lise M (1994) Phase II study on neoadjuvant hyperthermic-antiblastic perfusion with doxorubicin in patients with intermediate or high grade limb sarcomas. Cancer 73:2140–2146

Rossi CR, Foletto M, Di Filippo F, Vaglini M, Anza M, Azzarelli A, Pilati P, Mocellin S, Lise M (1999) Soft tissue limb sarcomas: Italian clinical trials with hyperthermic antiblastic perfusion. Cancer 86:1742–1749

Rossi CR, Mocellin S, Pilati P, Foletto M, Campana L, Quintieri L, De Salvo GL, Lise M (2005) Hyperthermic isolated perfusion with low-dose tumor necrosis factor alpha and doxorubicin for the treatment of limb-threatening soft tissue sarcomas. Ann Surg Oncol 12:398–405

Ruegg C, Yilmaz A, Bieler G, Bamat J, Chaubert P, Lejeune FJ (1998) Evidence for the involvement of endothelial cell integrin alphaVbeta3 in the disruption of the tumor vasculature induced by TNF and IFN-gamma. Nat Med 4:408–414

Santinami M, Deraco M, Azzarelli A, Cascinelli F, Chiti A, Costagli V, Inglese MG, Manzi R, Quagliolo V, Rebuffoni G, Santoro N, Vaglini M (1996) Treatment of recurrent sarcoma of the extremities by isolated limb perfusion using tumor necrosis factor alpha and melphalan. Tumori 82:579–584

Seynhaeve AL, Hoving S, Schipper D, Vermeulen CE, de Wiel-Ambagtsheer G, van Tiel ST, Eggermont AM, Ten Hagen TL (2007) Tumor necrosis factor alpha mediates homogeneous distribution of liposomes in murine melanoma that contributes to a better tumor response. Cancer Res 67:9455–9462

Shiu MH, Hilaris BS, Harrison LB, Brennan MF (1991) Brachytherapy and function-saving resection of soft tissue sarcoma arising in the limb. Int J Radiat Oncol Biol Phys 21:1485–1492

Sijens PE, Eggermont AM, van Dijk PV, Oudkerk M (1995) 31P magnetic resonance spectroscopy as predictor of clinical response in human extremity sarcomas treated by single dose TNF-alphamelphalanmelphalan isolated limb perfusion. NMR Biomed 8:215–224

Stam TC, Swaak AJ, de Vries MR, ten Hagen TL, Eggermont AM (2000) Systemic toxicity and cytokine/acute phase protein levels in patients after isolated limb perfusion with tumor necrosis factor-alpha complicated by high leakage. Ann Surg Oncol 7:268–275

Stehlin JS Jr (1969) Hyperthermic perfusion with chemotherapy for cancers of the extremities. Surg Gynecol Obstet 129:305–308

Stotter A (1992) Comparison of amputation with limb-sparing operations for adult soft tissue sarcoma of the extremity. Ann Surg 216:615–616

Sugarman BJ, Aggarwal BB, Hass PE, Figari IS, Palladino MA Jr, Shepard HM (1985) Recombinant human tumor necrosis factor-alpha: effects on proliferation of normal and transformed cells in vitro. Science 230:943–945

Suit HD, Proppe KH, Mankin HJ, Wood WC (1981) Preoperative radiation therapy for sarcoma of soft tissue. Cancer 47:2269–2274

Swaak AJ, Lienard D, Schraffordt Koops H, Lejeune FJ, Eggermont AM (1993) Effects of recombinant tumour necrosis factor (rTNF-alpha) in cancer. Observations on the acute phase protein reaction and immunoglobulin synthesis after high dose recombinant TNF-alpha administration in isolated limb perfusions in cancer patients. Eur J Clin Invest 23:812–818

ten Hagen TL, Eggermont AM, Lejeune FJ (2001) TNF is here to stay—revisited. Trends Immunol 22:127–129

Thijssens KM, van Ginkel RJ, Pras E, Suurmeijer AJ, Hoekstra HJ (2006) Isolated limb perfusion with tumor necrosis factor alpha and melphalan for locally advanced soft tissue sarcoma: the value of adjuvant radiotherapy. Ann Surg Oncol 13:518–524

Thom AK, Alexander HR, Andrich MP, Barker WC, Rosenberg SA, Fraker DL (1995) Cytokine levels and systemic toxicity in patients undergoing isolated limb perfusion with high-dose tumor necrosis factor, interferon gamma, and melphalan. J Clin Oncol 13:264–273

Thompson JF, Gianoutsos MP (1992) Isolated limb perfusion for melanoma: effectiveness and toxicity of cisplatin compared with that of melphalan and other drugs. World J Surg 16:227–233

Thompson JF, Eksborg S, Kam PC, Ingvar C, Yau DF, Lai DT, Ramzan I (1996) Determinants of acute regional toxicity following isolated limb perfusion for melanoma. Melanoma Res 6:267–271

van der Veen AH, de Wilt JH, Eggermont AM, van Tiel ST, Seynhaeve AL, ten Hagen TL (2000) TNF-alpha augments intratumoural concentrations of doxorubicin in TNF-alpha-based isolated limb perfusion in rat sarcoma models and enhances anti-tumour effects. Br J Cancer 82:973–980

van Etten B, de Vries MR, van IMG, Lans TE, Guetens G, Ambagtsheer G, van Tiel ST, de Boeck G, de Bruijn EA, Eggermont AM, ten Hagen TL (2003a) Degree of tumour vascularity correlates with drug accumulation and tumour response upon TNF-alpha-based isolated hepatic perfusion. Br J Cancer 88:314–319

van Etten B, van Geel AN, de Wilt JH, Eggermont AM (2003b) Fifty tumor necrosis factor-based isolated limb perfusions for limb salvage in patients older than 75 years with limb-threatening soft tissue sarcomas and other extremity tumors. Ann Surg Oncol 10:32–37

van Ginkel RJ, Thijssens KM, Pras E, van der Graaf WT, Suurmeijer AJ, Hoekstra HJ (2007) Isolated limb perfusion with tumor necrosis factor alpha and melphalan for locally advanced soft tissue sarcoma: three time periods at risk for amputation. Ann Surg Oncol 14:1499–1506

van Horssen R, Ten Hagen TL, Eggermont AM (2006) TNF-alpha in cancer treatment: molecular insights, antitumor effects, and clinical utility. Oncologist 11:397–408

Vrouenraets BC, Klaase JM, Kroon BB, van Geel BN, Eggermont AM, Franklin HR (1995) Long-term morbidity after regional isolated perfusion with melphalan for melanoma of the limbs. The influence of acute regional toxic reactions. Arch Surg 130:43–47

Vrouenraets BC, Eggermont AM, Hart AA, Klaase JM, van Geel AN, Nieweg OE, Kroon BB (2001) Regional toxicity after isolated limb perfusion with melphalan and tumour necrosis factor-alpha versus toxicity after melphalan alone. Eur J Surg Oncol 27:390–395

Watanabe N, Niitsu Y, Umeno H, Kuriyama H, Neda H, Yamauchi N, Maeda M, Urushizaki I (1988) Toxic effect of tumor necrosis factor on tumor vasculature in mice. Cancer Res 48:2179–2183

Wieberdink J, Benckhuysen C, Braat RP, van Slooten EA, Olthuis GA (1982) Dosimetry in isolation perfusion of the limbs by assessment of perfused tissue volume and grading of toxic tissue reactions. Eur J Cancer Clin Oncol 18:905–910

17 Management of Locally Recurrent Soft Tissue Sarcoma after Prior Surgery and Radiation Therapy

Peter Hohenberger and Matthias H.M. Schwarzbach

Abstract Surgery and radiation therapy are the standard for local tumour control in the treatment of soft tissue sarcoma. Sarcoma recurrence within a previously irradiated area is one of the most problematic therapeutic challenges in soft tissue tumours. Any information on previous therapy needs to be available in detail. In case of recurrent sarcoma not amenable to surgical resection with wide and clear margins, a multimodality therapy needs to be applied. The armamentarium usually looks for a neoadjuvant downstaging of the sarcoma by radiotherapy, chemo-radiotherapy or isolated limb perfusion with all of those strategies bearing benefits, but also specific risks. The potential of repeated radiotherapy and the modality that can be used (intraoperative radiotherapy, brachytherapy) needs to be carefully evaluated. The pathologist saves these major problems in intraoperative frozen section histology or resection margins and thus needs to be aware of the type of cancer cells potentially present within the resection specimen. Plastic and reconstructive surgery to cover the area of re-resection with viable and well-v tissue is absolutely crucial to prevent lymphatic fistula. Thus, adequate treatment of those specific situations usually involves postoperative physiotherapy and a specific rehabilitation, which is extremely important.

Peter Hohenberger (✉)
Divison of Surgical Oncology
and Thoracic Surgery
Department of Surgery
University Hospital Mannheim
Theodor Kutzer Ufer 1-3
68167 Mannheim
Germany
E-mail: peter.hohenberger@chir.ma.uni-heidelberg.de

17.1 Introduction

Radiation therapy is a major weapon in the therapeutic armamentarium for soft tissue sarcoma whether used pre- or postoperatively. However, despite combined modality treatment, 10%–25% of sarcomas recur locally (Ballo et al. 2007). Even in the most recent reports on T1 sarcoma (less than 5 cm in size and located at the superficial fascia level) the local recurrence rate is 12.5% (Pisters et al. 2007). When discussing local treatment for the relapse, the problem of function preservation and local disease control is raised a second time. In the absence of systemic metastasis, the primary aim of treatment is radical surgical resection; amputation is sometimes recommended in those situations.

Limb-preserving surgery is usually preferred as the local disease status has often been reported to be of limited impact on overall survival. It is argued that low-grade tumours may recur often locally without threat to the patient's survival (Trovik et al. 2000). On the other hand, high-grade tumours usually are accompanied by systemic metastasis either synchronous to local recurrence or developing after a short time lapse rendering these patients eligible for systemic treatment strategies. Also, in initially low-grade soft tissue sarcoma, local recurrences develop to intermediate- or high-grade tumours.

17.2
Treatment Options

The standard of care in soft tissue sarcoma adds external beam radiation therapy to high-grade tumours as an adjuvant measure (Yang et al. 1998). In case of recurrence of a sarcoma within the irradiation field it seems logical that it should be necessary to look for even more aggressive therapy, otherwise tumour control cannot be achieved. Thus, combined modality therapies without radiotherapy or including special delivery of irradiation have been evaluated. In principle, the following (combination) treatments can be applied:

- Re-excision alone
- Re-excision combined with brachytherapy or intraoperative radiotherapy (IORT)
- Isolated limb perfusion with rhTNF-α and melphalan followed by resection
- Systemic chemotherapy followed by resection
    - Systemic chemotherapy plus deep wave hyperthermia

Only a few studies exist evaluating the management of locally recurrent tissue sarcoma after prior surgery and radiation therapy, and institutional series often include only a small number of patients or summarize heterogeneous disease situations treated with different therapeutic strategies. Torres and colleagues reported the management of 62 consecutive patients who had undergone resection and external beam radiation for a primary sarcoma and who presented with an isolated first local recurrence in the irradiation fields (Torres et al. 2007). Of this cohort, 25 patients were treated by wide local excision of the recurrence alone, whereas another 37 patients were treated with additional irradiation of 45–64 Gy. Out of those 37 patients, 33 received their radiotherapy by afterloading brachytherapy. The authors compared the treatment outcome in both groups and concluded that conservative surgery alone was able to control tumour growth in the minority of patients only. However, treatment intensification with additional radiotherapy did not improve the outcome but was associated with an increase in complication rate. Limb amputation was more common in the subgroup of patients with extremity re-irradiation, with more than one-third of the patients losing their limb, whereas only 11% of the "surgery only" group faced this fate. Resection with clear surgical margins (R0-resection) was associated with improved local control rates and represented the most important single contributor to local control in multivariate analysis ($p<0.001$). Five-year distant metastasis-free survival was 65% and 73%, respectively. It is noteworthy that reconstructive plastic surgery had to be performed in 33 patients, with those in the additional radiotherapy group more likely to undergo reconstructive plastic surgery vs the wide local excision group.

Further experience has been gained by retrospective analysis of 26 patients undergoing perioperative brachytherapy in the 1990s for recurrence of tissue sarcoma. All cases showed a recurrence within a previously irradiated field. The treatment of choice was Ir-192-guided wired brachytherapy to surgical tumour excision with negative intraoperative frozen section margins. External beam radiotherapy applied earlier ranged from 30 to 70 Gy, whereas the mean dose of radiation added by brachytherapy was 47.2 Gy with a range of 11–50 Gy. As in other studies, half of the patients required a tissue transfer to provide adequate wound healing from unirradiated tissue. Despite this, 5 patients suffered from significant wound complications including osteonecrosis. Unfortunately, half of the patients also developed a tumour recurrence, 9 patients with local relapse and another 4 with distant metastases during a median follow-up of 16 months (Pearlstone et al. 1999). The authors concluded that by this treatment strategy local control could be achieved in the majority of patients, who otherwise would have required more radical surgical procedures. Further experience has been reported from Toronto in a group of 25 patients (Catton et al. 1996). This group was much more heterogeneously composed, with 2 patients treated with palliative intent due to systemic relapse, 7 patients undergoing amputation, while 11 patients underwent limb-sparing resection of the tumour without irradiation. Of these, 7 patients relapsed and 5 of them underwent a combination of repetitive surgery and re-irradiation. The local control rate for patients treated with excision alone was 36%, whereas all patients showed local disease control at additional re-irradiation. In this latter group, 60% of the patients experienced significant post-irradiation wound healing complications. The authors concluded that combination of limb-sparing surgery with irradiation provides superior local control to local re-excision alone. Systemic relapse was a significant problem in the overall group of patients, and 72 of the patients had a history of intralesional excision in their initial intervention, suggesting inappropriate initial management of their disease.

Lans et al. reported on the treatment of 29 patients undergoing isolated limb perfusion for recurrent sarcoma in irradiation fields of 62–70 Gy (Lans et al. 2005). Of those patients, 6 showed a complete remission of the tumour (with a 100% necrosis), whereas 15 patients showed between 50% and 90% necrosis in the resection specimen. Only 9 patients did not show major influence of this pretherapeutic measure. The R0-resection rate was 78%, resulting in a limb salvage rate of 65%.

All other treatment options mentioned in the paragraph above have not been reported in more than a summary of single case reports and with prospective and standardized evaluation.

17.3
Problems for Surgery Encountered with Previous Radiotherapy

A combination of radiation and surgical resection of soft tissue sarcomas might result in major problems in wound healing. Out of a large series of more than 200 patients after preoperative radiotherapy, Bujko et al. (1993) reported uneventful wound healing in 63% of the patients only, whereas the remaining group of patients suffered from wound dehiscence, infection, seroma formation and even skin graft breakdown (Bujko et al. 1993). The amputation rate in early series was 3%. Preoperative irradiation is known to increase wound morbidity in comparison to postoperative radiotherapy. In the Canadian randomized trial, the wound complication rate was 35% in patients after preoperative radiotherapy compared with 17% in the postoperative group (O'Sullivan et al. 2002). However, even in those patients receiving postoperative adjuvant radiotherapy, it can be shown that irradiation results in significantly worse limb strength, increased oedema formation, decreased range of motion and lower quality of life scores (Yang et al. 1998; Davis et al. 2002, 2005). Radiotherapy primarily affects wound healing due to decreased collagen formation. Wound healing is a complex process that shows different phases of inflammatory reaction of the wounding with deposition of fibrin. This is followed by a proliferation phase with active proliferation of fibroblasts and synthesis of collagen and mucopolysaccharides, and finally results in a maturation phase, the scar (Springfield 1993). Radiotherapy affects the healing process by suppressing the proliferation phase and diminishing collagen production; radiation damage to the microvasculature becomes particularly evident after irradiation. Wound healing is mediated by polypeptide growth factors released from inflammatory cells (PDGF-β, FGF). The wound breaking strength of irradiated wounds is compromised at least for 1 year postoperatively (Cannon et al. 2006). At the time of a surgical re-resection for recurrence sarcoma in an irradiation field, the tissue areas are characterized by radiation-induced fibrosis. It is often very problematic to delineate the extent of sarcoma recurrence in the radiation field, and rather wide margins of excision therefore need to be approached to avoid incomplete resection with tumour cells at the resection margin. As a result, major parts of the vascular compartment bearing the tumour need to be excised, resulting in devascularized bone or neural tissues (Lin et al. 1998). Often, oedema formation results in long-lasting fluid accumulation in such resection areas. "These surgical wounds result in complex and less-than-satisfactory implant geometry" (Torres et al. 2007). Consequently, the probability of developing significant complications rises in parallel to the dose of previous and/or additional radiotherapy.

As shown in the literature reported, radiation therapy in the context of the treatment of the primary sarcoma results in major wound healing problems. Wound rupture following postoperative radiotherapy for sarcoma may develop even 2–3 weeks of the completing adjuvant radiotherapy, thus 2 to 3 treatments after initial resection (Fig. 17.1). Local problems encountered by radiotherapy in combination with surgery are even more prominent following extensive sarcoma excision, including bone periosteal removal. An analysis of 9 patients developing a femoral fracture in an area of previous radiation and surgery showed that all had undergone periosteal excision (Lin et al. 1998). The risk of fracture was 29% at 5 years; mainly females are threatened from this complication.

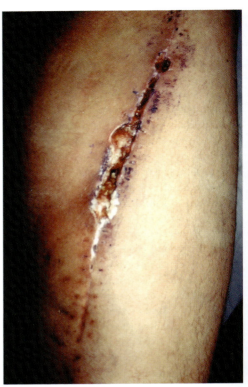

Fig. 17.1 Wound rupture following postoperative adjuvant radiotherapy for a soft tissue sarcoma of the right thigh developing after 48 Gy. Primary wound healing had been uneventful and irradiation had started at day 28 postoperatively

As a late effect, extensive tissue fibrosis might occur, particularly in special types of radiotherapy looking to control sarcomas of the subcutaneous tissues or in patients with low body mass index and thin layer of subcutaneous fat (Fig. 17.2). Particularly neutron therapy put these patients at increased risk due to the fact that dose distribution was close to 100% at the skin and subcutaneous area, whereas at 3 cm depth to the subfascial areas the dose decreased rapidly to less than 50%. Tissue fibrosis

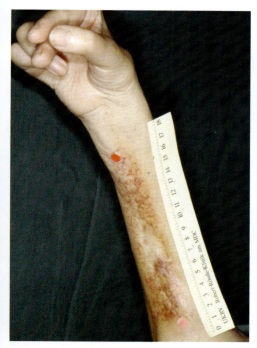

Fig. 17.2 Late effects of adjuvant radiotherapy for soft tissue sarcoma of the forearm. Using neutron therapy, there was complete fibrosis of the subcutaneous tissue and of the tendons to flexor muscles, leading to fixation of the fingers in flexed position (female, 66 years). Irradiation dose had been 45 Gy

also might involve destruction of tendons and nerves.

An immunohistochemical analysis of radiation-induced non-healing dermal wounds showed a decreased expression of vascular endothelial growth factor (VEGF), fibroblast growth factor (FGF) and VEGF associated with decreased wound breaking strength (Riedel et al. 2005). Despite an increased expression of the collagenases matrix metalloproteinase (MMP)-2 and MMP-9, the decreased expression of angiogenic compounds seems to be the second biggest factor after the involvement of fibroblasts' collagen production, since microvessel density remains undisturbed.

17.4
Practical Management of In-Field Sarcoma Recurrence

Tumours suspected of representing sarcoma regrowth and newly arising within the former sarcoma bed and irradiation field should always be proved by biopsy and be examined by an experienced pathologist. Availability of the original sarcoma tumour block is of major importance, as sometimes scar formation with spindle cell proliferation can mimic remnants of sarcoma tissue. On the other hand, infiltration by inflammatory cells with a high cell turnover and showing mitoses could wrongly lead to the assumption of spotted sarcoma recurrence, a skip-metastasis or multifocal disease. Comparison of the immunohistochemical profile of the primary tumour and the presumed recurrence is helpful for a unanimous decision. In case of resection of sensory or motor nerves as a part of the excision of the primary tumour, development of neuroma formation within the scar area could also result in misinterpretation.

Detailed information on the radiation field should be available to clearly depict whether the recurrence is within the field of radiotherapy, at the border of the radiation field or only close to the field of radiation. Detailed work-up of these factors influences the judgement about the biological behaviour of the tumour and its aggressiveness with respect to the previous histological grading, but is also of major influence on the planning of a surgical re-excision (Fig 17.3a–c). The higher the radiation dose already applied, the more a recommendation must be made to excise the complete irradiation field and fill it up by a pedicled or free tissue flap in order to provide wound healing for non-involved tissue. Therefore, a radiation oncologist should assist the surgeon in marking the irradiation field and its dosages on the patient's skin based on the preparatory CT scans. Also, the depth of irradiation is important to know prior to re-excision – how deep the soft tissues were destroyed by previous radiotherapy.

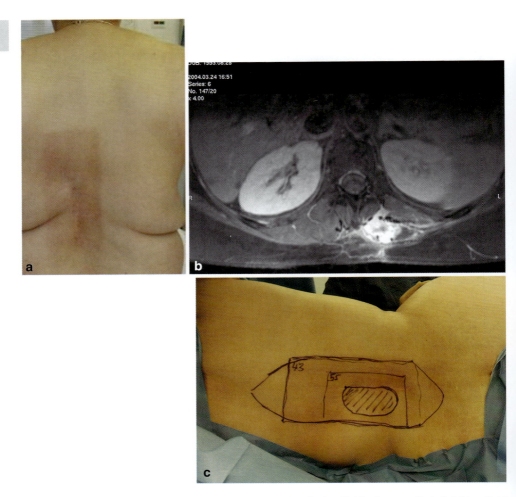

Fig. 17.3 a Sarcoma recurrence within the irradiation field 9 months after resection of the primary tumour with positive resection margins (grade 3 myxofibrosarcoma, female, 51 years). **b** Magnetic resonance image (MRI) of the tumour recurrence within the irradiation field (T1-weighted image). **c** Details of the irradiation field after so-called shrinking-field technique applying 43 Gy to the whole tumour field with a boost to 55 Gy to the centrally located R1-resection area. Depicted are the margins of re-excision and the preoperative delineation of the radiation field

17.5 Treatment Decisions in Surgical Re-intervention

The basic decision has to be made about whether a pure surgical re-excision with adequate margins is possible, or whether a combined treatment modality is required to devitalize the sarcoma, enabling a resection with small margins of clearance. In high-grade lesions, systemic chemotherapy can be of value. Some typical scenarios are discussed below.

In case of a sarcoma recurrence amenable to complete surgical excision within an irradiation field, extensive preoperative work-up needs to be done to plan adequately for wound coverage (Fig. 17.4a–g). Dependent on the damage of the soft tissues due to radiation dose and radiation source used, a simple pedicled muscle flap might be a nearly perfect solution. It is important to involve the plastic reconstructive surgeon early and make him part of the therapeutic team at the initial treatment planning. Troubleshooting for wound breakdown by plastic reconstructive surgery at the stage of an infected re-excision wound or one already abscessed clearly is of adverse influence on the results of reconstructive repair. In the case shown, a fibrosarcoma developed within an irradiation field 26 years after combined surgery and radiotherapy for cancer of the uterine cervix with abscess formation of the anterior abdominal wall. All areas of the tumour and infection had to be resected. The MRI (Fig. 17.4b) depicts a combined destruction of the abdominal wall by fibrosis due to radiotherapy and multiple abscesses in the "hot spots" of radiotherapy. The secondary sarcoma although biopsy-proven, could not be delineated. As a consequence, the indication was taken to excise the whole previous area of radiotherapy. The following complete resection of both rectus abdominis and obliquus abdominis muscles and a multilayer solution for the reconstruction of the abdominal wall had to be created. For closure of the abdomen and to prevent hernia formation, a Gore-Tex DualMesh (W.L. Gore and Associates, Newark, DE) was used. This allograft shows almost no resistance to bacterial challenge, so a free myocutaneous latissimus dorsi flap with microvascular anastomosis to the external iliac artery and vein of the right side was used for coverage. The muscle parts of the latissimus dorsi not covered by the skin island were grafted with an Integra (Integra LifeSciences, Plainsboro, NJ) bilayer skin replacement system using a collagen matrix covered with polyurethane. After 14 days after coverage of the latissimus dorsi muscle, the silicone outer layer of the Integra mesh could be removed, clearly showing granulation tissue below covering the muscle in close vicinity to a well-nourished skin island. The granulation area was covered with an epidermal skin graft resulting in multilayer reconstruction of the abdominal wall without herniation.

17.6
Indication for Multimodal Re-treatment

In case of recurrent sarcoma not amenable to surgical resection with wide and clear margins, a multimodality therapy needs to be applied. The armamentarium usually looks for a neoadjuvant downstaging of the sarcoma by radiotherapy, chemo-radiotherapy or isolated limb perfusion with all of those strategies bearing benefits, but also specific risks (Hohenberger and Wysocki 2008). In the specific setting of sarcoma recurrence in an irradiation field, isolated limb perfusion (ILP) remains a treatment of choice, if available. The proportion of complete tumour remissions proved by histology reliably ranges from 15% to 25% with another 40%–60% of the patients showing greater than 80%–90% necrosis in the resection specimen (Eggermont et al. 1996; Gutman et al. 1997; Noorda et al. 2003). This treatment can contribute to a downstaging of the recurrent sarcoma without adding additional toxicity to the region to be re-operated and without additional compromising wound healing problems (P. Hohenberger, A. Herrmann, C. Kettelhack, P.U. Tunn, et al., submitted). The scarce data available on limb perfusion following irradiation did not show less efficacy (Lans et al. 2005). Particularly in areas with very limited possibilities to get clear margins, such as the groin and popliteal fossa, looking to a necrotic tumour remnant for resection seems to be more advantageous than trying to get clear margins from extensive resection (Fig. 17.5). Tumours arising close to neurovascular bundles should always be resected together with the vessels, if there is any doubt about the tumour extension to the vessel wall. Often, due to the scar formation of radiotherapy, neither contrast-enhanced CT scans nor DCE-MRI can

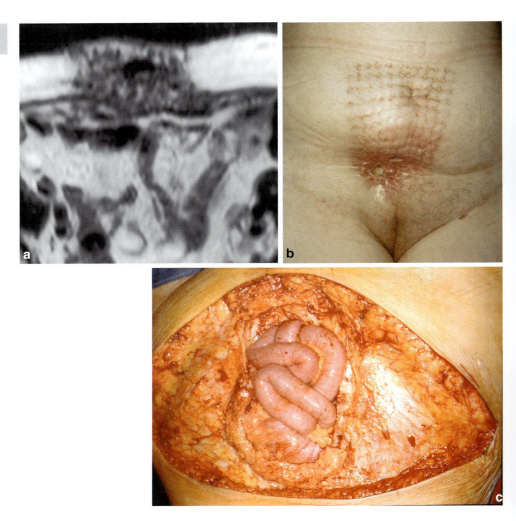

Fig. 17.4 a Fibrosarcoma developing in an irradiation field after so-called Lochblenden radiotherapy for prior cervical cancer (female, 78 years) with abscess formation. **b** This MR image depicts combined destruction of the abdominal wall by late sequelae of radiotherapy, infection and secondary sarcoma. **c** Intraoperative picture after complete resection of the whole irradiation field including the abdominal wall. **d** Reconstruction of the central part of the abdominal wall by use of a W.L. Gore and Associates (Newark, DE) DualMesh to prevent adhesion formation. **e** Coverage of the allograft with a free myocutaneous latissimus dorsi myocutaneous flap with microvascular anastomoses to the external iliac artery and vein. The muscle parts of the flap are grafted with Integra (Integra LifeSciences, Plainsboro, NJ), a bi-layer skin replacement system of basal collagen matrix covered with silicone. **f** Status after regeneration of the dermal skin layer and removal of the silicone outer layer. **g** Status 3 months after coverage of the granulation with an epidermal skin graft

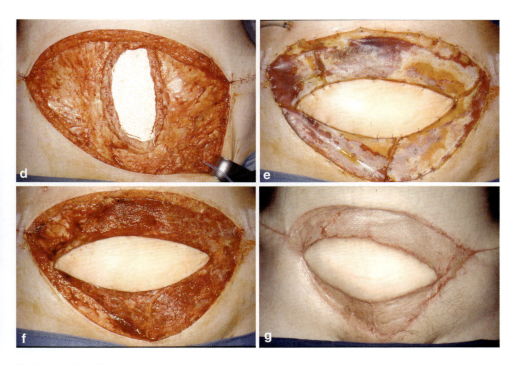

Fig. 17.4 (continued)

discriminate vessel wall invasions by sarcoma from a tumour extension close to the vessel. Intravascular ultrasound might be an additional help through high-resolution (17.5 MHz or even 20 MHz) intravascular probes (Hünerbein et al. 2007). Usually such a tumour location with previous irradiation requires complete clearing of the compartment of the joint including vessel replacement by autologous vein grafts and additional tissue coverage by three microvascular flaps (Fig. 17.5c).

In large sarcoma recurrences of high grade, preoperative systemic chemotherapy could be an option to be pursued in many selected cases. There are no prospective randomized studies available evaluating the use of new adjuvant systemic chemotherapy in the setting of the primary tumour. The only study had to be closed after completion of phase II due to low accrual (Gortzak et al. 2001). Limb salvage in this study was achieved in 88%. No general recommendation to use a preoperative combination of adriamycin and ifosfamide can be given; however, this regimen produces the best tumour remission rates. As there is no proof of postoperative adjuvant chemotherapy to be of value in this group of patients, it should be strongly considered in grade III lesions exceeding a tumour size of 5 cm, as it adds an additional modality to the otherwise limited therapeutic armamentarium.

In specific subtypes such as myxoid and round cell liposarcoma (MRCLS) with proven translocation, the use of trabectedin (Yondelis®) could result in a specific tumour growth arrest initially followed by myxoid degeneration and shrinkage. This approach has been very recently introduced, and at present has been

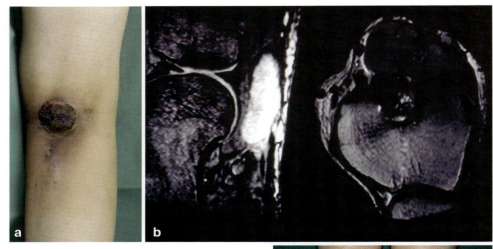
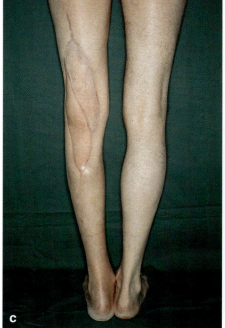

Fig. 17.5 a Sarcoma recurrence arising in the poplitea fossa 26 months after excision of the primary tumour and local irradiation of 56 Gy photon bean therapy (male 59 years). **b** CT image of a the subcutaneous extension of sarcoma recurrence in a similar case of relapse arising in the popliteal fossa after radiotherapy. **c** Final status 24 months after complex treatment of the sarcoma recurrence with isolated limb perfusion using Beromun® (Boehringer Ingelheim, Ingelheim, Germany) and melphalan, followed by complete dissection of the popliteal fossa including vessel resection of replacement by contralaterally saphenous vein graft and coverage with a myocutaneous latissimus dorsi flap, and with microvascular pedicle to the superficial popliteal artery and vein

proved effective in this tumour type only (Grosso et al. 2007). Studies are on the way evaluating the use of the drug in other sarcoma subtypes. At present, the response rate to be expected is beyond 50% with very low toxicity. This could also contribute to a less radical procedure that does not compromise wound healing postoperatively.

The use of combined chemotherapy with deep-wave hyperthermia has been first reported to be effective in sarcoma nearly a decade ago. Most recently, the results of a prospective randomized neoadjuvant study (EORTC 62961-ESHO) have been presented showing that in greater than 5 cm, high-grade, deep and extra-compartmentally located sarcoma, the addition of deep wave hyperthermia significantly improves response rate, R0-resection, and disease-free survival of the patients (Issels et al. 2007). Hyperthermia is established by putting the patient into an electromagnetic ring-antenna system allowing for the establishment of the defined field of regional hyperthermia, heating the area of the sarcoma to 42.5°C. Maintaining this temperature for 90 min results in significant changes in tumour blood flow and lowers the interstitial fluid pressure. A phase II study reported already in 2001 in locally advanced primary or recurrent high-risk soft tissue sarcoma showed a complete histological necrosis in 10% of the patients and greater than 75% necrosis in another 20% (Issels et al. 2001). When available, deep-wave hyperthermia adds a rather non-toxic treatment modality potentially improving the access of systemic chemotherapy to the tumour and, by this method, exploring a maximum of cytotoxic treatment to a sarcoma recurrence.

17.7 Conclusion

Sarcoma recurrence within a previously irradiated area is one of the most problematic therapeutic challenges in soft tissue tumours. It is absolutely mandatory that a multidisciplinary treatment team sees such patients. Any information on previous therapy needs to be available in detail. The therapeutic approach usually is not unidimensional. Whether preoperative measures of downstaging, such as limb perfusion, systemic chemotherapy and deep-wave hyperthermia, can be applied and make sense with respect to tumour grading and subtype needs to be carefully explored (Hohenberger and Wysocki 2008). The potential of repeated radiotherapy and the modality that can be used (intraoperative radiotherapy, brachytherapy) needs to be very carefully evaluated. The pathologist saves these major problems in intraoperative frozen section histology or resection margins and thus needs to be aware of the type of cancer cells potentially present within the resection specimen. Plastic and reconstructive surgery to cover the area of re-resection with viable and well-nourished tissue is absolutely crucial. Avoiding dead spaces in the resection area is a must to prevent lymphatic fistula. Thus, adequate treatment of those specific situations usually involves at least five different disciplines, with postoperative physiotherapy and rehabilitation also playing an extremely important role.

References

Ballo MT, Zagars GK, Pollock RE, Benjamin RS, Feig BW, Cormier JN, Hunt KK, Patel SR, Trent JC, Beddar S, Pisters PW (2007) Retroperitoneal soft tissue sarcoma: an analysis of radiation and surgical treatment. Int J Radiat Oncol Biol Phys 67:158–163

Bujko K, Suit HD, Springfield DS, Convery K (1993) Wound healing after preoperative radiation for sarcoma of soft tissues. Surg Gynecol Obstet 176:124–134

Cannon CP, Ballo MT, Zagars GK, Mirza AN, Lin PP, Lewis VO, Yasko AW, Benjamin RS, Pisters PW (2006) Complications of combined modality treatment of primary lower extremity soft-tissue sarcomas. Cancer 107:2455–2461

Catton C, Davis A, Bell R, O'Sullivan B, Fornasier V, Wunder J, McLean M (1996) Soft tissue sarcoma of the extremity. Limb salvage after failure of combined conservative therapy. Radiother Oncol 41:209–214

Davis AM, O'Sullivan B, Bell RS, Turcotte R, Catton CN, Wunder JS, Chabot P, Hammond A, Benk V, Isler M, Freeman C, Doddard K, Bezjak A, Kandel RA, Sadura A, Day A, James K, Tu D, Pater J, Zee B (2002) Function and health status outcomes in a randomized trial comparing preoperative and postoperative radiotherapy in extremity soft tissue sarcoma. J Clin Oncol 20:4472–4477

Davis AM, O'Sullivan B, Turcotte R, Bell R, Catton C, Chabot P, Wunder JS, Hammond A, Benk V, Kandel R, Goddard K, Freeman C, Sadura A, Zee B, Day A, Tu D, Pater J (2005) Canadian Sarcoma Group; NCI Canada Clinical Trial Group Randomized Trial. Late radiation morbidity following randomization to preoperative versus postoperative radiotherapy in extremity soft tissue sarcoma. Radiother Oncol 75:48–53

Eggermont AM, Schraffordt Koops H, Klausner JM, Kroon BB, Schlag PM, Lienard D, van Geel AN, Hoekstra HJ, Meller I, Nieweg OE, Kettelhack C, Ben-Ari G, Pector C, Lejeune FJ (1996) Isolated limb perfusion with tumor necrosis factor and melphalan for limb salvage in 186 patients with locally advanced soft tissue extremity sarcomas. The cumulative multicenter European experience. J Clin Oncol 14:2653–2665

Gortzak E, Azzarelli A, Buesa J, Bramwell VH, van Coevorden F, van Geel AN, Ezzat A, Santoro A, Oosterhuis JW, van Glabbeke M, Kirkpatrick A, Verweij J (2001) A randomised phase II study on neo-adjuvant chemotherapy for 'high-risk' adult soft-tissue sarcoma. Eur J Cancer 37:1096–1103

Grosso F, Jones RL, Demetri GD, Judson IR, Blay JY, Le Cesne A, Sanfilippo R, Casieri P, Collini P, Dileo P, Spreafico C, Stacchiotti S, Tamborini E, Tercero JC, Jimeno J, D'Incalci M, Gronchi A, Fletcher JA, Pilotti S, Casali PG (2007) Efficacy of trabectedin (ecteinascidin-743) in advanced pretreated myxoid liposarcomas: a retrospective study. Lancet Oncol 8:595–602

Gutman M, Inbar M, Lev-Shlush D, Abu-Abid S, Mozes M, Chaitchik S, Meller I, Klausner JM (1997) High dose tumor necrosis factor-alpha and melphalan administered via isolated limb perfusion for advanced limb soft tissue sarcoma results in a >90% response rate and limb preservation. Cancer 79:1129–1137

Hohenberger P, Wysocki WM (2008) Neoadjuvant treatment of locally advanced soft tissue sarcoma of the limbs: which treatment to choose? Oncologist 13:175–186

Hünerbein M, Hohenberger P, Stroszczynski C, Bartelt N, Schlag PM, Tunn PU (2007) Resection of soft tissue sarcoma of the lower limb after evaluation of vascular invasion with intraoperative intravascular ultrasonography. Br J Surg 94:168–173

Issels R, Abdel-Rahman S, Wendtner C, alk MH, Kurze V, Sauer H, Aydemir U, Hiddemann W (2001) Neoadjuvant chemotherapy combined with regional hyperthermia (RHT) for locally advanced primary or recurrent high-risk adult soft-tissue sarcomas (STS) of adults: long-term results of a phase II study. Eur J Cancer 37:1587–1589

Issels RD, Lindner LH, Wust P, Hohenberger P, Jauch KW, Daugaard S, Mansmann U, Hiddemann W, Blay JY, Verweij J (2007) Regional hyperthermia (RHT) improves response and survival when combined with systemic chemotherapy in the management of locally advanced, high grade soft tissue sarcomas (STS) of the extremities, the body wall and the abdomen: a phase III randomised prospective trial (EORTC-ESHO intergroup trial). Proc Am Soc Clin Oncol 25:10009

Lans TE, Grünhagen DJ, deWilt JH, van Geel AN, Eggermont AM (2005) Isolated limb perfusions with tumor necrosis factor and melphalan for locally recurrent soft tissue sarcoma in previously irradiated limbs. Ann Surg Oncol 12:406–411

Lin PP, Schupak KD, Boland PJ, Brennan MF, Healey JH (1998) Pathologic femoral fracture after periosteal excision and radiation for the treatment of soft tissue sarcoma. Cancer 82:2356–2365

Noorda EM, Vrouenraets BC, Nieweg OE, van Coevorden F, van Slooten GW, Kroon BBR (2003) Isolated limb perfusion with tumor necrosis factor-alpha and melphalan for patients with unresectable soft tissue sarcoma of the extremities. Cancer 98:1483–1490

O'Sullivan B, Davies AM, Turcotte R, Bell R, Catton C, Chabot P, Wunder J, Kandel R, Goddard K, Sadura A, Pater J, Zee B (2002) Preoperative versus postoperative radiotherapy in soft-tissue sarcoma of the limbs: a randomised trial. Lancet 359:2235–2241

Pearlstone DB, Janjan NA, Feig BW, Yasko AW, Hunt KK, Pollock RE, Lawyer A, Horton J, Pisters PW (1999) Re-resection with brachytherapy for locally recurrent soft tissue sarcoma arising in a previously radiated field. Cancer J Sci Am 5:26–33

Pisters PW, Pollock RE, Lewis VO, Yasko AW, Cormier JN, Respondek PM, Feig BW, Hunt KK, Lin PP, Zagars G, Wei C, Ballo MT (2007) Long-term results of prospective trial of surgery alone with selective use of radiation for patients with T1 extremity and trunk soft tissue sarcomas. Ann Surg 246:675–681

Riedel F, Philipp K, Sadick H, Goessler U, Hörmann K, Verse T (2005) Immunohistochemical analysis of radiation-induced non-healing dermal wounds of the head and neck. In Vivo 19:343–350

Springfield DS (1993) Surgical wound healing. Cancer Treat Res 1993 67:81–89

Temple CL, Ross DC, Magi E, DiFrancesco M, Kurien E, Temple WJ (2007) Preoperative chemoradiation and flap reconstruction provide high local control and low wound complication rates for patients undergoing limb salvage surgery for upper extremity tumors. J Surg Oncol 95:135–141

Torres MA, Ballo MT, Butler CE, Feig BW, Cormier JN, Lewis VO, Pollock RE, Pisters PW, Zagars GK (2007) Management of locally recurrent soft-tissue sarcoma after prior surgery and radiation therapy. Int J Radiat Oncol Biol Phys 67:1124–1129

Trovik CS, Bauer HC, Alvegård TA, Anderson H, Blomquist C, Berlin O, Gustafson P, Saeter G, Wallöe A (2000) Surgical margins, local recurrence and metastasis in soft tissue sarcomas: 559 surgically-treated patients from the Scandinavian Sarcoma Group Register. Eur J Cancer 36:710–716

Wust P, Hildebrandt B, Sreenivasa G, Rau B, Gellermann J, Riess H, Felix R, Schlag PM (2002) Hyperthermia in combined treatment of cancer. Lancet Oncol 3:487–497

Yang JC, Chang AE, Baker AR, Sindelar WF, Danforth DN, Topalian SL, DeLaney T, Glatstein E, Steinberg SM, Merino MJ, Rosenberg SA (1998) Randomized prospective study of the benefit of adjuvant radiation therapy in the treatment of soft tissue sarcomas of the extremity. J Clin Oncol 16:197–203

Management of Vascular Involvement in Extremity Soft Tissue Sarcoma

Ashish Mahendra, Yair Gortzak, Peter C. Ferguson, Benjamin M. Deheshi, Thomas F. Lindsay, and Jay S. Wunder

Abstract Advances in adjuvant treatment protocols and improvements in imaging techniques have helped improve the limb-salvage rate for extremity soft tissue sarcomas to approximately 95%. Moreover, improvements in operative techniques have enabled successful limb-salvage surgery to be performed even in the face of vascular invasion or encasement by tumor. En bloc resection of major vascular structures with the tumor and reconstruction with reversed saphenous vein grafts, femoral venous grafts, or synthetic grafts has proved to be a feasible option in limb-salvage surgery. However, the surgical oncologist and patient should be aware that although overall function is only slightly worse after these procedures, individual functional results are less predictable. In addition, procedures requiring vascular resection and reconstruction are associated with an increased risk of complications, including amputation.

Jay S. Wunder (✉)
University Musculoskeletal Oncology Unit
Mount Sinai Hospital
476-600 University Avenue
Toronto, ON M5G 1X5, Canada
E-mail: jwunder@mtsinai.on.ca

18.1 Introduction

Limb-salvage surgery has become the standard of care in the surgical management of most patients with extremity soft tissue sarcomas. With the use of adjuvant chemotherapy, radiation protocols, or both, as well as advanced imaging techniques, adequate margins can be obtained in most cases without the need for radical resection or amputation. The current concept for local management of soft tissue sarcomas of the extremities consists of either a wide excision of the tumor with an adequate surgical margin alone, or a less-than-wide or more marginal excision together with adjuvant treatment. It has been demonstrated that when a less-than-wide yet adequate surgical margin is combined with adjuvant radiation therapy, there is no difference in local disease-free status or the survival rate between limb-salvage procedures and amputations.

One of the theoretical roadblocks to limb-salvage surgery is neurovascular involvement by the tumor. Soft tissue sarcomas can be safely resected when adjacent to major blood vessels by longitudinally splitting the adventitia opposite the tumor, thereby preserving a rim of "normal" tissue in the vessel–tumor interface. Prior experience from our multidisciplinary sarcoma group has shown that even a planned microscopically positive margin against one or more critical structures (e.g., major vessel, nerve, or bone) following resection of a soft issue sarcoma in combination with (neo-) adjuvant radiotherapy is associated with a low risk of local recurrence (Gerrand et al. 2001; Clarkson et al. 2005). If a soft tissue sarcoma arises directly from the vessel wall, then vascular resection is inevitable. Furthermore, if a soft tissue sarcoma infiltrates or surrounds vascular structures, then too the vessels will require resection. Therefore, it is generally accepted that when it is impossible to achieve a wide or even marginal resection margin with major vessel preservation, vascular resection may be indicated. This is also supported by several studies showing that limb salvage combined with vascular reconstruction offers rates of local tumor control and overall survival that are comparable to amputation (Ghert et al. 2005; Leggon et al. 2001; Hohenberger et al. 1999).

Reports in the literature have also shown that resection of major peripheral nerves in conjunction with resection of extremity soft tissue sarcomas particularly of the lower extremity, does not preclude an acceptable functional outcome (Brooks et al. 2002; Bickels et al. 2002; Fuchs et al. 2001). However, disabling limb edema and ultimately amputation are frequent complications of limb-salvage procedures requiring resection of major blood vessels without vascular repair. More recently, resection of major vessels followed by vascular reconstruction has been found to be technically feasible and successful, with an amputation rate of approximately 10% (Nishinari et al. 2006a; Ghert et al. 2005; Hohenberger et al. 1999).

In contrast to the revascularization for atheromatous occlusive diseases, there have been relatively few reports on vascular reconstruction following resection for extremity soft tissue sarcomas. Reconstruction following resection of a major artery is generally recommended while the value of venous reconstruction in extremity tumor surgery remains more controversial.

The functional results of such extensive attempts at limb salvage with vascular reconstruction have been carefully addressed in only a few studies in the literature. Postoperative edema, the risk of vascular graft thrombosis, wound-healing complications, and occasionally the concomitant need for major peripheral nerve resection can all potentially add to the morbidity of the procedure thus limiting function of the salvaged extremity and at times leading to delayed amputation (Nishinari et al. 2006a; Ghert et al. 2005; Koperna et al. 1996).

18.2
Indications for Vascular Resection and Reconstruction in Extremity Soft Tissue Sarcoma

Most patients who would be considered satisfactory candidates for limb-preserving surgery for extremity soft tissue sarcoma should also be considered for vascular resection and reconstruction when involvement of major arterial or venous blood vessels is identified. Vascular involvement may be either primary (i.e., primary vascular origin such as leiomyosarcoma) or secondary, such as when a soft tissue sarcoma infiltrates or encases major blood vessels. In cases with secondary vascular involvement, vessel resection is only required when the tumor has either completely encased or partially encircled the vessel. If the area of vessel wall infiltration is limited, rarely a partial or limited resection can be performed leaving the uninvolved portion of the vessel in continuity followed by a "patch" type of repair. If the tumor is adjacent to, but not infiltrating the wall of a main vessel, then vascular resection can usually be avoided by leaving the vascular adventitia as a margin with the tumor (Gerrand et al. 2001; Ghert et al. 2005). However, one particular scenario of vascular encasement deserves further consideration when the tumor is a low-grade liposarcoma (i.e., lipoma-like liposarcoma, well-differentiated liposarcoma). In the extremity, this particular tumor subtype is generally considered to be more indolent and tends to be treated more like a lipoma than a typical sarcoma (Kooby et al. 2004; Kubo et al. 2006). Only with a low-grade liposarcoma encircling a major vessel may it be reasonable to consider "bivalving" the tumor to extirpate the vessel intact and avoid the potential morbidity associated with vascular reconstruction, particularly for older patients with medical comorbidities. However, this type of treatment plan should only be undertaken in the context of a multidisciplinary approach, and should probably be performed in conjunction with (neo-) adjuvant radiotherapy (Fig. 18.1a–e).

Resection of any major artery is an indication for reconstruction. However, the indications for venous reconstruction following vascular resection in extremity soft tissue sarcoma are less clear-cut and depend on the clinical setting, the surgeon's preference and the findings at the time of surgery (Nishinari et al. 2006a; Schwarzbach et al. 2005; Kawai et al. 1996).

18.3
Patient Workup

The presence of clinical signs and symptoms indicative of vascular compromise is uncommon in patients with extremity soft tissue sarcomas and is not considered to be a reliable indicator of vascular involvement. Evidence of edema or claudication is rare in these patients. The diagnosis of major vascular involvement by a soft tissue sarcoma is usually established by cross-sectional magnetic resonance (MR) or computed tomography (CT) imaging. Such a sarcoma may arise from the involved vessel wall or infiltrate or encase the major blood vessels.

Proper workup of the patient with a soft tissue sarcoma of the extremity is essential in order to formulate a successful treatment plan. Local and systemic staging by imaging is usually followed with a tissue diagnosis by appropriate biopsy. Once involvement of major vessels is identified, it becomes critical to determine the extent of vascular resection required and consider possible methods of vascular reconstruction including assessment of donor sites. Local anatomical factors including both the length and diameter of vascular conduits required for reconstruction and the potential for local wound-healing complications are important considerations.

For extremity sarcoma patients requiring vascular resection and reconstruction the preoperative workup should be standardized. This would include:

– History

This would include smoking, diabetes mellitus, hypertension and renal failure, elevated serum lipid levels.

– Physical examination

Peripheral pulses, evaluation of tumor size and location, venous markings (varicose veins, evidence of chronic venous insufficiency) and limb edema need to be assessed. A similar examination is performed on the unaffected limb.

– Vascular lab

Peripheral arterial Doppler is used to determine the ankle-brachial index (ABI) and evidence of preexistent disease such as atherosclerosis. A venous Doppler scan on the affected limb is performed to rule out deep vein thrombosis (DVT) and assess the patency of deep and superficial veins (e.g., common femoral, superficial femoral, deep femoral, popliteal, tibial, and saphenous

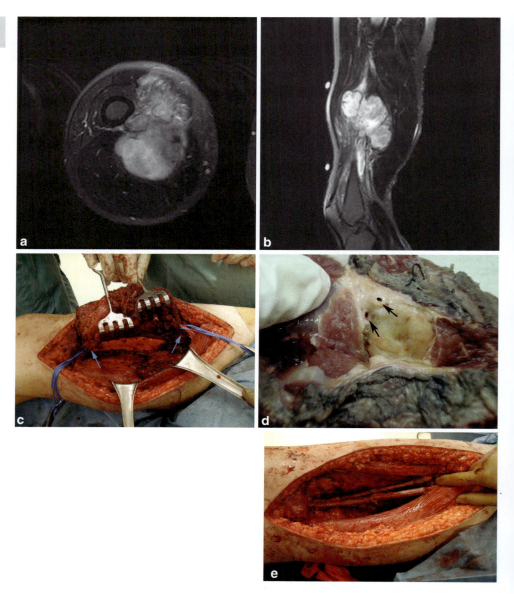

Fig. 18.1 Synovial sarcoma encasing the distal third of the femoral vessels. **a, b** Axial and sagittal T2-weighted fast spin echo magnetic resonance images (MRI) with fat suppression show a large lobulated and high-signal heterogeneous mass involving the medial quadriceps, adductors, and surrounding both the femoral artery and vein. **c** Intraoperative photograph showing the tumor subperiosteally elevated from the medial femur. The superficial femoral vessels are marked proximally and distally by vessel loops (*arrows*). **d** Cross-section of the gross specimen showing the vessels (*arrows*) surrounded circumferentially by tumor. **e** Intraoperative photograph showing reconstruction of the vascular defect in the femoral artery and vein using a graft from the contralateral superficial femoral vein

veins). Venous ultrasound on the unaffected limb (donor leg) can be performed to assess the femoral and saphenous veins for size compatibility and suitability for harvest.

-Length of vascular resection and graft selection

Estimation of resection length is based on the preoperative MRI scan and aids in identifying the appropriate donor site. An estimate of graft length and suitable width can be made at this stage. This is useful information because the segment of superficial femoral vein that can be harvested lies between the popliteal vein distally and the profunda vein proximally. In adults this is approximately 30 cm long (but is influenced by the height of the patient and his or her leg length) and 4–8 mm in diameter, although it usually dilates an additional 1 mm under arterial pressure (Dorweiler et al. 2001; Cardozo et al. 2002). A key consideration for the vascular surgeon is the spasm and resultant shortening of vessels in the recipient bed after tumor and vascular resection. Spasm is more significant in younger patients and the use of local papaverine helps in reducing the spasm that results in a narrowed and shortened vessel. Any significant discrepancy between graft length and length of vascular resection can have a detrimental effect on success of the vascular reconstruction, as too long a graft can kink while a short graft is even worse as it can tear under tension.

In the past, a traditional workup of patients with extremity sarcomas prior to contemplating limb-sparing surgery included arteriography. Although uncommon, conventional angiography can be associated with substantial morbidity, including access site hematoma, pseudoaneurysm, dissection, and arterial occlusion (Meyerson et al. 2002). We do not routinely use angiography in these cases since the information available from the vascular lab and preoperative high-quality cross-sectional imaging studies with enhancement such as CT or MR angiograms usually provides sufficient data for clinical decision-making. Recent reports of intravascular ultrasound during surgery or three-dimensional MRI with contrast raise the possibility of additional studies that can guide the surgeon in these cases (Hünerbein et al. 2007).

18.4
Surgical and Functional Outcome

We recently conducted a study at our center of the surgical and functional outcomes in patients with extremity soft tissue sarcoma requiring vascular resection and reconstruction. In this investigation, we used demographic, tumor, and treatment-specific criteria to individually match our sample of 19 patients who underwent limb-salvage surgery with vascular resection and reconstruction for a soft tissue sarcoma of the extremity to 38 patients who underwent similar procedures without requiring vascular reconstruction. We were also able to individually match 6 of the vascular reconstruction patients to 6 limb-salvage patients who did not require a vascular procedure, to directly compare functional outcome (Ghert et al. 2005).

We found that patients who required vascular resection and reconstruction were significantly more likely to require a muscle transfer for wound closure, and experience a wound complication, deep venous thrombosis, and clinically significant limb edema. Although uncommon, these patients were also at greater risk for ultimately requiring a secondary amputation. The functional outcome following vascular reconstruction was not significantly worse at 1 year after treatment, although clinically significant limb edema was both more frequent and more severe in this group of patients. It is important to note that in this study the majority of patients in each treatment group received preoperative radiotherapy. This may be related to the higher wound-healing complication rate in the patients requiring vascular resection. However, the clinical benefits associated with preoperative radiation may also help explain why the functional results are as good as they are in this group of patients.

18.4.1
Amputation Risk

Reports in the literature as early as 1977 described vascular resection and reconstruction in the setting of soft tissue sarcoma of the extremity. A review of pooled data from the literature and two other recent reports indicates that 10 (8.4%; range; 0%–25%) of 119 patients who underwent vascular reconstruction for a soft tissue sarcoma of the extremity ultimately required an amputation (Leggon et al. 2001; Hohenberger et al. 1999; Bonardelli et al. 2000).

In our study, 3 (16%) of 19 vascular reconstruction patients required amputation, compared with only 1 (3%) of 38 in the matched limb-salvage control group. This indicates the high-risk nature of this procedure. The higher risk for amputation in patients undergoing vascular reconstruction is multifactorial and is at least partially related to the technical aspects of vascular repair, its physiologic impact on the limb, and the notably higher rate of wound-associated morbidity.

18.4.2
Use of Muscle Flaps

In our study, it was interesting to note that a higher rate of muscle flap coverage in this group of patients did not decrease the wound complication rate. This same lack of effect of muscle flaps on decreasing wound complications after preoperative radiation for extremity sarcomas has been reported previously in a randomized clinical trial (O'Sullivan et al. 2002).

18.4.3
Wound Complications

Of the vascular reconstruction patients in this study, 68% experienced a wound complication. This was significantly higher than the control group, which had a wound complication rate of 36%–similar to the preoperative radiation arm in a previously reported randomized clinical trial comparing preoperative vs postoperative external beam radiation and surgical resection for extremity soft tissue sarcoma (O'Sullivan et al. 2002).

The literature also reports a high rate of postoperative wound complications in patients undergoing vascular reconstruction. Although major wound complications have been reported to occur in 15%–20% of these cases, a review of the pooled data in the literature included both bone and soft tissue sarcomas and reported 43 complications (46%) in 92 patients. These complications included wound dehiscence, hematoma, and swelling (Leggon et al. 2001; Hohenberger et al. 1999). The wound complication rate in our investigation was higher but also included complications that required nonoperative management, such as prolonged deep wound packing (O'Sullivan et al. 2002). Furthermore, management of the bone sarcomas included in the pooled data would have utilized radiotherapy infrequently, thereby skewing the results toward fewer wound-healing complications.

18.4.4
Postoperative Limb Edema and DVT

Procedures involving resection of major vessels imply the loss of more collateral vessels and disruption of additional lymphatic drainage channels, which further impairs wound perfusion and increases postoperative edema. Another contributory factor is the extent of muscle resection. Deep venous thrombosis in vascular reconstruction patients may also be a contributing factor for limb edema and amputation. However, in the vascular repair patients who were matched for comparing functional outcome, postoperative limb edema was not associated with the occurrence of deep venous thrombosis. A significantly greater proportion of patients in the vascular reconstruction group did develop deep venous thrombosis in this study, although the risk varied according to the postoperative anticoagulation protocol. Currently all patients with an arterial and venous reconstruction are managed with low-dose IV heparin for 48–72 h postoperatively. If bleeding is not encountered then full-dose IV heparin or low-molecular-weight heparin is administered and followed eventually with warfarin. We routinely treat venous and arterial reconstruction patients for 1 year with prophylactic anticoagulation. Deep vein thrombosis was more than twice as likely to occur in patients with vascular repair if they were treated with prophylactic or low dose anticoagulation compared with full dose anticoagulation (Ghert et al. 2005). As a result, we now treat these patients with prophylactic anticoagulation for only a short time immediately following surgery, and initiate full-dose anticoagulation as early as possible postoperatively. Although no complications in this study could be directly attributed to wound hematoma, it must be recognized that prophylactic and especially full-dose anticoagulation may play a role in the high incidence of wound-healing complications in these cases. However, the benefits of anticoagulation in minimizing thromboembolic disease and ensuring graft patency likely outweigh any potential detrimental effects on wound healing.

18.4.5
Risk of Local Recurrence

Extensive vascular involvement by extremity sarcoma raises a major concern regarding not only the risk of local recurrence after limb-salvage surgery, but also the potential increased risk for metastatic disease. In general, patients presenting with extremity sarcoma complicated by vascular involvement are at a higher risk of requiring amputation for primary definitive management, and only a well-defined subset are eligible for limb-salvage procedures. However, there was only one local recurrence in the 19 patients treated with vascular reconstruction in our series, which supports the oncological safety of this approach.

Similar local recurrence rates have been reported by other groups (Nishinari et al. 2006a; Baxter et al. 2007; Schwarzbach et al. 2005; Koperna et al. 1996; Bonardelli et al. 2000).

18.4.6
Risk of Systemic Disease

A higher proportion of patients in the vascular reconstruction group in our study presented with systemic disease (32% vs 8%). When patients presenting with localized disease were considered separately, however, there was no difference in metastasis-free survival between the two treatment groups. In our series of 19 vascular reconstruction patients, 11 (58%) were alive without evidence of disease at a mean of 47 months follow-up, which is almost identical to pooled data from the literature for patients undergoing similar procedures (Ghert et al. 2005; Nishinari et al. 2006a; Schwarzbach et al. 2005; Koperna et al. 1996; Bonardelli et al. 2000).

18.4.7
Functional Outcome

Functional outcome of patients who undergo limb-salvage surgery with vascular reconstruction has been described only briefly in the literature. Leggon et al. (2001) reported that 76% of a group of 58 patients pooled from the literature had a "functional limb." Bonardelli et al. (2000) reported on function of 7 patients after vascular reconstruction using the Musculoskeletal Tumor Society Rating Scale, a clinician-completed assessment of impairment, and reported good results in 6 patients and fair results in 1. Koperna et al. (1996) found good or excellent results in 9 of 13 patients using the same rating system (Fig. 18.2a–d).

Our group previously showed that the main determinants of functional outcome after limb-salvage surgery and radiotherapy for soft tissue sarcoma are tumor size, wound complications,

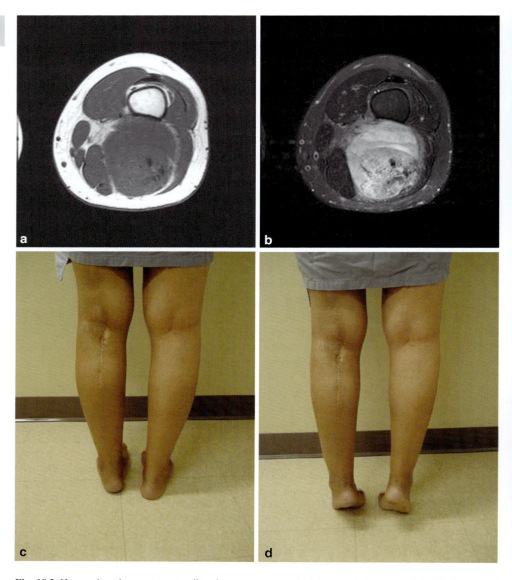

Fig. 18.2 Hemangiopericytoma surrounding the popliteal vessels. **a, b** Axial T1- and axial T2-weighted fast spin echo MRI with fat suppression shows a large heterogeneous sarcoma in the posterior calf extending into the popliteal space and surrounding the popliteal vessels. **c, d** The patient's limb 7 years following treatment. She has mild but persistent distal edema, and hyperpigmentation of the treatment region related to adjuvant radiation. However, she has regained full range of motion of the knee, plays multiple sports including those requiring running, and has no functional limitations. She considers herself to have an excellent result

and motor nerve sacrifice (Davis et al. 2000). In our study, while considering functional outcome between patients who underwent vascular reconstruction and those who did not, strict matching criteria were used, including similar tumor size, wound complications, and preoperative

Toronto Extremity Salvage Scores (TESS). We ensured that none of the patients had motor nerve sacrifice so that the functional comparison would specifically address the issue of vascular reconstruction. Patients in these groups were not matched for the timing of radiation because functional outcome at 1 year after treatment is more closely related to wound-complication status (Davis et al. 2002). We used the TESS, which is a reliable patient-derived measure of physical disability developed specifically for the extremity sarcoma population. TESS evaluates the patients' perceptions of difficulty with activities of daily living, mobility, work, and recreation and has been systematically validated. Overall, we found that patients with similar demographics, tumor size and location, treatment, complications, and preoperative function had only slightly lower postoperative TESS scores at 1 year if they underwent vascular resection and reconstruction. Although the difference in TESS evaluation was not statistically significant in our study, previous work has shown that the magnitude of change we identified is likely to be clinically meaningful. Applying this degree of change to the individual patient matches in our study suggests that one vascular reconstruction patient had better postoperative function, two had similar function, and three had worse function than patients who did not require vascular procedures. It is interesting that the functional difference between the two groups was not greater even though the vascular reconstruction patients had more frequent and severe limb edema after treatment. It must be emphasized that this functional comparison is based on two very closely matched patient groups. Because complications including deep venous thrombosis and limb edema are much more frequent overall in patients who require vascular repair, these patients are more likely to have a worse functional outcome (Ghert et al. 2005). Recent experience using a more aggressive early anticoagulation protocol reduced the incidence of DVT and may help prevent long-term edema in these patients. Consideration must also be given to the contralateral limb where vein harvesting may impact functional recovery as well.

18.5
Vascular Outcome

18.5.1
Arterial Reconstruction

The long-term patency of arterial reconstruction has been reported to be 45%–91% at 5 years following resection for lower extremity soft tissue sarcomas (Schwarzbach et al. 2005; Nishinari et al. 2006b). Even in patients with late graft occlusion, the limbs are usually preserved without ischemic symptoms because of the development of collateral circulation (Matsushita et al. 2001). Thus, the long-term limb-salvage rate is good, and amputation is rarely required if the tumor does not recur.

18.5.2
Venous Reconstruction

Simultaneous venous reconstruction with arterial grafting has been recommended in patients who have undergone resection of major vessels for tumor to prevent massive intractable edema in the early postoperative period (Fortner et al. 1977). However, a proportion of venous grafts likely become occluded soon after surgery. Furthermore, edema following venous resection alone or after graft occlusion can often be treated by leg elevation and elastic support. In comparison, venous reconstruction following vascular trauma has been associated with excellent long-term results and less risk of amputation (Rich 1982; Phifer et al. 1984). This may be related in part to the shorter length of the venous interposition grafts required in most trauma scenarios compared to patients with tumors. In addition, patients with tumors likely have had more opportunity for development of collateral venous channels during tumor development and prior to treatment (Fig. 18.3a–g).

Interestingly, however, venous occlusion following vascular reconstitution has a less obvious effect on failure of limb salvage in patients undergoing venous resection for tumor. Accordingly, many surgeons do not perform venous reconstruction in these cases. Some authors have described patients with mild to moderate edema that was adequately treated with elastic support. Matsushita et al. (2001) evaluated chronic venous disease on the basis of standard vascular surgery criteria in patients of extremity soft tissue sarcoma following venous reconstruction. Only mild clinical disease was found in most of their patients. However, clinically significant edema was identified in patients who underwent complete resection of the proximal adductor muscles together with both the superficial and the deep femoral veins. Thus, it may be reasonable to presume that the deep femoral vein and surrounding muscles constitute an important source for the formation of collateral femoral venous circulation. Patients undergoing resection of both the superficial and the deep femoral vein with the adductor muscles are at highest risk for development of chronic venous disease. These patients should be considered as possible candidates for simultaneous venous reconstruction.

At our center we now routinely reconstruct major veins even if sufficient adductor muscles and the long saphenous vein have been preserved. We feel that the surgical and functional outcome is already compromised by several factors beyond our control such as loss of muscles, lymphatics, use of radiation and wound-healing complications. By not reconstructing the vein, we might be introducing yet another variable with potential negative impact on functional outcome.

18.5.3 Type of Vascular Graft

Cross-sectional imaging and studies from the vascular lab provide adequate details related to the extent of vascular resection and the size of graft required. We now often use the contralateral superficial femoral vein as the donor. Several studies of this technique have shown no significant additional donor limb morbidity compared to the more common use of the saphenous vein (Cardozo et al. 2002; Dorweiler et al. 2001). An important consideration favoring use of the superficial femoral vein is to avoid donor–recipient size mismatch, which can be a major issue if long lengths of saphenous vein are used as the donor vessel (Bell et al. 2005; McKay et al. 2007).

A review of the literature suggests that synthetic vascular grafts can also be used safely and effectively in these cases (Schwarzbach et al. 2005; Adelani et al. 2007). However, we

---

Fig. 18.3 Leiomyosarcoma arising from the common femoral vein. **a** Axial T1-weighted MRI image through the right proximal thigh shows a large mass adjacent to the femoral vessels with effacement of the femoral vein (*arrow*). **b** Coronal T2-weighted fast spin echo MRI image of the right proximal thigh with fat suppression demonstrates a heterogeneous mass arising from the common femoral vein and displacing laterally the femoral artery (*arrow*). Tumor within the lumen of the vein is evident immediately distal to the arrow. **c, d** Intraoperative photographs show the femoral artery marked with vessel loops (**c**) and dissected free of the tumor (**d**) which is arising from the common femoral vein (*arrows*). The intravascular component of the tumor is evident within the vein. **e** The tumor has been resected, and the proximal and distal ends of the femoral vein are marked by vessel clamps. **f** Cross-section view of the resected specimen shows the tumor arising from the wall of the femoral vein. The vessel lumen is being held open by a clamp. **g** The femoral vein was reconstructed using the contralateral superficial femoral vein to avoid a size mismatch

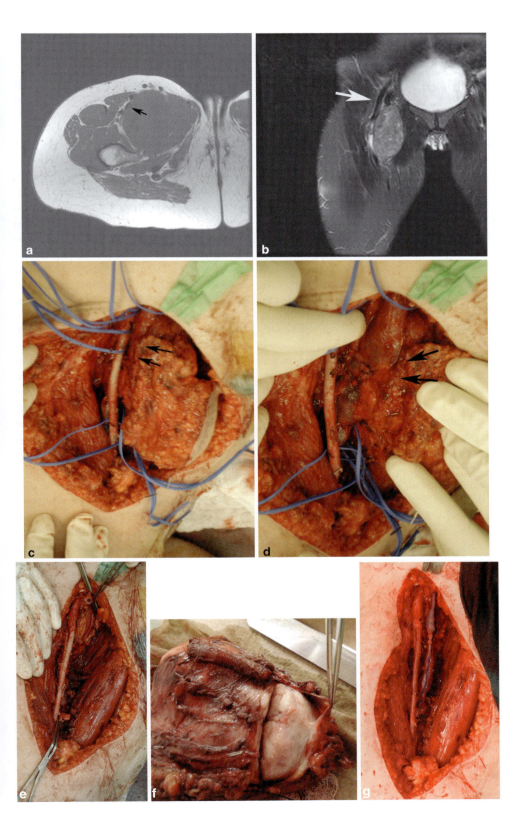

try to avoid using synthetic vascular grafts whenever possible in patients with extremity soft tissue sarcoma because of the higher incidence of wound problems, and the long-term excellent outcomes using autogenous grafts (Nishinari et al. 2006a, b; Leggon et al. 2001).

18.6 Effects of Radiotherapy

Adjuvant radiotherapy in cases of extremity soft tissue sarcoma with vascular reconstruction may have the potential for adverse effects such as graft occlusion or arterial blowout. Several studies on the late effects of radiotherapy on carotid vessels in patients with head and neck cancers have shown a significant correlation between radiotherapy dose and carotid artery atheromatous disease (Carmody et al. 1999; Dorresteijn et al. 2005). A radiation dose exceeding 50 Gy is associated with higher-grade vessel wall abnormalities (Martin et al. 2005). Similarly, a significantly higher risk of death due to ischemic heart disease has been reported for patients treated with mantle radiation for Hodgkin's lymphoma (Swerdlow et al. 2007). There is no known similar direct correlation between radiotherapy and development of in-field atherosclerosis in extremity sarcomas, possibly due to the paucity of literature.

The following case study exemplifies the potential for postoperative radiation-induced atherosclerosis. A 55-year-old man presented to a vascular surgeon with a history of one block claudication but no night or rest pain. He had no history of smoking, hypertension, or diabetes. The patient had been treated for a sarcoma in the right groin 14 years previously by resection and high dose 66-Gy postoperative radiation. At the time of sarcoma surgery no vascular resection was required. On physical examination the patient had extensive scarring and fibrosis in his right groin making the femoral pulse difficult to feel, and no distal pulses were palpable. The patient's leg was chronically swollen to the mid-calf, this being his norm, and he controlled this with surgical support stockings. The vascular lab study demonstrated patent external iliac and common femoral vessels with a severe proximal superficial femoral artery stenosis with a peak systolic velocity of 438 cm/s. The ABI on the right leg was 0.56 vs 1.31 on the left leg. An angiogram (Fig. 18.4a) demonstrated a diseased proximal superficial femoral artery which was successfully treated with angioplasty and stenting (Fig. 18.4b). The patient's symptoms resolved and he no longer suffers from claudication. He regained his popliteal pulse and the ABI has increased to 0.99. He remains asymptomatic 6 months after therapy.

Although preoperative radiation is associated with a higher risk of wound-healing complications compared to postoperative treatment (O'Sullivan et al. 2002), local anatomy should be considered when making recommendations about multidisciplinary management for a specific patient. When radiation dose and field size issues are considered, the preoperative approach has benefits. This would apply specifically to the upper extremity where wound complications are uncommon. Such an approach is especially relevant in the upper arm so that the adjacent lung, shoulder joint, and axillary contents may be protected by the smaller preoperative radiotherapy treatment volume. In addition, a lower radiotherapy dose of 50 Gy to the axillary vessels, brachial plexus, and adjacent tissues is likely safer in the long term. Our group's experience has shown that although the preoperative radiotherapy protocol may be detrimental to function very early—at 6 weeks following surgery—due to a higher risk of wound complications, function becomes comparable between treatment groups at subsequent assessments up to 1 year after surgery (Davis et al. 2002). By 2 years post-treatment, patients who receive postoperative radiation tend to have worse fibrosis, stiffness, edema, and overall functional outcomes (Davis et al. 2005). The factors to be

18 Management of Vascular Involvement in Extremity Soft Tissue Sarcoma

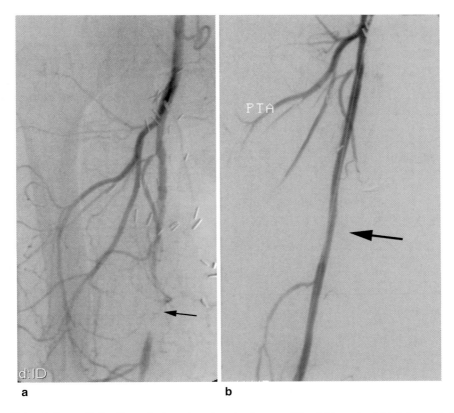

Fig. 18.4 a, b Post-radiation femoral artery stenosis. **a** Angiogram of the right proximal thigh demonstrates a short superficial femoral artery occlusion (*arrow*), patent profunda femoris artery, and multiple clips from the previous sarcoma resection. **b** Recanalized superficial femoral artery after angioplasty and stenting (*arrow*)

considered in deciding the timing of radiotherapy in such cases would include the anatomical site and proximity to radiosensitive structures, tumor size, the risk and consequence of complications, and the mode of wound reconstruction. Although we could not identify a specific study describing the effect of radiation on vessel walls in extremity sarcomas, the head and neck cancer literature clearly demonstrates a direct correlation between increasing radiation dose and the extent of vessel wall damage. Thus, the decision to accept increased short-term morbidity from wound-healing complications which are more common following lower dose and smaller field preoperative radiotherapy must be balanced against the potential longer term side effects of larger radiation doses and volumes associated with postoperative radiotherapy. Also, a major postoperative wound complication in a patient who was to receive postoperative radiotherapy has the potential to delay the start of adjuvant therapy or even prevent postoperative radiotherapy altogether, and this could definitely compromise the oncologic outcome.

Summary

The goal of combined surgery and radiotherapy in treating patients with soft tissue sarcoma is to achieve cure, both locally and systemically, and enhance function. Even the difficult situation of vascular involvement by sarcoma can now frequently be managed without amputation and with a good expected functional result. Preoperative and postoperative radiation approaches achieve similarly high levels of local control for extremity soft tissue sarcoma, but are associated with different short- and long-term benefits in this patient population.

References

Adelani MA, Holt GE, Dittus RS, Passman MA, Schwartz HS (2007) Revascularization after segmental resection of lower extremity soft tissue sarcomas. J Surg Oncol 95:455–460

Baxter BT, Mahoney C, Johnson PJ, Selmer KM, Pipinos II, Rose J, Neff JR (2007) Concomitant arterial and venous reconstruction with resection of lower extremity sarcomas. Ann Vasc Surg 21:272–279

Bell CL, Ali AT, Brawley JG, D'Addio VJ, Modrall JG, Valentine RJ, Clagett GP (2005) Arterial reconstruction of infected femoral artery pseudoaneurysms using superficial femoral-popliteal vein. J Am Coll Surg 200:831–836

Bickels J, Wittig JC, Kollender Y, Kellar-Graney K, Malawer MM, Meller I (2002) Sciatic nerve resection: is that truly an indication for amputation? Clin Orthop Relat Res 399:201–204

Bonardelli S, Nodari F, Maffeis R, Ippolito V, Saccalani M, Lussardi L, Giulini S (2000) Limb salvage in lower extremity sarcomas and technical details about vascular reconstruction. J Orthop Sci 5:555–560

Brooks AD, Gold JS, Graham D, Boland P, Lewis JJ, Brennan MF, Healey JH (2002) Resection of the sciatic, peroneal, or tibial nerves: assessment of functional status. Ann Surg Oncol 9:41–47

Cardozo MA, Frankini AD, Bonamigo TP (2002) Use of superficial femoral vein in the treatment of infected aortoiliofemoral prosthetic grafts. Cardiovasc Surg 10:304–310

Carmody BJ, Arora S, Avena R, Curry KM, Simpkins J, Cosby K, Sidawy AN (1999) Accelerated carotid artery disease after high-dose head and neck radiotherapy: is there a role for routine carotid duplex surveillance? J Vasc Surg 30:1045–1051

Clarkson PW, Griffin AM, Catton CN, O'Sullivan B, Ferguson PC, Wunder JS, Bell RS (2005) Epineural dissection is a safe technique that facilitates limb salvage surgery. Clin Orthop Relat Res 438:92–96

Davis AM, Sennik S, Griffin AM, Wunder JS, O'Sullivan B, Catton CN, Bell RS (2000) Predictors of functional outcomes following limb salvage surgery for lower-extremity soft tissue sarcoma. J Surg Oncol 73:206–211

Davis AM, O'Sullivan B, Bell RS, Turcotte R, Catton CN, Wunder JS, Chabot P, Hammond A, Benk V, Isler M, Freeman C, Goddard K, Bezjak A, Kandel RA, Sadura A, Day A, James K, Tu D, Pater J, Zee B (2002) Function and health status outcomes in a randomized trial comparing preoperative and postoperative radiotherapy in extremity soft tissue sarcoma. J Clin Oncol 20:4472–4477

Davis AM, O'Sullivan B, Turcotte R, Bell R, Catton C, Chabot P, Wunder J, Hammond A, Benk V, Kandel R, Goddard K, Freeman C, Sadura A, Zee B, Day A, Tu D, Pater J; Canadian Sarcoma Group; NCI Canada Clinical Trial Group Randomized Trial (2005) Late radiation morbidity following randomization to preoperative versus postoperative radiotherapy in extremity soft tissue sarcoma. Radiother Oncol 75:48–53

Dorresteijn LD, Kappelle AC, Scholz NM, Munneke M, Scholma JT, Balm AJ, Bartelink H, Boogerd W (2005) Increased carotid wall thickening after radiotherapy on the neck. Eur J Cancer 41:1026–1030

Dorweiler B, Neufang A, Schmiedt W, Oelert H (2001) Autogenous reconstruction of infected arterial prosthetic grafts utilizing the superficial femoral vein. Thorac Cardiovasc Surg 49:107–111

Fortner JG, Kim DK, Shiu MH (1977) Limb-preserving vascular surgery for malignant tumors of the lower extremity. Arch Surg 112:391–394

Fuchs B, Davis AM, Wunder JS, Bell RS, Masri BA, Isler M, Turcotte R, Rock MG (2001) Sciatic nerve resection in the thigh: a functional evaluation. Clin Orthop Relat Res 34–41

Gerrand CH, Wunder JS, Kandel RA, O'Sullivan B, Catton CN, Bell RS, Griffin AM, Davis AM (2001) Classification of positive margins after resection of soft-tissue sarcoma of the limb predicts the risk of local recurrence. J Bone Joint Surg Br 83:1149–1155

Ghert MA, Davis AM, Griffin AM, Alyami AH, White L, Kandel RA, Ferguson P, O'Sullivan B, Catton CN, Lindsay T, Rubin B, Bell RS, Wunder JS (2005) The surgical and functional outcome of limb-salvage surgery with vascular reconstruction for soft tissue sarcoma of the extremity. Ann Surg Oncol 12:1102–1110

Hohenberger P, Allenberg JR, Schlag PM, Reichardt P (1999) Results of surgery and multimodal therapy for patients with soft tissue sarcoma invading to vascular structures. Cancer 85:396–408

Hünerbein M, Hohenberger P, Stroszczynski C, Bartelt N, Schlag PM, Tunn PU (2007) Resection of soft tissue sarcoma of the lower limb after evaluation of vascular invasion with intraoperative intravascular ultrasonography. Br J Surg 94:168–173

Kawai A, Hashizume H, Inoue H, Uchida H, Sano S (1996) Vascular reconstruction in limb salvage operations for soft tissue tumors of the extremities. Clin Orthop Relat Res 332:215–222

Kooby DA, Antonescu CR, Brennan MF, Singer S (2004) Atypical lipomatous tumor/well-differentiated liposarcoma of the extremity and trunk wall: importance of histological subtype with treatment recommendations. Ann Surg Oncol 11:78–84

Koperna T, Teleky B, Vogl S, Windhager R, Kainberger F, Schatz KD, Kotz R, Polterauer P (1996) Vascular reconstruction for limb salvage in sarcoma of the lower extremity. Arch Surg 131:1103–1107

Kubo T, Sugita T, Shimose S, Arihiro K, Ochi M (2006) Conservative surgery for well-differentiated liposarcomas of the extremities adjacent to major neurovascular structures. Surg Oncol 15:167–171

Leggon RE, Huber TS, Scarborough MT (2001) Limb salvage surgery with vascular reconstruction. Clin Orthop Relat Res 387:207–216

Martin JD, Buckley AR, Graeb D, Walman B, Salvian A, Hay JH (2005) Carotid artery stenosis in asymptomatic patients who have received unilateral head-and-neck irradiation. Int J Radiat Oncol Biol Phys 63:1197–1205

Matsushita M, Kuzuya A, Mano N, Nishikimi N, Sakurai T, Nimura Y, Sugiura H (2001) Sequelae after limb-sparing surgery with major vascular resection for tumor of the lower extremity. J Vasc Surg 33:694–699

McKay A, Motamedi M, Temple W, Mack L, Moore R (2007) Vascular reconstruction with the superficial femoral vein following major oncologic resection. J Surg Oncol 96:151–159

Meyerson SL, Feldman T, Desai TR, Leef J, Schwartz LB, McKinsey JF (2002) Angiographic access site complications in the era of arterial closure devices. Vasc Endovascular Surg 36:137–144

Nishinari K, Wolosker N, Yazbek G, Zerati AE, Nishimoto IN (2006a) Venous reconstructions in lower limbs associated with resection of malignancies. J Vasc Surg 44:1046–1050

Nishinari K, Wolosker N, Yazbek G, Zerati AE, Nishimoto IN, Puech-Leão P (2006b) Arterial reconstructions associated with the resection of malignant tumors. Clinics 61:339–344

O'Sullivan B, Davis AM, Turcotte R, Bell R, Catton C, Chabot P, Wunder J, Kandel R, Goddard K, Sadura A, Pater J, Zee B (2002) Preoperative versus postoperative radiotherapy in soft-tissue sarcoma of the limbs: a randomised trial. Lancet 359:2235–2241

Phifer TJ, Gerlock AJ Jr, Vekovius WA, Rich NM, McDonald JC (1984) Amputation risk factors in concomitant superficial femoral artery and vein injuries. Ann Surg 199:241–243

Rich NM (1982) Principles and indications for primary venous repair. Surgery 91:492–496

Schwarzbach MH, Hormann Y, Hinz U, Bernd L, Willeke F, Mechtersheimer G, Böckler D, Schumacher H, Herfarth C, Büchler MW, Allenberg JR (2005) Results of limb-sparing surgery with vascular replacement for soft tissue sarcoma in the lower extremity. J Vasc Surg 42:88–97

Swerdlow AJ, Higgins CD, Smith P, Cunningham D, Hancock BW, Horwich A, Hoskin PJ, Lister A, Radford JA, Rohatiner AZ, Linch DC (2007) Myocardial infarction mortality risk after treatment for Hodgkin disease: a collaborative British cohort study. J Natl Cancer Inst 99:206–214

19 Current Concepts in the Management of Retroperitoneal Soft Tissue Sarcoma

Matthias H.M. Schwarzbach and Peter Hohenberger

Abstract Soft tissue sarcomas (STS) in the retroperitoneum are usually diagnosed at the late stages. Surgery is the mainstay of treatment. The technique of resection is standardized. After dissection of the retroperitoneal blood vessel, a retroperitoneal plane of dissection adjacent to the spinal foramina is established in between the layers of the abdominal wall. Complete resection with tumor-free resection margins is the primary goal in retroperitoneal sarcoma surgery. Preoperative assessment of pathoanatomical growth patterns with respect to retroperitoneal vascular structures—as well as to visceral and retroperitoneal organs—influences surgical strategies and thus the surgical outcome. Blood vessel replacement and a multivisceral en bloc approach improve the quality of resection. Blood vessel involvement is stratified in type I (arterial and venous involvement), type II (arterial involvement), type III (venous involvement), and type IV (no vascular involvement). Adjuvant and neoadjuvant treatment options (chemotherapy, targeted therapy, and radiation therapy) are currently being investigated. A prospective randomized phase III trial has shown a positive effect of neoadjuvant chemotherapy combined with regional hyperthermia in disease-free survival, response rate, and local control. Subsets of liposarcomas (myxoid and round cell type) are selectively responsive to novel drugs, such as trabectedin, a DNA-binding agent. Radiotherapy is applied in higher-grade locally advanced retroperitoneal STS. The optimal technique of delivering radiotherapy remains to be determined. The restricted number of patients with retroperitoneal STS and unsatisfying results in local tumor control and long-term survival indicate the need for multi-institutional cooperative studies. An international effort is required to improve the evidence level on multimodal treatment algorithms.

Matthias H.M. Schwarzbach (✉)
Department of Surgery
University Clinic of Mannheim
University of Heidelberg
Theodor Kutzer Ufer 1-3
68167 Mannheim, Germany
E.mail: Matthias.schwarzbach@chir.ma.uni-heidelberg.de

19.1 Introduction

Soft tissue sarcomas (STS) located in the retroperitoneum have been challenging surgeons and oncologists for decades. The retroperitoneum contains the aorta and the vena cava, which can be involved by retroperitoneal sarcomas (Arii et al. 2003; Babatasi et al. 1998; Chiche et al. 2003; Dong et al. 1998; Dzsinich et al. 1992; Hollenbeck et al. 2003; Ridwelski et al. 2001; Schwarzbach et al. 1997; Schwarzbach et al. 2006; Zheng et al. 1998). Besides blood vessels, retroperitoneal organs such as the kidneys, the spleen, and the pancreas are often affected by the expansive tumor growth (Ferrario and Karakousis 2003; Heslin et al. 1997; Lewis et al. 1998; Wente et al. 2007; Willeke et al. 1995). Although tumors emerge in the space behind the peritoneal cavity, expansion to abdominal organs is common. Here the bowel as well as the peritonealized organs are jeopardized (Schwarzbach et al. 2006; Wente et al. 2007). Retroperitoneal STS furthermore do sometimes expand to the thorax, lungs, and heart. The main reasons for extensive organ and blood vessel involvement in diverse anatomic compartments (retroperitoneum, abdomen, and thorax) are the expansive as well as infiltrative tumor growth (Schwarzbach et al. 2006; Wente et al. 2007). STS do not come to the attention of the patient until they are large (Weiss and Goldblum 2001). Small retroperitoneal STS are rarely seen and even extensive tumors may present with only minimal symptoms (Weiss and Goldblum 2001). Most retroperitoneal STS are liposarcomas, leiomyosarcomas, or malignant fibrous histiocytomas (Weiss and Goldblum 2001). The specimen can weigh several kilograms at the time of surgery. The macroscopic aspect of these large tumors is often heterogeneous. Local recurrence without distant metastasis is a common cause of sarcoma-related death in patients with retroperitoneal STS (Stojadinovic et al. 2002). Local control is therefore the most important treatment requirement. Surgery is the mainstay of treatment (Lewis and Benedetti 1997; Weiss and Goldblum 2001; Willeke et al. 1995). Radiotherapy, which is applied especially in higher-grade retroperitoneal STS, has the disadvantage of the toxicity to normal adjacent structures such as bowel or kidney (Brennan 2002). In contrast, effective adjuvant chemotherapy regimens remain to be identified.

19.2 Definitions Referring to Retroperitoneal Sarcomas

Primary tumor is defined as the initially diagnosed mass, including previously performed biopsy or incompletely resected lesions within 12 weeks after initial diagnosis. *Locally recurrent disease* is defined as the development of a mass of the same histological subtype following prior complete resection. The clinical setting in which tumors originate from the vessel wall is considered *primary blood vessel involvement* (Schwarzbach et al. 2005b, 2006). A tumor invading or embracing the blood vessel wall is referred to as *secondary vessel involvement* (Schwarzbach et al. 2005b, 2006). *Complete resection* is defined as the removal of all macroscopic disease, subdivided into complete resection with histologically negative margins and histologically positive margins. *Incomplete resection* (debulking) is defined as the removal of more than half of the tumor mass, otherwise surgery is considered to be *exploration/biopsy*. A resection is called *multivisceral* if one or more organs adherent to the tumor were resected.

19.3 Diagnostic Requirements in Retroperitoneal Sarcomas

Clinical evaluation of retroperitoneal STS include high-resolution computed tomography (CT) and/or magnetic resonance imaging (MRI). Organ and vascular involvement is characterized at best with the latter imaging modalities (Schwarzbach et al. 1997, 2005b, 2006; Weiss and Goldblum 2001). MRI and CT have largely replaced invasive arteriography and cavography. Ultrasound can be used for additional vascular evaluation (Doppler and duplex sonography). Besides radiological examinations, a preoperative histopathological diagnosis is important for oncological management. The need for histological specification has different justifications. STS need to be separated from malignant lymphomas or germ cell tumors. A false diagnosis can lead to an inadequate oncological approach. Furthermore, treatment of STS in the retroperitoneum is not only based on the pathoanatomical finding but on the histopathological type and tumor grade. Fine-needle aspiration (FNA) is relatively atraumatic and can be used to sample retroperitoneal masses under CT guidance (Weiss and Goldblum 2001). However, the use of FNA is limited because even experienced cytopathologists are often unable to discern the grade and type of an aspirate. Better results with respect to histopathological assessment are achieved by image-guided core-needle biopsy or open biopsy. The site of biopsy has to be chosen individualized according to the pathoanatomical situation and regional tumor viability. Trans-abdominal biopsy should be avoided and the canal of puncturing the lesion should be from the back or behind the colon. The area of tissue sampling should avoid necrosis and is best taken from viable tumor tissue. Surrogate markers for viable tumor tissue are (1) tissue perfusion, as detected on MRI or sonographic imaging, and (2) metabolic activity as presented on the positron emission tomography (PET) images. Semiquantitative PET imaging is especially good at supplying complementary metabolic information. The standardized uptake value (SUV) allows indirect assessment of the tumor grade in soft tissue sarcoma (Schwarzbach et al. 2000, 2005a). STS with a high SUV are more likely to be high-grade lesions than those with a low uptake. In this setting a high-grade STS has to be presumed. Nuclear medicine techniques are also used to assess the renal function. Patients with poor kidney function have to be critically assessed for the type of surgery to be performed (e.g., renal auto transplantation).

19.4
Vascular Involvement

Vascular involvement of retroperitoneal STS, as in extremity STS, is not uncommon (Schwarzbach et al. 2005b, 2006). Around 16% of the patients treated for retroperitoneal sarcoma by surgery present with blood vessel involvement (Schwarzbach et al. 2006). Primary vascular involvement is usually associated with leiomyosarcomas originating in the muscular wall of the blood vessels (Schwarzbach et al. 1997, 2006; Ockert et al. 2004). Malignant vascular tumors, which can also originate within blood vessels such as the angiosarcoma, are hardly ever seen in patients with primary retroperitoneal STS (Leowardi et al. 2005; Schwarzbach et al. 2006). Secondary vascular involvement is caused by diverse histopathological types (Hormann 2006; Schwarzbach et al. 2006). In our own analysis, two-thirds of the retroperitoneal STS with vascular involvement secondarily involve blood vessels and about one-third primarily originates in the blood vessel wall (consecutive series of surgical cases, Schwarzbach et al. 2006). The majority of patients with secondary vascular involvement are diagnosed with microscopic infiltration of the blood vessels (64.7%; Schwarzbach et al. 2006). The high rate of microscopic blood vessel infiltration clearly delineates that blood vessel resection is mandatory not only in patients with primary but also secondary blood vessel involvement. Vascular involvement by retroperitoneal STS has been systematized as follows (Hormann 2006; Schwarzbach et al. 2006; Fig. 19.1a, b). Lesions that involve major arterial and venous blood vessels in the

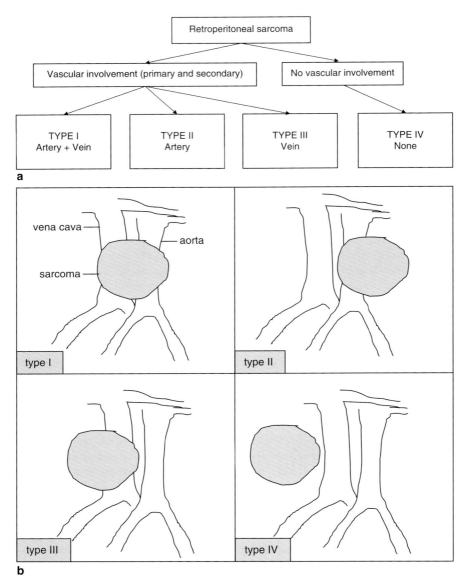

Fig. 19.1 a Classification of vascular involvement in patients with retroperitoneal soft tissue sarcoma (from Schwarzbach et al. 2006). **b** Schematic illustration of the different types of vascular involvement by retroperitoneal soft tissue sarcoma. The aorta and the vena cava are used as examples for arterial and venous blood vessel involvement in the retroperitoneum

retroperitoneum are defined as type I. STS with a tumor growth affecting the aorta or other major arterial blood vessels are defined as type II. Tumors that selectively involve venous blood vessels are defined as type III. In case STS show no vascular disease, type IV is diagnosed. Primary and secondary vascular involvement cannot be differentiated preoperatively and moreover

Table 19.1 Histopathological evaluation of surgical specimen in 25 patients concerning vascular and organ involvement of retroperitoneal soft tissue sarcoma (from Schwarzbach et al. 2006)

	Total (n=25)	Percentage (%)
Primary vascular involvement	8	32%
Vascular origin	8	32%
Artery (type II)	1	4%
Vein (type III)	7	28%
Secondary involvement	17	68%
Vascular infiltration	11	44%
Artery and vein (type I)	4	16%
Artery (type II)	1	4%
Vein (type III)	6	24%
Vascular encasement	6	24%
Artery and vein (type I)	0	0%
Artery (type II)	3	12%
Vein (type III)	3	12%

implies a similar surgical treatment algorithm (en bloc resection of the diseased blood vessels). Therefore both entities are classified together. Our own analysis has shown that type III is by far the most common type in the retroperitoneum (64% of the cases; type I, 16%; type II, 20%; see Tables 19.1 and 19.2). Besides the vena cava, the aorta is the most commonly involved retroperitoneal blood vessel (Tables 19.1 and 19.2; Arii et al. 2003; Babatasi et al. 1998; Chiche et al. 2003; Dong et al. 1998; Dzsinich et al. 1992; Hollenbeck et al. 2003; Ridwelski et al. 2001; Schwarzbach et al. 1997, 2006; Zheng et al. 1998).

19.5
Surgical Therapy in Localized Soft Tissue Sarcomas of the Retroperitoneum

The surgical approach to retroperitoneal STS usually requires a transperitoneal approach using a midline (Fig. 19.2a) or a transverse incision (Weiss and Goldblum 2001). Retroperitoneal approaches via the flank, as are often used for nephrectomy, do not allow adequate visualization and safe resection. The surgical technique in retroperitoneal STS has been outlined by Storm and Mahvi (1991). The initial maneuver is dependent on the tumor location and invasion of its surroundings. If the retroperitoneal compartment needs to be taken out, the dissection begins beyond the obliquus internus muscle and needs to reach the plane of dissection from the major retroperitoneal blood vessels (Fig. 19.2b). Subsequently, a retroperitoneal plane of dissection adjacent to the spinal foramina is established in between the layers of the abdominal wall musculature. Organs that lie in between the tumor and the resection plane have to be removed together with the specimen (Alvarenga et al. 1991; Ferrario and Karakousis 2003; Jaques et al. 1990; Karakousis et al. 1995). Kidney and the bowel invasion often require en bloc resection. Right or left sided colectomy, resection of the tail or the head of the pancreas, liver resection, or resection of the spleen are other common procedures of monobloc resection of retroperitoneal STS (Fig. 19.2c; Wente et al. 2007).

Table 19.2 Review of the literature. Clinicopathological data and results in patients undergoing surgery for retroperitoneal soft tissue sarcoma involving major blood vessels

Author		Cohort		Histopathological and clinical tumor characteristics					Vascular reconstruction (region/method)			Clinical results			
Reference	Years studied	No. of patients/ STS		Histology	Grade	Size (cm)	Primary/ recurrent tumor	Type	Graft location	Arterial repair	Venous repair	Morbidity/ mortality	Follow-up	Arterial/ venous patency	Local/ distant recurrence	Survival
Dzsinich et al. 1992	1957–1990	13/13		13 LMS	-[b]	-[b]	12/1	1 type I 12 type III	6 IVC 1 IV 1 IA	1	2 ePTFE BP 1 Dacron patch 1 venous BP 3 suture	2/13 (15%)/ 1/13 (7.5%)	-[b]	-[b] 5/7 (71%)	2/13 (15%)/ 5/13 (38%)	5/13 (38%)[c]
Dong et al. 1998	1990–1997	11/9		5 LMS 1 FS 1 MS 1 MP 1 MM 1 seminoma 1 CA		12–30		11 type III	9 IVC 1 IVC+RV 1 RV	0	Suture[a] Anastomosis[a] Ligation[a]	3/11 (27%)/ 0/11 (0%)	6	All repairs patent	-[b]	11/11 (100%)[c]
Babatasi et al. 1998	-[b]	3/3		3 LMS	3 h.g.		3/0	1 type II 1 type III 1 atrial	1 IVC 1 PA	1 synthetic BP	1 venous BP 1 HT	0/3 (0%)/ 0/3 (0%)		1/1 (100%)/ 1/1 (100%)	1/3 (33%)/ 1/3 (33%)	1/3 (33%)[c]
Zheng et al. 1998	-[b]	25/13		6 LMS 4 LS 1 NFS 2 FS 1 teratoma 11 benign	-[b]	-[b]	-[b]	-[b]	12 IA 8 IV 6 IVC 3 AO 7 others	7 suture 6 ven./syn.BP 3 anastomosis 1 ligation	8 suture 5 vein/synth.BP 5 anastomosis 4 ligation	0/25 (0%)/ 0/25 (0%)		16/16 (100%)/ 18/18 (100%)		25/25 (100%)[c]
Ridwelski et al. 2001	1993–1999	5/5		5 LMS	2 lg. 2 ig. 1 -[b]	5–7	5/0	5 type III	4 IVC 1 inoperable	-[b]	3 ePTFE patch -[b]	0/5 (0%)/ 0/5 (0%)	-[b]	3/3 (100%)	0/5 (0%)/ 2/5 (40%)	3/5 (60%)[c]
Arii et al. 2003	1990–2001	11/1		1 LMS 3 HCC 4 CC 3 metastasis	-[b]	3–15	8/3	11 type III	11 hep. IVC	0	11 ePTFE	1/11 (9%)/ 0/11 (0%)	-[b]	11/11 (100%)	6/11 (55%)/ 2/11 (18%)	25.5%[d]

Hollenbeck et al. 2003	1982–2002	25/25	25 LMS	25 h.g.	12	25/0	21 type III	21 IVC	11 ligation 7 suture 2 ePTFE BP 1 venous patch	4/25 (16%)/ 2/25 (8%)	24	—[b] —[b]	7/25 (33%)/ 10/25 (48%)	33%[d] 33%[d]
Chiche et al. 2003	1990–2000	5/5	1 LMS 1 MHE 2 intimal 1 —[b]	5 type II		5/0	5 type II	5 AO 2 AO/SMA	6 synthetic BP 1 venous BP	2/5 (40%)/ 1/5 (20%)	—[b]	6/7 (86%)/ —[b]	0/5 (0%)/ 1/5 (20%)	8%[d]
Schwarzbach et al. 2006	1988–2004	25/25	12 LMS 4 LS 2 MFH 2 CCS 5 STS 5 STS 5 STS	2 l.g. 5 i.g. 17 h.g. 1 —[b]	10.5	18/7	4 type I 5 type II 16 type III	11 IVC 3 IV 2 SMV 6 AO 3 IA 3 IA 3 IA	6 Dacron BP 2 ePTFE BP 1 reinsertion 7 ePTFE BP 3 ePTFE patch 1 venous patch 2 Dacron BP 2 venoplasty 1 anastomosis 2 ligation	9/25 (36%)/ 1/25 (4%)	—[b]	8/9 (89%)	3/19 —[b]	37.7[d]

AO, aorta; BP, bypass; CA, carcinoma; CCS, clear cell sarcoma; DR, distant recurrence; ES, Ewing's sarcoma; FS, fibrous sarcoma; h.g., high grade; hep., hepatic; HT, heart transplantation; IA, iliac artery; i.g., intermediate grade; IV, iliac vein; IVC, inferior vena cava; l.g., low grade; LMS, leiomyosarcoma; LR, local recurrence; LS, liposarcoma; MFH, malignant fibrous histiocytoma; MHE, malignant hemangioendothelioma; MP, malignant paraganglioma; MS, malignant schwannoma; NFS, neurofibrosarcoma; PA, pulmonary artery; PT, primary tumor; RV, renal vein; SMA, superior mesenteric artery; SMV, superior mesenteric vein; STS, soft tissue sarcoma

[a]Numbers not reported

[b]Not specified

[c]Absolute number of survivors

[d]5-year survival rate

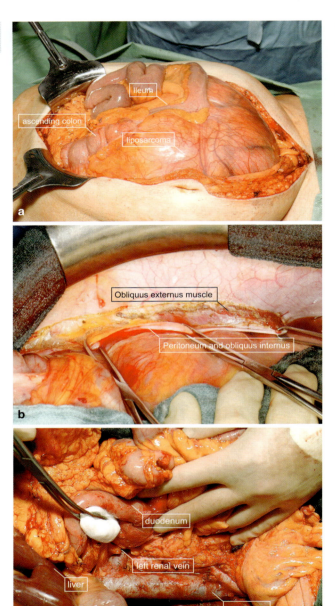

Fig. 19.2 a Intraoperative finding of a retroperitoneal liposarcoma after midline incision for abdominal exposure. The liposarcoma involves the ascending colon and the ileum. **b** lateral dissection plane; **c** Intraoperative finding after en bloc multivisceral resection (liposarcoma with ascending colon, ileum, kidney, and abdominal wall). Specimen; **d** cut specimen

The removal of adjacent or attached organs increases the chance for complete resection and thus the chance for survival. Dissecting between the tumor and the adjacent organs is technically feasible and can appear adequate during surgery. However, on microscopic analysis tumor invasion by infiltrative growth can be detected by the pathologist. Residual microscopic disease in

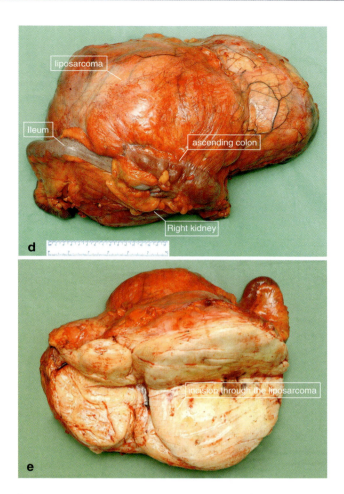

Fig. 19.2 (continued)

the dissected organs (e.g., the mesentery of the small bowel) might cause recurrence in the future. Therefore, whenever complete resection requires organ removal or organ resection surgeons should not be reluctant to do so, but rather prefer a multivisceral approach. In case surgery is carried out on type I, II or III STS blood vessel resection is inevitable (Table 19.2). We have suggested a resection algorithm for these retroperitoneal sarcomas (Fig. 19.3; Schwarzbach et al. 2006). With an adequate safety margin the aorta or iliac vessels should be replaced in type I and II STS. Arterial prosthesis such as the straight 16-mm Dacron graft is used for aortic replacement (for an example of a type II STS involving the aorta, see Fig. 19.4a, b).

In case of a type I and III STS, the vena cava or iliac vessels are resected. Replacement of venous blood vessels is currently performed whenever possible. On the level of the renal veins

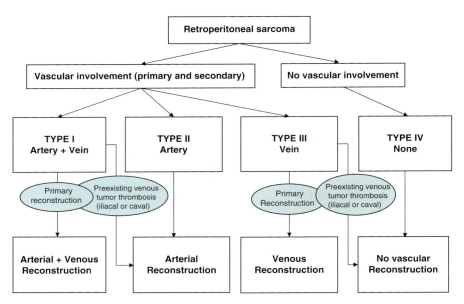

Fig. 19.3 Surgical algorithm according to the type of vascular reconstruction in patients with retroperitoneal soft tissue sarcoma. (Schwarzbach et al. 2006)

and above (retrohepatic) caval reconstruction is mandatory in most cases (Vollmar et al. 1973). An expanded polytetrafluoroethylene (ePTFE) prosthesis with ring enforcement can be implanted for repair (Schwarzbach et al. 2006). Below the renal veins, ligation of the vena cava or the iliac veins has been described below as a treatment option. (Vollmar et al. 1973). Ligation of the vena cava, the iliac veins, or the left renal vein is usually feasible without life-threatening consequences. However, lower limb edema, unpleasant venous congestion after surgery, and the squeal of chronic limb edema can be avoided by reconstruction even if thrombosis develops secondarily. More important intraoperatively bleeding from collateral vessels can be avoided. With aggressive surgical approaches and a willingness to resect adjacent organs, most retroperitoneal STS are nowadays amenable to complete resection. There are patients who develop a retroperitoneal STS that is adjacent to major retroperitoneal blood vessels but do not present with a blood vessel involvement (type IV STS adjacent to major blood vessels; Fig. 19.5). In these cases the surgical technique of choice is a subadventitial dissection of the vessel wall (Schwarzbach et al. 2006; Hormann 2006). A longitudinal incision of the blood vessel adventitia is carried out opposite to the STS. Then the dissected adventitia is left at the en bloc specimen.

Dissatisfying results with respect to resectability (30%–49%) were reported in the past (Alvarenga et al. 1991; Cody et al. 1981; McGrath et al. 1984; Pinson et al. 1989). Our review of the series published in the last decade present improved resectability rates ranging from 64% to 95% (Table 19.3). Ferrario and Karakousis reported excellent resectability rates in primary as well as recurrent retroperitoneal STS (Ferrario and Karakousis 2003). This analysis clearly indicates that both types of retroperitoneal STS can be resected completely in the majority of the patients. In case a complete resection is impossible the value of surgery is still unclear (Cody et al.

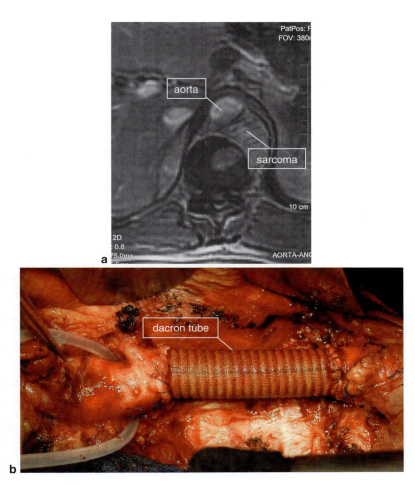

Fig. 19.4 a Magnetic tomography of a sarcoma involving the retroperitoneal aorta. **b** Reconstruction of the aorta with a straight 16-mm Dacron prosthesis. (Hormann 2006)

1981; Pinson et al. 1989; Stoeckle et al. 2001). Some authors report that incomplete resection of retroperitoneal STS is not associated with improved long-term survival rates compared to biopsy and subsequent nonsurgical treatment (Jaques et al. 1990; Kilkenny et al. 1996; Lewis et al. 1998). On the other hand Shibata et al. showed that debulking surgery in retroperitoneal liposarcoma prolongs survival (Shibata et al. 2001). The authors found a survival benefit in patients after incomplete resection with a median survival of 26 months compared to exploration alone with a median survival of 4 months. Besides that benefit, debulking surgery led to a palliation of symptoms, which was achieved in 75% of patients (Shibata et al. 2001). A metaanalysis on incomplete resection of retroperitoneal STS also revealed an improved survival time after debulking (Storm and Mahvi 1991). Tumor reductive surgery is therefore an option that should be discussed with the patient within multimodality treatment approaches.

Fig. 19.5 a, b MR-imaging of a malignant peripheral nerve sheath tumor (MPNST) in the retroperitoneum adjacent to the iliac blood vessels (type IV). **c** Intraoperative finding of the MPNST and dissection of the iliac blood vessels (subadventitial dissection) and the ureter. **d** Intraoperative finding after en-bloc resection. **e** Cut specimen with abdominal musculature and osseous structures (safety margin). **f** The MPNST is completely covered by the dissected muscle and bone

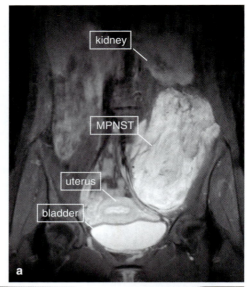

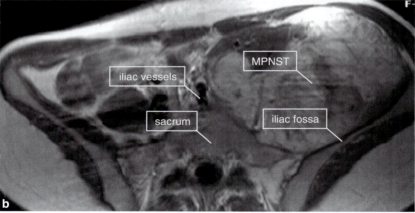

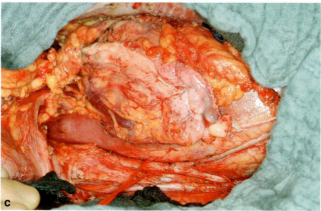

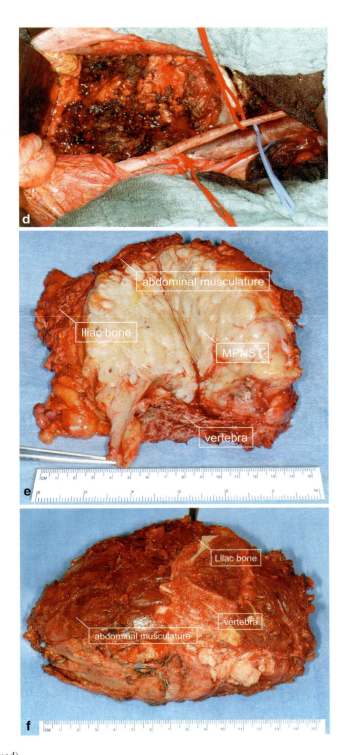

Fig. 19.5 (continued)

Table 19.3 Overview of the literature with respect to the recent series reporting 5-year and 10-year survival rates after complete resection of retroperitoneal soft tissue sarcoma

Reference	No. of patients	Complete resection	5-year overall survival	10-year overall survival
Lewis et al. 1998	231	80%	54%	35%
Stoeckle et al. 2001	145[a]	65%	49%	ND
Ferrario and Karakousis 2003	130	95%	60%	48%
Gronchi et al. 2004	167	88%	54%	27%
Hassan et al. 2004	99	78%	51%	36%
Erzen et al. 2005	102	95%	52%	36%
Pierie et al. 2006	103	64%	62%	52%
Chen et al. 2007	132	74%	ND	ND

ND, not determined
[a]National survey

19.6 Surgical Therapy in Metastasized Soft Tissue Sarcomas of the Retroperitoneum

The lungs are the most common site of distal recurrence in high-grade STS (Potter et al. 1985). In retroperitoneal STS the local recurrence is seen more often than distant recurrence (Stojadinovic et al. 2002). Concerning the time of recurrence, almost 80% of all recurrences after STS resection, including distant sites, become evident within 5 years after primary treatment. As is the case for patients with isolated local or regional recurrence, surgical treatment of pulmonary metastasis should be attempted when feasible (Weiss and Goldblum 2001). In patients with retroperitoneal STS with pulmonary lesions on plain radiography, CT imaging of the chest and either MR or CT imaging of the abdomen is necessary to rule out local recurrence and concomitant hepatic disease. Patients with extrapulmonary disease are not candidates for curative pulmonary metastasectomy, while patients eligible for pulmonary curative metastasectomy without any further site of recurrence undergo surgery. The 3-year disease-free survival rate after resection of isolated pulmonary metastasis was reported in a small series of 56 patients as 38% (Potter et al. 1985). Factors predicting outcome in patients with resectable pulmonary metastasis are a small number of metastases (fewer than three or four) on preoperative CT imaging, a long disease-free period from the primary treatment, and a long tumor doubling time (>40 days) (Putnam and Roth 1993). These factors were correlated at univariate analysis with longer postoperative survival. However, it should be noted that no single criterion must exclude any patient from resection, as even patients with several unfavorable factors are long-term survivors occasionally (Weiss and Goldblum 2001). The 5-year survival ranges from 10% to 35% after resection of pulmonary STS metastasis. Unlike osteosarcoma, it is unclear whether neoadjuvant chemotherapy is of benefit to the patients with resectable pulmonary disease (Skinner et al. 1992; Weiss and Goldblum 2001). Patients who achieve a partial response to chemotherapy but are left with one or several potentially resectable metastases should be considered for surgical resection. Conversion to a chemotherapy-induced partial response to a complete response by surgical resection of pulmonary metastasis can enhance the duration of response and is associated with a survival time equivalent to that obtained with complete response to chemotherapy alone (Weiss and Goldblum 2001). The occasional patient with one or several metastases not amenable to surgery can be treated effectively with local irradiation to consolidate the response to chemotherapy.

19.7
Prognosis

In completely resected retroperitoneal sarcomas, Ferrario and Karakousis found a 5-year survival of 65% for patients with primary tumors and of 53% for patients referred with local recurrence (Ferrario and Karakousis 2003). Local control is higher for patients who underwent surgery for primary STS compared to those who were treated for local recurrence (Ferrario and Karakousis 2003). Local recurrence rates in general are high and believed to be a major cause of death in patients with retroperitoneal STS (Alvarenga et al. 1991; Hassan et al. 2004; Karakousis et al. 1995; Kilkenny et al. 1996; Lewis et al. 1998; Stoeckle et al. 2000; van Dahlen et al. 2001; Jones et al. 2002; Ferrario et al. 2003). The probability for local relapse increases with the size of the sarcomas (5-year local recurrence rate: 19.2% in tumors <10 cm and 47.8% in tumors >20 cm; Gronchi et al. 2004). Besides that histologic margin, tumor grade, and histologic type are under discussion as other factors predicting local failure. After complete tumor resection, the major determinant of overall survival is the histologic grade of the tumor. After 10 years about 42% of the patients with completely resected tumors are alive (Weiss and Goldblum 2001). The corresponding 10-year survival rate for high-grade sarcomas is 11% (Weiss and Goldblum 2001). In Table 19.3, the overall survival rates after complete resection (tumor control and survival) of recent surgical series (over the past decade) are presented.

19.8
Chemotherapy and Radiation Therapy

The role of adjuvant and neoadjuvant chemotherapy in the treatment of retroperitoneal STS remains to be defined. Divergent results indicate that chemotherapy in the neoadjuvant and adjuvant setting should not be offered to patients except in clinical studies. At present different prospective trials are being undertaken. At the American Society of Clinical Oncology (ASCO) meeting 2007 Issels et al. presented the results of a prospective multicenter trial [European Organisation for Research and Treatment of Cancer (EORTC) 62961 phase III trial] on neoadjuvant chemotherapy combined with regional hyperthermia in high-grade STS (Issels et al. 2007). Non-extremity STS were included. Primary endpoints were local progression-free survival and disease-free survival. The objective response rate was a secondary endpoint. In this first phase III trial, chemotherapy (etoposide, ifosfamide, and adriamycin) with regional hyperthermia presented with improved disease-free survival, local progression-free survival, and objective response rate compared to chemotherapy alone. In histological subgroups of STS, innovative therapies might play an important role in the future. Myxoid and round cell liposarcoma (MRCLS) are associated with a specific chromosomal translocation resulting in an FUS/CHOP fusion protein in most of the cases (Aman et al. 1992; Crozat et al. 1993; Schwarzbach et al. 2004; Willeke et al. 1998). In these liposarcomas a new agent, trabectedin (ecteinascidin 743; ET-741; Yondelis, PharmaMar, USA), is selectively efficient in devitalization of tumor tissue (change of tissue density and shrinkage) (Grosso et al. 2007). Trabectedin is a novel DNA-binding agent, originally derived from a murine tunicate and now produced synthetically (Schöffski et al. 2007; Trabectedin 2006). Positive results have been observed in a compassionate-use program of five Italian institutions (Grosso et al. 2007). In the Italian study an overall response rate of 51% in advanced myxoid liposarcoma was observed for trabectedin as a second-line treatment. Therefore, prospective studies have been suggested to investigate trabectedin in the neoadjuvant setting in MRCLS (currently under evaluation). In adult patients without a curative surgical option, chemotherapy represents the best currently available palliative treatment. Objective tumor regression and relief of symptoms can be achieved in a significant number of patients (Weiss and Goldblum 2001). The most effective cytotoxic agents used are doxorubicin and ifosfamide besides others (methotrexate, vincristine, cisplatin, dactinomycin, and dacarbazine). In locally advanced nonoperable or metastasized STS, the EORTC 62012 trial offers treatment in a randomized phase III trial. The study is accessible for retroperitoneal STS. Among malignant fibrous histiocytoma (MFH), liposarcoma, and pleomorphic rhabdomyosarcoma, other histologic subtypes can be included. The important inclusion criteria are no radiotherapy for the index lesion and no prior chemotherapy in the advanced settings. Randomization is made for receiving Adriamycin (doxorubicin) or doxorubicin and ifosfamide. One study (EORTC trial 62061) offers a randomization of advanced or metastatic STS (including the retroperitoneum) to either brostallicin (PNU-166196A) versus doxorubicin as a first-line chemotherapy.

Most of the studies comparing patients who received radiotherapy for retroperitoneal STS with those who did not clearly delineate the indicatory preselection: patients with higher-grade tumors (intermediate-grade and high-grade lesions) and marginal resection received adjuvant treatment, while those with low-grade tumors and clear margin did not. This preselection reflects the multimodal treatment algorithm that is currently adopted in most of the oncological institutions in the treatment of retroperitoneal STS throughout Europe and North America (Weiss and Goldblum 2001). A prospective randomized clinical trial of intraoperative radiotherapy has shown an improvement toward local tumor control in retroperitoneal sarcoma (Sindelar et al. 1993). Other recent studies combining preoperative radiotherapy with brachytherapy reported promising results during short-term follow-up (Jones et al. 2002). However, despite aggressive surgical resection, local disease progression was a significant component determining a patient's prognosis and did not seem to improve (Ballo et al. 2007). Single institution series report on major problems of toxicity handling and R0 resection rates around 50% only (Caudle et al. 2007). The major problem is the lack of a well-defined study of adequate patient numbers, and transatlantic cooperation might be required to answer these questions (Pisters 2007).

Some retrospective studies have not supported the use of adjuvant radiation therapy in retroperitoneal sarcoma (Heslin et al. 1997; Kinsella et al. 1988; Mäkela et al. 2000). The ideal method of delivering radiotherapy either as neoadjuvant alone, neoadjuvant combined with intraoperative radiotherapy, or postoperatively remains to be determined (Willeke et al. 1995). Attention has turned to preoperative multimodality approaches. Radiosensitizers have been successfully administered along with external beam radiotherapy prior to resection. Preoperative therapy is advantageous because the patient is able to withstand the treatment effects, potentially minimizing the effect on normal healthy structures and allowing initially unresectable tumors to be completely excised (Weiss and Goldblum 2001). Tumor shrinkage and devitalization are believed to improve resectability and local tumor control. Due to the lack of prospective multi-institutional trials and the overall rareness retroperitoneal STS, the ideal treatment algorithm concerning radiotherapy has to be established.

Summary

Multivisceral en bloc resection with or without blood vessel replacement is the primary treatment of localized retroperitoneal STS. The standardization of the surgical strategy and a classification of vascular involvement improve the surgical approach and thus the quality of resection. Localized primary as well as locally recurrent retroperitoneal STS are resectable nowadays in the majority of the cases. In retroperitoneal liposarcoma debulking surgery can be beneficial to the patient, and patients with solitary pulmonary metastasis have to be evaluated for curative resection. Radiotherapy is used in higher-grade tumors and in case of marginal resections. The optimal way of delivering radiation therapy has not been identified yet. Chemotherapy combined with regional hyperthermia is a promising modality in the neoadjuvant setting within multimodal therapy concepts. Novel molecular inhibitors such as trabectedin show promising results in specific histological subgroups (myxoid and round cell liposarcoma). Due to the rarity of the disease, internationally based clinical trials are required.

References

Alvarenga JC, Ball AB, Fisher C, Fryatt I, Jones L, Thomas JM (1991) Limitations of surgery in the treatment of retroperitoneal sarcoma. Br J Surg 78:912–916

Aman P, Ron D, Mandahl N, Fioretos T, Heim S, Arheden K, Willen H, Rydholm A, Mitelman F (1992) Rearrangement of the transcription factor gene CHOP in myxoid liposarcomas with t(12;16)(q13;p11). Genes Chromosomes Cancer 5:278–285

Arii S, Teramoto K, Kawamura T, Takamatsu S, Sato E, Nakamura N, Iwai T, Mori A, Tanaka J, Imamura M (2003) Significance of hepatic resection combined with inferior vena cava resection and its reconstruction with expanded polytetrafluoroethylene for treatment of liver tumors. J Am Coll Surg 196:243–249

Babatasi G, Massetti M, Agostini D, Gallateau F, Le Page O, Saloux E, Bhoyroo S, Grollier G, Potier JC, Khayat A (1998) Leiomyosarcoma of the heart and great vessels. Ann Cardiol Angiol 47:451–458

Ballo MT, Zagars GK, Pollock RE, Benjamin RS, Feig BW, Cormier JN, Hunt KK, Patel SR, Trent JC, Beddar S, Pisters PW (2007) Retroperitoneal soft tissue sarcoma: an analysis of radiation and surgical treatment. Int J Radiat Oncol Biol Phys 67:158–163

Brennan MF (2002) Editorial. Retroperitoneal sarcoma: time for a national trial. Ann Surg Oncol 9:324–325

Caudle AS, Tepper JE, Calvo BF, Meyers MO, Goyal LK, Cance WG, Kim HJ (2007) Complications associated with neoadjuvant radiotherapy in the multidisciplinary treatment of retroperitoneal sarcomas. Ann Surg Oncol 14:577–582

Chen C, Yin L, Peng CH, Cai Y, Li Y, Zhao R, Zhou H, Li H (2007) Prognostic factors of retroperitoneal sarcomas: analysis of 132 cases. Chin Med J 120:1047–1050

Chiche L, Mongredien B, Brocheriou I, Kieffer E (2003) Primary tumors of the thoracoabdominal aorta: surgical treatment of 5 patients and review of the literature. Ann Vasc Surg 17:354–364

Cody HS, Turnbull AD, Fortner JG, Hajdu SI (1981) The continuing challenge of retroperitoneal sarcomas. Cancer 47:2147–2152

Crozat A, Aman P, Mandahl N, Ron D (1993) Fusion of CHOP to a novel RNA-binding protein in human myxoid liposarcoma. Nature 363:640–644

Dong M, Liang F, Song S (1998) Resection and reconstruction of inferior vena cava and renal vein in surgical treatment of retroperitoneal tumors: a report of 11 cases. Zhonghua Wai Ke Za Zhi 36:23–25

Dzsinich C, Gloviczki P, van Heerden JA (1992) Primary venous leiomyosarcoma: a rare but lethal disease. J Vasc Surg 15:592–603

Erzen D, Sencar M, Novak J (2005) Retroperitoneal sarcoma: 25 years of experience with aggressive surgical treatment at the institute of Oncology, Ljubljana. J surg Oncol 91:1–9

Ferrario T, Karakousis CP (2003) Retroperitoneal sarcomas. Grade and survival. Arch Surg 138:248–251

Gronchi A, Casali PG, Fiore M, Mariani L, Lo Vullo S, Bertulli R, Colecchia M, Lozza L, Olmi P, Santinami M, Rosai J (2004) Retroperitoneal soft tissue sarcomas. Patterns of recurrence in

167 patients treated at a ingle institution. Cancer 100:2448–2455

Grosso F, Jones RL, Demetri GD, Judson IR, Blay JY, Le Cesne A, Sanfilippo R, Casieri P, Collini P, Dileo P, Spreafico C, Stacchiotti S, Tamborini E, Tercero JC, Jimeno J, Dincalci M, Gronchi A, Fletcher JA, Pilotti S, Casali PG (2007) Efficacy of trabectedin (ecteinascidin-743) in advanced pretreated myxoid liposarcomas: a retrospective study. Lancet Oncol 8:595–602

Hassan I, Park SZ, Donohue JH, Nagorney DM, Kai PA, Nasciemento AG, Schleck CD, Ilstrup DM (2004) Operative management of primary retroperitoneal sarcomas: a reappraisal of an institutional experience. Ann Surg 239:244–250

Heslin MJ, Lewis J, Nadler E, Newman E, Woodruff JM, Casper ES, Leung D, Brennan MF (1997) Prognostic factors associated with long-term survival for retroperitoneal sarcoma: implications for management. J Clin Oncol 15:2832–2839

Hollenbeck ST, Grobmyer SR, Kent KC, Brennan MF (2003) Surgical treatment and outcomes of patients with primary inferior vena cava leiomyosarcoma. J Am Coll Surg 197:575–579

Hormann Y (2006) Gefäßbeteiligung durch Weichteilsarkome. Inauguraldissertation der Medizinischen Fakultät Heidelberg der Ruprecht-Karls-Universität

Issels RD, Linder HL, Wust P, Hohenberger P, Jauch K, Daugaard S, Mansman U, Hiddemann W, Blay J, Verweij J (2007) Regional hyperthermia (RHT) improves response and survival when combined with systemic chemotherapy in the management of locally advanced, high grade soft tissue sarcomas (STS) of the extremities, the body wall and the abdomen: a phase III randomised prospective trial. J Clin Oncol, 2007 ASCO Annual Meeting Proceedings 25[June 20 Suppl]:10009

Jaques DP, Coit DG, Hajdu SI, Brennan MF (1990) Management of primary and recurrent soft tissue sarcoma of the retroperitoneum. Ann Surg 212:51–59

Jones JJ, Catton CN, O'Sullivan B, Couture J, Heisler RL, Kandel RA, Swallow CJ (2002) Initial results of a trial of preoperative external-beam radiation therapy and postoperative brachytherapy for retroperitoneal sarcoma. Ann Surg Oncol 9:346–354

Karakousis CP, Kontzoglou K, Driscoll DL (1995) Resectability of retroperitoneal sarcomas: a matter of surgical technique? Eur J Surg Oncol 21:617–622

Kilkenny JW, Bland KI, Copeland EM (1996) Retroperitoneal sarcoma: the University of Florida experience. J Am Coll Surg 182:329–332

Kinsella TJ, Sindelar WF, Lack E, Glatstein E, Rosenberg SA (1988) Preliminary results of a randomized study of adjuvant radiation therapy in resectable adult retroperitoneal soft tissue sarcomas. J Clin Oncol 6:18–25

Leowardi C, Hinz U, Hormann Y, Wente MN, Mechtersheimer G, Willeke F, Böckler D, Friess H, Allenberg JR, Herfarth C, Büchler MW, Schwarzbach MH (2005) Malignant vascular tumors: clinical presentation, surgical therapy, and long term prognosis. Ann Surg Oncol 12:1090–1101

Lewis JJ, Benedetti F (1997) Adjuvant therapy for soft tissue sarcomas. Surg Oncol Clin N Am 6:847–862

Lewis JJ, Leung D, Woodruff JM, Brennan MF (1998) Retroperitoneal soft-tissue sarcoma. Analysis of 500 patients treated and followed at a single institution. Ann Surg 228:355–365

Mäkela J, Kiviniemi H, Laitinen S (2000) Prognostic factors predicting survival in the treatment of retroperitoneal sarcoma. Eur J Surg Oncol 26:552–555

McGrath PC, Neifeld JP, Lawrence W Jr, DeMay RM, Kay S, Horsley JS 3rd, Parker GA (1984) Improved survival in following complete excision of retroperitoneal sarcomas. Ann Surg 200:200–204

Ockert S, Schumacher H, Boeckler D, Schwarzbach MH, Rotert H, Allenberg JR (2004) Intraluminal mass lesions of the thoracic aorta. Chirurg 11:41–48

Pierie JP, Betensky RA, Choudry U, Willett CG, Souba WW, Ott MJ (2006) Outcomes in a series of 103 retroperitoneal sarcomas. Eur J Surg Oncol 32:1235–1241

Pinson CW, ReMine SG, Fletcher WS, Braasch JW (1989) Long-term results with primary retroperitoneal tumors. Arch Surg 124:1168–1173

Pisters PW (2007) Retroperitoneal sarcomas—an SOS to colleagues in Europe. Ann Surg Oncol 14:1787–1789

Potter DA, Glenn J, Kinsella T, Glatstein E, Lack EE, Restrepo C, White DE, Seipp CA, Wesley R, Rosenberg SA (1985) Patterns of recurrence in patients with high grade soft-tissue sarcoma. J Clin Oncol 3:353–366

Putnam JB Jr, Roth JA (1993) Resection of sarcomatous pulmonary metastases. Surg Oncol Clin N Am 2:673

Ridwelski K, Rudolph S, Meyer F, Buhtz P, Burger T, Lippert H (2001) Primary sarcoma of the inferior vena cava: review of diagnosis, treatment, and outcomes in a case series. Int Surg 86:184–190

Schöffski P, Wolter P, Clement P, Sciot R, De Wever I, Wozniak A, Stefan C, Dumez H (2007) Trabectedin (ET-743): evaluation of its use in advanced soft-tissue sarcoma. Future Oncol 3:381–392

Schwarzbach MH, Willeke F, Hoffmann V, Mechtersheimer G, Otto G (1997) Leiomyosarcoma of the inferior vena cava. Dtsch Med Wochenschr 439–444

Schwarzbach MH, Dimitrakopoulou-Strauss A, Willeke F, Cardona S, Mechtersheimer G, Lehnert T, Strauss LG, Herfarth C, Büchler MW (2000) Clinical value of [18-F] fluorodeoxyglucose positron emission tomography imaging in soft tissue sarcomas. Ann Surg 231:380–386

Schwarzbach MH, Koesters R, Germann A, Mechtersheimer G, Geisbill J, Winkler S, Niedergethmann M, Ridder R, Buechler MW, von Knebel Doeberitz M, Willeke F (2004) Comparable transforming capacities and differential gene expression patterns of variant FUS/CHOP fusion transcripts derived from soft tissue liposarcomas. Oncogene 23:6798–6805

Schwarzbach MH, Hinz U, Dimitrakopoulou-Strauss A, Willeke F, Cardona S, Mechtersheimer G, Lehnert T, Strauss LG, Herfarth C, Büchler MW (2005a) Prognostic significance of preoperative [18-F] fluorodeoxyglucose (FDG) positron emission tomography (PET) imaging in patients with resectable soft tissue sarcomas. Ann Surg 241:286–294

Schwarzbach MH, Hormann Y, Hinz U, Bernd L, Willeke F, Mechtersheimer G, Böckler D, Schumacher H, Herfarth C, Büchler M, Allenberg JR (2005b) Results of limb-sparing surgery with vascular replacement for soft tissue sarcoma in the lower extremity. J Vasc Surg 42:88–96

Schwarzbach MH, Hormann Y, Hinz U, Leowardi C, Böckler D, Mechtersheimer G, Böckler D, Friess H, Büchler M, Allenberg JR (2006) Clinical results of surgery for retroperitoneal sarcoma with major blood vessel involvement. J Vasc Surg 44:46–55

Shibata D, Lewis JJ, Leung DH, Brennan MF (2001) Is there a role for incomplete resection in the management of retroperitoneal liposarcomas? J Am Coll Surg 193:373–379

Sindelar W, Kinsella T, Chen P, DeLaney TF, Tepper JE, Rosenberg SA, Glatstein E (1993) Intraoperative radiotherapy in retroperitoneal sarcomas. Final results of a prospective, randomized, clinical trial. Arch Surg 128:402–410

Skinner KA, Eilber FR, Holmes EC, Eckardt J, Rosen G (1992) Surgical treatment and chemotherapy for pulmonary metastasis from osteosarcoma. Arch Surg 127:1065–1070

Stoeckle E, Coindre JM, Bonvalot S, Kantor G, Terrier P, Bonichon F, Nguyen Bui B (2001) Prognostic factors in retroperitoneal sarcoma. A multivariate analysis of a series of 165 patients of the French Cancer Center federation Sarcoma group. Cancer 92:359–368

Stojadinovic A, Yeh A, Brennan MF (2002) Completely resected recurrent soft tissue sarcoma: primary anatomic site governs outcome. J Am Coll Surg 194:436–447

Storm FK, Mahvi DM (1991) Diagnosis and management of retroperitoneal soft tissue sarcoma. Ann Surg 214:2–10

Trabectedin (2006) Ecteinascidin 743, Ecteinascidin-743, ET 743, ET-743, NSC 684766. Drugs R D 7:317–328

van Dalen T, Hoekstra HJ, van Geel AN, van Coevorden F, Albus-Lutter C, Slootweg PJ, Hennipman A; Dutch Soft Tissue Sarcoma Group (2001) Locoregional recurrence of retroperitoneal soft tissue sarcoma: second chance of cure for selected patients. Eur J Surg Oncol 27:564–568

Vollmar J, Loeprecht H, Nadjafi AS (1973) Acute interruption of the inferior vena cava: ligature or reconstruction. Münch Med Wschr 21:978–985

Weiss SW, Goldblum JR (2001) Sarcomas in the retroperitoneum In: Weisss SW (ed) Enzinger and Weiss's soft tissue tumors, 4th edn. Mosby, St. Louis, pp 37–44

Wente M, Schwarzbach MH, Hinz U, Leowardi C, Mechtersheimer G, Krempien R, Egerer G, Friess H, Büchler M (2007) Perioperative outcome in sarcoma surgery. Langenbecks Arch Surg 392:83–93

Willeke F, Eble MJ, Lehnert T, Schwarzbach MH, Hinz U, Wannenmacher M, Herfarth C (1995) Intraoperative radiotherapy within the treatment of retroperitoneal soft tissue sarcoma. Chirurg 66:899–904

Willeke F, Ridder R, Mechtersheimer G, Schwarzbach MH, Duwe A, Weitz J, Lehnert T, Herfarth C, von Knebel Doeberitz M (1998) Analysis of FUS-CHOP fusion transcripts in different types of soft tissue liposarcoma and their diagnostic implications. Clin Cancer Res 4:1779–1784

Zheng W, Song S, Liang F (1998) Major blood vessel excision and reconstruction in the treatment of retroperitoneal neoplasms. Zhonghua Zhong Liu Za Zhi 20:225–227

20 Pulmonary Metastasectomy for Soft Tissue Sarcomas: Is It Justified?

Joachim Pfannschmidt, Hans Hoffmann, Thomas Schneider, and Hendrik Dienemann

Abstract Pulmonary metastases are common in patients following resection for soft tissue sarcoma. Pulmonary resection of metastatic soft tissue sarcomas is widely practiced in surgical oncology. No randomized phase III trials are available, and data for this review were retrieved only from retrospective studies. This article addresses the issues of patient selection, surgical technique, and adjuvant chemotherapy, and provides the surgical oncologist with a current review of pulmonary metastasectomy in metastatic soft tissue sarcoma. In summary, there is a substantial body of evidence demonstrating that resection of soft tissue pulmonary metastases can be performed safely and with a low mortality rate. For a subset of highly selected patients, the overall results of a 5-year actuarial survival rate ranged between 25% and 37.6%. These outcomes exceed those normally associated with metastatic soft tissue sarcoma and are well comparable with surgical resection for other malignancies.

20.1 Introduction

Soft tissue sarcomas of an extremity or the trunk metastasize to the lungs in approximately 20% of patients (Billingsley et al. 1999). These metastases do not always represent diffuse systemic disease, which may render the tumor inoperable. Many patients who develop distant metastases will have a limited number of isolated pulmonary metastases.

The probability for pulmonary metastatic spread depends on histopathology, site, size, depth of the location, recurrent disease, and the grade of the primary tumor (Kane 2004). Most commonly malignant fibrous histiocytoma (MFH), synovial sarcoma, and leiomyosarcoma develop pulmonary metastases (Table 20.1). High-grade soft tissue sarcomas tend to metastasize more frequently than low-grade sarcomas (Potter et al. 1986). Despite the apparent paradox of local resection for a systemic disease, however,

Joachim Pfannschmidt (✉)
Department of Surgery
Thoraxklinik Heidelberg
Amalienstr. 5
69126 Heidelberg, Germany
E-mail: Joachim.pfannschmidt@thoraxklinik-heidelberg.de

Table 20.1 Clinicopathologic features of reported pulmonary metastases from soft tissue sarcoma

	Casson et al. (1992)	Gadd et al. (1993)	Van Geel et al. (1996)	Billingsley et al. (1999)	Pfannschmidt et al. (2006b)	Canter et al. (2007)	Rehders et al. (2007)
Recruitment period	1981–1985	1983–1990	<1993	1982–1997	1996–2002	1990–2005	1991–2003
Selection of patients	Resected	Unresected and resected	Unresected and resected	Unresected and resected	Resected	Resected	Resected
Characteristics of patients	♂: 44 ♀: 25, median age 46y	♂: 82 ♀: 53, median age 55y	♂: NR ♀: NR, mean age 40y	♂: 367 ♀: 352, mean age 49y	♂: 27 ♀: 23, median age 51y	♂: 77 ♀: 61, median age 50y	♂: 33 ♀: 28, mean age 42y
Median follow-up	NR	12 mo	2.5 y	9.7 mo	34 mo	22 mo	mean: 60 mo
Postoperative mortality	1.5	NR	<0.5%	NR	0	NR	0
5-year survival (resected)	26	3y: 23 (CR)	38	37 (CR)	37.6	29	25
MFH	20	36	62	132	9	41	13
Synovial cell	7	30	59	98	8	34	5
Leiomyosarcoma	9	7	49	149	1	15	12
Liposarcoma	3	25	32	86	3	9	5
Fibrosarcoma	4	1	32	19	6		3
Rhabdomyosarcoma		9		25	10		1
Peripheral nerve tumor		7		36			6
Angiosarcoma		4		33			2
Chondrosarcoma	3	3		18	2		4
Spindle cell	3	9		20			
Alveolar soft part sarcoma	1			13			3
Neurogenic sarcoma					3		
Hemangiopericytoma					3		1
Ewing's sarcoma	4				2		
Other	14		21	90	3	39	6
Total	69	135	255	719	50	138	61

♂: total number of males ♀: total number of females; CR, complete resection; MO, months; NR, not reported; y, years

subsequent experience from several institutions have suggested that in selected cases indications for pulmonary metastasectomy in soft tissue sarcoma were appropriate. However, the benefit of chemotherapy in the treatment of pulmonary metastases in patients with soft tissue sarcoma is not considered a curative.

Since Weinlechner (1882) reported the first pulmonary resection (en bloc chest wall resection) for metastasizing soft tissue sarcoma in the 1880s, several case reports and unselected small series have been published. Alexander and Haight reported the results of a first series of 25 patients after resection of pulmonary metastases in 1947 (Alexander and Haight 1947). In the following years surgical treatment was considered only if the patient had a long disease-free interval following resection of the primary tumor, and had only a few lesions confined to one lung. The decision on whether a pulmonary metastasectomy might induce a benefit for the patient is still basically related to the criteria defined by Thomford et al. (1965).

The International Registry of Lung Metastases was established in 1991 and accrued 5,206 patients with lung metastasectomy of different tumor types (No authors listed 1997b). They noted that the probability of relapse was higher for sarcomas than for epithelial or germ cell tumors, and the 5-year survival rate for soft tissue sarcoma patients was lower than that for patients with osteosarcoma.

20.2
Clinical Features

Most patients with pulmonary metastases of soft tissue sarcoma remain relatively asymptomatic for long periods and are detected during follow-up. Most pulmonary metastatic disease is located subpleurally or in the periphery of the lung. Thus, symptoms related to bronchial or vascular invasion, such as cough, shortness of breath, and hemoptysis, is relatively uncommon. Pain related to localized chest wall invasion or spontaneous pneumothorax or hemothorax may be highly suggestive of pulmonary metastasis in patients with a history of soft tissue sarcoma (Putnam 2000).

Most patients presenting with metachronous detection of pulmonary lesions have metastases that compare to metastases developed synchronously with the primary tumor (Billingsley et al. 1999).

20.3
Radiology

Surveillance strategies are especially based on radiographic imaging for distant recurrence. The vast majority of recurrent disease in patients with soft tissue sarcoma will present within the first 2 to 5 years after therapy (Kane 2004). Flemming et al. (2001) retrospectively evaluated the added benefit of routine chest computed tomography (CT) as compared with chest radiograph alone for patients with initial T1 extremity soft tissue sarcoma. Pulmonary metastases were found in less than 1% of patients using the staging algorithm employing routine chest radiography vs the selective use of chest CT. Thus, using a surveillance staging algorithm along with routine chest CT has come into question and should be recommended only for patients with a high risk of developing lung metastases (Kane 2004).

In a patient with a history of soft tissue sarcoma, a new pulmonary lesion detected by chest radiograph is approximately ten times more likely to be a metastasis than a second primary cancer (Chao and Goldberg 2000). Helical CT is the most effective method of imaging pulmonary metastases and can detect nodules smaller than 5 mm. In a prospective study by Diederich et al. (1999) a sensitivity of 95% in detecting pulmonary lesions of 6 mm or greater was documented for helical CT, while nodules less than 6 mm were detected with 69% sensitivity. Margaritora et al. (2002) published a superior sensitivity of helical CT compared to high resolution CT. However, complete manual exploration by thoracotomy remains the procedure of choice for patients undergoing pulmonary metastasectomy because of the inherent limitations in preoperative radiological assessment of lung lesions smaller than 6 mm.

Magnetic resonance imaging (MRI) has limited use in the detection of pulmonary metastases. Compared with helical CT, Kersjes et al. (1997) found only 36% of the pulmonary nodules detected by helical CT. MRI is very useful to identify tumor invasion into mediastinal or chest wall structures (Downey 1999; Webb 1997). The role of positron emission tomography (PET) is still evolving. There are sparse reports on PET in lung metastasis. Lucas et al. (1998) compared the results of F-18 fluorodeoxyglucose (FDG) PET and chest CT for pulmonary metastases in 62 patients. For the identification of lung metastases, 70 comparisons showed that the sensitivity and specificity of FDG PET were 86.7% and 100%, respectively. Chest CT is more sensitive than FDG PET in detecting pulmonary metastases, with 100% sensitivity and 96.4% specificity, but 13 other sites of metastases were identified by FDG PET. The value of PET in preoperative staging lies in the identification on both local and distant recurrence of tumor in a one-step procedure (Pastorino et al. 2003). Iagaru and coworkers (2006) have noted that subcentimeter CT lesions should not be considered falsely positive if inactive on PET. Thus, a negative PET scan in the presence of suspicious CT findings in the chest cannot reliably exclude pulmonary metastases from soft tissue sarcoma.

20.4
Patient Selection

Patient selection for resection of lung metastases is based on individual patient and tumor characteristics. Only patients who meet the criteria for potentially curative operation should be included.

According to the Thomford criteria (Thomford et al. 1965), the preconditions valid for potentially curative operations for pulmonary metastasectomy, in general, are as follows:

1. The metastases seem to be technically resectable.
2. The general and functional risks are tolerable.
3. The primary tumor is controlled.
4. No extrathoracic lesions are detected.

These criteria are sufficiently liberal so as not to exclude patients who potentially benefit from resection of their metastases. However, there are further indications for partial or complete resection of pulmonary metastases in soft tissue sarcoma patients (Putnam 1998).

1. Establish a diagnosis
2. Evaluate residual disease after chemotherapy
3. Obtain tissue for tumor markers or immunohistochemical studies
4. Decrease tumor burden

The presence of extrathoracic spread in patients with lung metastasis is the main reason for exclusion from surgery. To determine whether the primary tumor is controlled or whether there are extrathoracic metastatic lesions CT, a bone scan, MRI, and PET are used in the assessment of patients with soft tissue sarcoma (Virgo et al. 2006). Recently Pastorino and coworkers (2003) reported on a series of 86 patients with different primary histologies and preoperative PET scan. With PET extrapulmonary metastases that modified the treatment plan were detected in over 20% of patients. Furthermore, mediastinal node metastases were detected with a sensitivity greater than CT by PET. Thus, it can be assumed that PET may play an important role in the selection of surgical candidates for lung metastasectomy in the future.

To rule out endobronchial metastatic spread, which may result in more extensive resection, routine preoperative bronchoscopy has been recommended, although endobronchial metastases are rare in soft tissue sarcoma (Sorensen 2004; Virgo et al. 2006).

Patients with pulmonary metastases may undergo multiple wedge resections as well as segmentectomy, lobectomy, or even, in highly selected patients, pneumonectomy for metastasectomy. The short- and long-term effects of pulmonary resection on cardiopulmonary function have to be considered prior surgery.

Patient selection for pulmonary metastasectomy should be based on good pulmonary function (Kick et al. 2005). The presence of associated comorbid conditions increases the risk of death and surgical complications. Several studies have evaluated the usefulness of preoperative exercise testing for predicting postoperative morbidity and mortality, leading to the British Thoracic Society (BTS 2001) and American College of Chest Physicians guidelines (Beckles et al. 2003) for selection of patients for lung cancer surgery, which are also appropriate to patients with pulmonary metastases.

20.5
Surgery

Anterior thoracotomy and posterolateral thoracotomy is the standard approach most commonly used in lung metastasectomy for unilateral disease or as staged thoracotomies for bilateral lesions. Sternotomy or a clamshell bilateral thoracotomy may offer less postoperative discomfort but can obviate exposure problems in the posterior aspects of the lungs and for systemic mediastinal lymph node dissection. However, sternotomy is the preferred approach for many surgeons in commonly bilateral metastatic pulmonary lesions, such as sarcomas (Roth et al. 1986; Pastorino et al. 1990). Bilateral exploration and careful bi-manual palpation of both lungs in unilateral disease versus a unilateral approach and surveillance of the contralateral site by helical CT is under discussion.

Nakajima and colleagues (2007) demonstrated, examining patients with pulmonary metastases of colorectal origin, that pulmonary nodules smaller than 5 mm in diameter that were detected by helical CT were often not pulmonary metastases. Finger palpation detects more nonmetastatic pulmonary nodules during the operation but is also limited in the detection of small nodules. The number of pulmonary metastases detected by finger palpation may range between the number detected by preoperative CT and the true number of metastatic pulmonary nodules. Waters et al. (1998) analyzed a dog model and found many small metastatic nodules being misdiagnosed by CT and also being missed by finger palpation because they are often less than 1 mm in diameter.

In the study by Roth et al. (1986) the finding and removal of contralateral disease in patients preoperatively presumed to have only unilateral disease did not influence survival. Thus, after preoperative assessment of unilateral metastatic disease, many authors make a case for open manual pulmonary examination with the use of unilateral thoracotomy to approach the metastatic lesion, and to follow-up the contralateral side by helical CT scan (Dienemann et al. 1998; Younes et al. 2002). The recent advances in CT and PET technology improve the ability for detection of lung metastases and support an observant surgical strategy for the nondiseased lung.

In adoption of the recommended procedures in surgical oncology and especially for lung cancer it has been recommended to perform a systematic lymph node dissection as a standard procedure for pulmonary metastasectomy (Dominguez-Ventura and Nichols 2006; Pfannschmidt et al. 2006a). Kamiyoshihara and coworkers (1998), in a retrospective study of 28 patients undergoing pulmonary metastasectomy, suggested that local recurrence seemed to decrease when a mediastinal lymph node dissection was performed. Thus, systematic lymph node dissection is considered as diagnostic as well as an element of complete surgical resection in pulmonary metastasectomy by many thoracic surgeons.

On the other hand, it has been argued that the low incidence of nodal involvement of sarcomas calls into question the need for a systemic mediastinal lymph node dissection in every patient undergoing pulmonary metastasectomy (Putnam 2000). Thus, lymph node involvement has not been analyzed for prognostic significance in most studies, and lymph node dissection was carried out only in cases when node enlargement was detected either intraoperatively or by a CT chest scan (Casson et al. 1992; Inoue et al. 2000; Saito et al. 2002).

Unfortunately, the limited efficiency of adjuvant chemotherapy in the treatment of primary soft tissue sarcoma to reduce the risk of distant metastases (Gortzak et al. 2001) makes the need for pulmonary metastasectomy more compelling. So far, surgery remains a major issue for patients with metastatic disease even in cases where positive mediastinal lymph nodes can be anticipated.

Postoperative mortality is infrequently reported, with a rate between 0.0% (Rehders et al. 2007; Pfannschmidt et al. 2006b; van Geel et al. 1996; Casson et al. 1992) and 1.5% (Casson et al. 1992; No authors listed 1997b) in patients undergoing their first operation (Table 20.1). In patients after metastasectomy for recurrent disease, a 3% mortality has been reported (Weiser et al. 2000). The low rate of operative deaths attests to the safety of the operation in this population of patients, who are generally in good health otherwise.

Most frequently, postoperative dysrhythmia and impaired bronchial cleaning with pneumonia and atelectasis have been reported after pulmonary metastasectomy (Vogt-Moykopf et al. 1994). For patients who have received preoperative chemo- or radiotherapy there is a specific risk of postoperative pulmonary complications.

20.6
Video-Assisted Thoracic Surgery

Management of isolated metastatic deposits to the lungs and the role of video-assisted thoracic surgery (VATS) techniques have been considered controversial. VATS has been proved to provide good surgical access, minimize postoperative pain, shorten hospital stay, and improve long-term quality of life in comparison to open thoracotomy (Ketchedjian et al. 2006). The inability to perform a detailed bimanual palpation of the lung for occult lesions and completely resect all macroscopic metastases has been considered an inherent weakness in this approach. In a prospective trial by McCormack and colleagues (1996) the study was abandoned after analysis of 18 patients due to a 56% failure rate of a CT scan and video-assisted thoracic surgery to detect all pulmonary lesions. But this study was conducted with older CT scan generations and, it may be argued, if the newer helical CT scans would have been used, more lesions may have been identified.

Although helical CT has been shown to improve detection of pulmonary nodules compared to conventional CT, there are still limitations in the sensitivity for lesions of less than 6 mm. Studies from Diederich et al. (1999), Margaritora et al. (2002), Ambrogi et al. (2000), and Kayton et al. (2006) still identified pulmonary metastases by palpation being missed at helical CT scan; on the other hand, Watanabe et al. (1998) reported that the accuracy of preoperative CT evaluation was 92% when the number of metastatic nodules was one or two.

In recent years some authors (Nakajima et al. 2001; Ketchedjian et al. 2006) have favored the VATS approach for resection of lung metastases based on careful patient selection by high-resolution spiral-CT scans.

Lin et al. (1999) reported on 99 potentially curative resections of lung metastases with long-term survival comparable with historical results by an open approach. Mutsaerts et al. (2002) reported similar long-term survival in patients after VATS metastasectomy in comparison to open thoracotomy. The retrospective nature of the available data on pulmonary metastasectomy and the role of VATS led the Cancer and Leukemia Group B (CALGB 9336) to undertake a randomized trial of open thoracotomy versus VATS for pulmonary metastases. Unfortunately, the study was closed in 2000 due to poor accrual.

20.7
Prognostic Factors

Most consistently, several different factors have been shown to influence prognosis after pulmonary metastasectomy: patient demographics (i.e., age and gender), primary tumor characteristics (i.e., TNM, stage, histology, origin), lung metastases (i.e., number, size, laterality, type of resection, thoracic lymph node involvement, completeness of resection), and timing of metastases (i.e., disease-free interval) (Table 20.2).

No randomized trials comparing surgical resection versus no surgery have ever been conducted; therefore, Aberg (1997) and Fey and Rauch (2001) speculated that improved survival after metastasectomy may be related solely to favorable patient selection.

This review discusses a series of retrospective studies with patients undergoing removal of pulmonary metastases from a primary soft tissue sarcoma at different international institutions published in the English literature from 1990 to 2007. To ensure that the reviewed surgical series reflected the outcomes for patients treated with modern surgical, anesthetic, medical, and diagnostic care techniques, we have restricted our qualitative analysis to surgical series with a recruitment period no later than 1980. There should be a reporting of at least 50 patients into each study (Table 20.1). Three of the reviewed articles retrieved data mainly from the Memorial Sloan-Kettering Cancer Center Database (Billingsley et al. 1999; Canter et al. 2007; Gadd et al. 1993).

20.7.1
Overall Survival

All studies reported overall 5-year survival as between 25% and 37.6% for all patients undergoing resection of pulmonary metastases (Table 20.1). It has been shown that the most important and constant favorable prognostic factor for long-term survival is a complete surgical resection of all pulmonary metastases (No authors listed 1997b). A complete resection is considered an R0 resection (negative microscopic margins), and an incomplete resection represents an R1 resection (positive microscopic margins) or an R2 resection (positive gross margins).

The presence of occult metastatic disease seems to be the reason for recurrent pulmonary disease. Nonetheless, there are some individual patients who may benefit from incomplete resection because even if they proved to be unresectable in entirety, they had a lesser tumor burden left behind. Metastasectomy as a cytoreductive strategy for treatment of pulmonary metastases in breast cancer has been discussed and may also play a role in other malignancies (Bathe et al. 1999).

It is commonly stated that radicality is a prognostic factor for long-term survival in patients with pulmonary metastasectomy of soft tissue sarcoma that can achieve 5-year survival rates of 52.7% (Pfannschmidt et al. 2006b). In the group of patients with an incomplete resection, prognosis is well compared to patients who did not undergo a pulmonary metastasectomy (Jablons et al. 1989).

Of all surgical procedures the most common procedure reported was wedge resection or segmentectomy because 80% pulmonary metastases

Table 20.2 Favorable prognostic factors (multivariate analysis)

	Casson et al. (1992)	Gadd et al. (1993)	Van Geel et al. (1996)	Billingsley et al. (1999)	Pfannschmidt et al. (2006)	Canter et al. (2007)	Rehders et al. (2007)
Age	No	No	<40 y	>50 y	No	No	No
Histology	MFH unclassified sarcomas (unfavorable)	Rhabdomyosarcoma extraskeletal osteosarcoma (unfavorable)	No	Liposarcoma (unfavorable) malign. peripheral nerve tumor (unfavorable)	No	No	No
Location primary	NR	NR	No	No	NR	No	No
Grading	NR	No	Grade I,II	Low grade	No	No	No
Repeat resection	NR	NR	NR	NR	No	NR	No
DFI	No	No	<30 mo	<12 mo	No	<12 mo (dss)	No
Extend of resection	No	No	NR	NR	No	NR	No
Complete resection	Yes	Yes	Yes	Yes	Yes	Yes (dss)	No
Number of lesions	<4 nodules	No	No	No	No	No	No
Maximum tumor size	NR	No	NR	NR	NR	No	NR
TDT	>40 d	NR	NR	NR	NR	NR	NR
Laterality	No	No	No	No	NR	NR	No
Chemotherapy	NR	No	NR	No	No	No (dss)	No

d, days; dss, disease-specific survival; mo, months; NR, not reported; TDT, tumor doubling time; DFI, disease-free interval; y, years

20 Pulmonary Metastasectomy for Soft Tissue Sarcomas: Is It Justified?

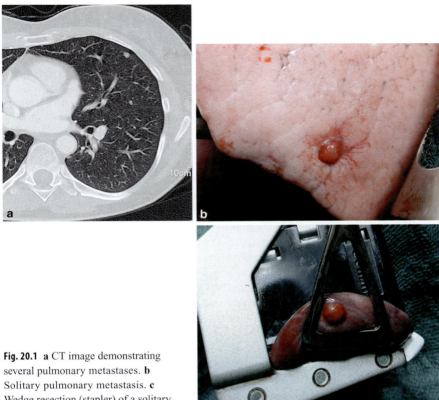

Fig. 20.1 **a** CT image demonstrating several pulmonary metastases. **b** Solitary pulmonary metastasis. **c** Wedge resection (stapler) of a solitary pulmonary metastasis

are localized peripherally (Fig. 20.1a–c). Lobectomy, and in selected cases even pneumonectomy, is indicated for centrally located or multilobular lesions. Rusch (1995) recommended resection of metastases by taking a circumferentially 0.5- to 1.0-cm margin of normal lung tissue in all directions. Since the 1990s, laser technique was applied for parenchyma-sparing pulmonary resection of multiple lung metastases and also in soft tissue sarcoma patients (Rolle et al. 2006). Although there is limited experience in the use of modern laser devices, analysis of long-term survival disclosed no statistically significant differences between different types of resections i.e., conventional resection, lobectomy, or laser resection (Mineo et al. 2001).

In the reviewed articles, the number of pulmonary resections by a laser device was not specifically reported. In the analysis for prognostic relevance, type of resection did not influence long-term survival.

In general, sex was not a significant prognostic factor. In the reporting of van Geel et al. (1996) and Billingsley et al. (1999) an age of greater than 40 or 50 years was identified as an ominous prognosticator. So far age has not been found to be statistically related to prognosis in most other publications.

Furthermore, upon statistical analysis of different clinical parameters: re-resection, extent of resection, maximum tumor size, laterality, and additional chemotherapy, appear to have no significant effect on long-term prognosis.

Variance between the different published series on 5-years survival data may be related to the fact that soft tissue sarcomas include a wide spectrum of different histological types. Pastorino et al. (1989), Casson et al. (1992), Gadd et al. (1993), and Billingsley et al. (1999) reported that 5-year survival has been shown to correspond with histological type. Billingsley and coworkers (1999) found unfavorable tumor biology in patients with pulmonary metastases originating from liposarcoma and malignant peripheral nerve tumors. Extraskeletal osteosarcomas in the studies by Gadd et al. (1993) and unclassified sarcomas in the analysis by Casson et al. (1992) were poor prognostic indicators. The frequency of high-grade lesions within each of the histological categories further influenced long-term prognosis in the comprehensive studies published by Billingsley et al. (1999) and van Geel et al. (van Geel et al. 1996). No statistical significance differentiating survival was seen on histological parameters in the studies by van Geel et al. (1996), Pfannschmidt et al. (2006b), Canter et al. (2007), and Rehders et al. (2007).

The disease-free interval between the resection of the primary tumor and pulmonary metastasectomy was confirmed to be a prognostic factor in multivariate analysis in the studies by van Geel and coworkers (1996), Billingsley et al. (1999), and Canter et al. (2007). The median disease-free interval for patients being treated by metastasectomy was reported between 10.3 months and 25.8 months (Canter et al. 2007; Pfannschmidt et al. 2006b; Gadd et al. 1993; Rehders et al. 2007). Improved outcome was associated with patients presenting with metachronous detection of pulmonary lesions and a disease-free interval (DFI) over 12 months (Billingsley et al. 1999; Canter et al. 2007) or 30 months (van Geel et al. 1996). Most patients were selected for pulmonary metastasectomy with a limited number of pulmonary metastases, the median being between 1 and 3 metastases in most studies (Canter et al. 2007; Gadd et al. 1993; Pfannschmidt et al. 2006b; Rehders et al. 2007).

Casson et al. (1992) found postthoracotomy survival to be associated with the number of nodules detected by CT preoperatively. Multivariate analysis found that patients having 4 and more nodules seen by CT scan had a significantly worse prognostic outcome.

Discordant results have been published on the prognostic value of tumor doubling time (TDT). Only observed in the reviewed article by Casson and colleagues (1992) and a report by Putnam et al. (1984), tumor doubling time seems debatable, if it may play a role for survival in patients diagnosed with pulmonary metastases of soft tissue sarcoma origin. Chojniak and Younes (2003) presented an analysis of growth rate in patients with pulmonary metastases of different malignoma origin by CT scan. They found an individual and unpredictable growing pattern for every independent lesion. Most likely TDT reflects such biological factors as tumor growth properties and vascular supply. The best method to quantify the variation of tumor doubling time in the preoperative workup is by two consecutive CT scans. If this parameter is considered as relevant in decision making for pulmonary metastasectomy, tumor growth of pulmonary metastases can be calculated. Casson et al. (1992) found the best prognosis for tumors with a tumor doubling time of at least 40 days.

The presence or absence of thoracic lymph node metastasis is discussed as a single important factor for estimating the prognosis in pulmonary metastasectomy for most extrapulmonary malignancies (Dominguez-Ventura and Nichols 2006; Ercan et al. 2004; Pfannschmidt et al. 2006a). The pattern of metastasis of most primary sarcomas is hematogenous; lymph node metastases are uncommon, except for synovial sarcoma, MFH, rhabdomyosarcoma, and angiosarcoma (Ariel 1988).

Pfannschmidt et al. (2006b) reported on patients with lung metastases of soft tissue sarcoma with a tendency for pulmonary lymphatic spread, but they compromised in settling on a small histological subgroup with high-grade rhabdomyosarcoma and MFH.

Routine systematic mediastinal and hilar lymph node dissection contemporary with pulmonary metastasectomy has not been uniformly performed in many thoracic surgical centers and was reported vaguely or not at all in many of the reports. Only in the studies reported by Jablons et al. (1989), and Pfannschmidt et al. (2006b) survival was found to be worse in patients with intrathoracic lymph node involvement of soft tissue sarcoma compared to patients without nodal metastases, but there was no statistical significance in univariate analysis.

20.7.2
Recurrent Pulmonary Metastases

After complete resection of pulmonary metastases from soft tissue sarcoma pulmonary re-recurrence is common, with a reported re-recurrence rate between 45% and 83% (Billingsley et al. 1999; Casson et al. 1992; van Geel et al. 1996). There are limited data concerning the management of patients with pulmonary re-recurrence. Treatment options include systemic therapy, surveillance, and re-resection, but in the absence of effective nonsurgical treatment, re-exploration is often considered. Liebl et al. (2007) reported that patients who underwent at least one repeat resection showed a significantly improved 5-year survival rate than patients with a single resection. This may be strongly related to a highly selective subset of patients with favorable tumor biology and therefore resectable disease.

Weiser et al. (2000) noted a median survival for 86 patients with soft tissue sarcoma undergoing pulmonary re-resection of 42.8 months (5-year survival: 36%), Liebl et al. (2007) reported on 19 patients and a median survival of 22 months, and Casson et al. (1992) on 34 patients and a median survival of 28 months. Weiser et al. (2000) described metastasis size, metastasis number by CT, and primary tumor histological grade in patients considered for repeat pulmonary metastasectomy as independent prognostic parameters for long-term survival.

Patients with complete resection had a significantly better outcome than those incompletely resected; thus, complete surgical resection is most warranted even in pulmonary re-resection.

These factors help stratify patient outcomes following re-resection. We do not use them to exclude patients from re-resection but rather determine which patients derive the least benefit from re-resection and may therefore be candidates for additional therapy.

20.7.3
Perioperative Chemotherapy

The role of chemotherapy in the treatment of patients with soft tissue sarcoma remains to be elucidated. A metaanalysis by the Sarcoma Meta-analysis Collaboration provided evidence that adjuvant doxorubicin-based chemotherapy significantly improve the recurrence-free survival and showed a trend toward improved overall survival ([no authors listed] 1997a).

There are limited data in the literature on how best to integrate metastasectomy with chemotherapy, primary indication, and adjuvant systemic therapy.

The most recent attempt has been made by the European Organization for Research and Treatment of Cancer (EORTC-Protocol 62933) with a randomized multicenter trial on metastasectomy alone versus induction chemotherapy followed by metastasectomy and a targeted sample size of 340 patients. Started in 1996, this trial was closed due to poor accrual in November 2000.

Although in some centers perioperative chemotherapy has been a standard therapy for metastatic soft tissue sarcomas, a lack of prospective randomized trials has made it unclear whether or not the therapy improves survival. Nevertheless, Pastorino and colleagues (1989) reported an improvement in 3-year survival after 1984 when chemotherapy was introduced to the surgical treatment of pulmonary metastases in soft tissue sarcoma, but selection bias may be an objective in this study. In a study by Lanza et al. (1991), which was conducted before 1990, and therefore no patients received ifosfamide, they found no survival benefit in 26 patients with neoadjuvant chemotherapy.

Data from the Memorial Sloan-Kettering Cancer Center Sarcoma Database on 138 patients being treated with pulmonary metastasectomy were analyzed concerning the impact of perioperative chemotherapy in 53 patients (Canter et al. 2007). In the contemporary study period from 1990 to 2005, doxorubicin–ifosfamide chemotherapy was established as the most active regimen in the treatment. Comparison between the perioperative chemotherapy cohort and the surgery-alone cohort with respect to the predominant clinicopathological characteristics were similar; there was also a statistically significant difference in age between the groups. The median postmetastasis disease-specific survival was 24 months in patients who were treated with surgery and chemotherapy compared with 33 months in patients who were treated with surgery alone ($p=0.19$). In 38 patients treated with neoadjuvant chemotherapy, no association was noted between the radiographic response to preoperative chemotherapy and postmetastasis survival. The authors concluded that neoadjuvant or adjuvant chemotherapy had minimal if any impact on postmetastasis overall survival or disease-specific survival. However, it must be recognized that the sample size of this study was small and may be underpowered to detect small, but even clinically relevant, differences.

20.8
Future Directions

Unfortunately, the majority of patients will have unresectable disease, and chemotherapy remains their only option in soft tissue sarcoma stage IV. Despite the ability of systemic chemotherapy to induce tumor shrinkage in 35%–50% of patients, rendering the primary tumor amenable for subsequent optimal local treatment, systemic therapy has not had a major impact on the survival of these patients ([no authors listed] 1997a; Chang et al. 1988; Glenn et al. 1985; Lerner et al. 1987). However, the rationale—systemic treatment for patients who are at high risk of developing micrometastatic spread and also to select out the patients for pulmonary metastasectomy—will be more effectively assessed in future studies when more effective substances become available. Unfortunately the EORTC-Study 62933 has been closed and a unique chance to evaluate the value of additive chemotherapy has been missed.

Isolated lung perfusion has been investigated as an alternative method for delivering high-dose chemotherapy to the lungs while minimizing systemic toxicities.

In patients with pulmonary metastases who are surgically unresectable, isolated lung perfusion for pulmonary metastases is an experimental technique, providing an opportunity to dose intensify local chemotherapy, while minimizing systemic toxicity and avoiding toxic drug metabolism through the liver and kidneys. Trials in a limited number of patients with soft tissue sarcoma have shown this method to be safe, feasible, and reproducible (Burt et al. 2000). Even feasibility of isolated lung perfusion for resectable lung metastases has been evaluated in a phase I trial. However, the clinical value and efficacy of lung perfusion techniques remains at present unclear (Johnston et al. 1995).

20.9 Conclusions

The surgical treatment of pulmonary metastases from soft tissue sarcoma is an established technique in the interdisciplinary concept of oncological therapy. The retrospective nature of the studies is subjected to bias and often fail to provide information on relevant potential prognostic parameters.

In summary, there is a substantial body of evidence from retrospective case series demonstrating that resection of pulmonary metastases by soft tissue sarcoma histology can be performed safely with a low mortality rate.

For a subset of highly selected patients, the overall results of a 5-year actuarial survival rate ranged between 25% and 37.6%.

These data reinforce the view that, with proper patient selection under consideration of established prognostic factors, long-term survival with pulmonary metastasectomy is possible.

It is commonly stated that radicality is a prognostic factor for long-term survival, while Sex, distribution of the pulmonary metastases, repeat pulmonary resection, and additional chemotherapy has not been reported to be significant prognostic factors of survival so far. Technical aspects of pulmonary metastasectomy, such as the best surgical approach, the role of minimally invasive techniques, laser techniques, and mediastinal lymphadenectomy are still not clearly determined. Furthermore, the DFI was shown to be a significant prognostic factor in three studies, but in the majority the DFI did not affect long-term survival. Another interesting result is the finding that 5-year survival of patients may be influenced by histological characteristics: histology and grading of the tumor.

Randomized trials comparing pulmonary metastasectomy versus nonsurgical treatment modalities are now impossible because the retrospective data are strong enough to make randomization impossible. There will never be a trial comparing surgery with medical therapy unless better chemotherapeutic agents are developed.

To improve the outcome for patients with pulmonary metastatic soft tissue sarcoma, strategies based on intensive systemic chemotherapy, new molecular targeted therapeutic regimen, and the combination with pulmonary metastasectomy is a promising research direction and should be evaluated.

References

(1997a) Adjuvant chemotherapy for localised resectable soft-tissue sarcoma of adults: meta-analysis of individual data. Sarcoma Meta-analysis Collaboration. Lancet 350:1647–1654

(1997b) Long-term results of lung metastasectomy: prognostic analyses based on 5206 cases. The International Registry of Lung Metastases. J Thorac Cardiovasc Surg 113:37–49

Aberg T (1997) Selection mechanisms as major determinants of survival after pulmonary metastasectomy. Ann Thorac Surg 63:611–612

Alexander J, Haight C (1947) Pulmonary resection for solitary metastatic sarcomas and carcinomas. Surg Gynecol Obstet 85:129–146

Ambrogi V, Paci M, Pompeo E, Mineo TC (2000) Transxiphoid video-assisted pulmonary metastasectomy: relevance of helical computed tomography occult lesions. Ann Thorac Surg 70:1847–1852

Ariel IM (1988) Incidence of metastases to lymph nodes from soft-tissue sarcomas. Semin Surg Oncol 4:27–29

Bathe OF, Kaklamanos IG, Moffat FL, Boggs J, Franceschi D, Livingstone AS (1999) Metastasectomy as a cytoreductive strategy for treatment of isolated pulmonary and hepatic metastases from breast cancer. Surg Oncol 8:35–42

Beckles MA, Spiro SG, Colice GL, Rudd RM (2003) The physiologic evaluation of patients with lung cancer being considered for resectional surgery. Chest 123:105S–114S

Billingsley KG, Burt ME, Jara E, Ginsberg RJ, Woodruff JM, Leung DH, Brennan MF (1999) Pulmonary metastases from soft tissue sarcoma: analysis of patterns of diseases and postmetastasis survival. Ann Surg 229:602–610

British Thoracic Society (2001) BTS guidelines: guidelines on the selection of patients with lung cancer for surgery. Thorax 56:89–108

Burt ME, Liu D, Abolhoda A, Ross HM, Kaneda Y, Jara E, Casper ES, Ginsberg RJ, Brennan MF (2000) Isolated lung perfusion for patients with unresectable metastases from sarcoma: a phase I trial. Ann Thorac Surg 69:1542–1549

Canter RJ, Qin LX, Downey RJ, Brennan MF, Singer S, Maki RG (2007) Perioperative chemotherapy in patients undergoing pulmonary resection for metastatic soft-tissue sarcoma of the extremity: a retrospective analysis. Cancer 110:2050–2060

Casson AG, Putnam JB, Natarajan G, Johnston DA, Mountain C, McMurtrey M, Roth JA (1992) Five-year survival after pulmonary metastasectomy for adult soft tissue sarcoma. Cancer 69:662–668

Chang AE, Kinsella T, Glatstein E, Baker AR, Sindelar WF, Lotze MT, Danforth DN, Jr Sugarbaker PH, Lack EE, Steinberg SM (1988) Adjuvant chemotherapy for patients with high-grade soft-tissue sarcomas of the extremity. J Clin Oncol 6:1491–1500

Chao C, Goldberg M (2000) Surgical treatment of metastatic pulmonary soft-tissue sarcoma. Oncology 14:835–841

Chojniak R, Younes RN (2003) Pulmonary metastases tumor doubling time: assessment by computed tomography. Am J Clin Oncol 26:374–377

Diederich S, Semik M, Lentschig MG, Winter F, Scheld HH, Roos N, Bongartz G (1999) Helical CT of pulmonary nodules in patients with extrathoracic malignancy: CT-surgical correlation. Am J Roentgenol 172:353–360

Dienemann H, Hoffmann H, Trainer C, Muley T (1998) Lung metastases: tumor reduction as an oncologic concept [in German]. Langenbecks Arch Chir Suppl Kongressbd 115:138–142

Dominguez-Ventura A, Nichols FC 3rd (2006) Lymphadenectomy in metastasectomy. Thorac Surg Clin 16:139–143

Downey RJ (1999) Surgical treatment of pulmonary metastases. Surg Oncol Clin N Am 8:341

Ercan S, Nichols FC 3rd, Trastek VF, Deschamps C, Allen MS, Miller DL, Schleck CD, Pairolero PC (2004) Prognostic significance of lymph node metastasis found during pulmonary metastasectomy for extrapulmonary carcinoma. Ann Thorac Surg 77:1786–1791

Fey MF, Rauch D (2001) Metastasectomy—a direct therapeutic effect or an illusion due to patient selection? [in German]. Ther Umsch 58:726–731

Fleming JB, Cantor SB, Varma DG, Holst D, Feig BW, Hunt KK, Patel SR, Benjamin RS, Pollock RE, Pisters PW (2001) Utility of chest computed tomography for staging in patients with T1 extremity soft tissue sarcomas. Cancer 92:863–868

Gadd MA, Casper ES, Woodruff JM, McCormack M, Brennan MF (1993) Development and treatment of pulmonary metastases in adult patients with extremity soft tissue sarcoma. Ann Surg 218:705–712

Glenn J, Kinsella T, Glatstein E, Tepper J, Baker A, Sugarbaker P, Sindela W, Roth J, Brennan M, Costa J (1985) A randomized, prospective trial of adjuvant chemotherapy in adults with soft tissue sarcomas of the head and neck, breast, and trunk. Cancer 55:1206–1214

Gortzak E, Azzarelli A, Buesa J, Bramwell VH, van Coevorden F, van Geel AN, Ezzat A, Santoro A, Oosterhuis JW, van Glabbeke M, Kirkpatrick A, Verweij J (2001) A randomised phase II study on neo-adjuvant chemotherapy for 'high-risk' adult soft-tissue sarcoma. Eur J Cancer 37:1096–1103

Iagaru A, Chawla S, Menendez L, Conti PS (2006) 18F-FDG PET and PET/CT for detection of pulmonary metastases from musculoskeletal sarcomas. Nucl Med Commun 27:795–802

Inoue M, Kotake Y, Nakagawa K, Fujiwara K, Fukuhara K, Yasumitsu T (2000) Surgery for pulmonary metastases from colorectal carcinoma. Ann Thorac Surg 70:380–383

Jablons D, Steinberg SM, Roth J, Pittaluga S, Rosenberg SA, Pass HI (1989) Metastasectomy for soft tissue sarcoma. Further evidence for efficacy and prognostic indicators. J Thorac Cardiovasc Surg 97:695–705

Johnston MR, Minchen RF, Dawson CA (1995) Lung perfusion with chemotherapy in patients with unresectable metastatic sarcoma to the lung or diffuse bronchioloalveolar carcinoma. J Thorac Cardiovasc Surg 110:368–373

Kamiyoshihara M, Hirai T, Kawashima O, Ishikawa S, Morishita Y (1998) The surgical treatment of metastatic tumors in the lung: is lobectomy with mediastinal lymph node dissection suitable treatment? Oncol Rep 5:453–457

Kane JM 3rd (2004) Surveillance strategies for patients following surgical resection of soft tissue sarcomas. Curr Opin Oncol 16:328–332

Kayton ML, Huvos AG, Casher J, Abramson SJ, Rosen NS, Wexler LH, Meyers P, LaQuaglia MP (2006) Computed tomographic scan of the chest underestimates the number of metastatic lesions in osteosarcoma. J Pediatr Surg 41:200–206

Kersjes W, Mayer E, Buchenroth M, Schunk K, Fouda N, Cagil H (1997) Diagnosis of pulmonary metastases with turbo-SE MR imaging. Eur Radiol 7:1190–1194

Ketchedjian A, Daly B, Luketich J, Fernando HC (2006) Minimally invasive techniques for managing pulmonary metastases: video-assisted thoracic surgery and radiofrequency ablation. Thorac Surg Clin 16:157–165

Kick J, Schelzig H, Heinecke A, Forster R (2005) Resection of lung metastases—risk or chance? Zentralbl Chir 130:534–538

Lanza LA, Putnam JB, Benjamin RS, Roth JA (1991) Response to chemotherapy does not predict survival after resection of sarcomatous pulmonary metastases. Ann Thorac Surg 51:219–224

Lerner HJ, Amato DA, Savlov ED, DeWys WD, Mittleman A, Urtasun RC, Sobel S, Shiraki M (1987) Eastern Cooperative Oncology Group: a comparison of adjuvant doxorubicin and observation for patients with localized soft tissue sarcoma. J Clin Oncol 5:613–617

Liebl LS, Elson F, Quaas A, Gawad KA, Izbicki JR (2007) Value of repeat resection for survival in pulmonary metastases from soft tissue sarcoma. Anticancer Res 27:2897–2902

Lin JC, Wiechmann RJ, Szwerc MF, Hazelrigg SR, Ferson PF, Naunheim KS, Keenan RJ, Yim AP, Rendina E, DeGiacomo T, Coloni GF, Venuta F, Macherey RS, Bartley S, Landreneau RJ (1999) Diagnostic and therapeutic video-assisted thoracic surgery resection of pulmonary metastases. Surgery 126:636–641

Lucas JD, O'Doherty MJ, Wong JC, Bingham JB, McKee PH, Fletcher CD, Smith MA (1998) Evaluation of fluorodeoxyglucose positron emission tomography in the management of soft-tissue sarcomas. J Bone Joint Surg Br 80:441–447

Margaritora S, Porziella V, D'Andrilli A, Cesario A, Galetta D, Macis G, Granone P (2002) Pulmonary metastases: can accurate radiological evaluation avoid thoracotomic approach? Eur J Cardiothorac Surg 21:1111–1114

McCormack PM, Bains MS, Begg CB, Burt ME, Downey RJ, Panicek DM, Rusch VW, Zakowski M, Ginsberg RJ (1996) Role of video-assisted thoracic surgery in the treatment of pulmonary metastases: results of a prospective trial. Ann Thorac Surg 62:213–216

Mineo TC, Ambrogi V, Tonini G, Nofroni I (2001) Pulmonary metastasectomy: might the type of resection affect survival? J Surg Oncol 76:47–52

Mutsaerts EL, Zoetmulder FA, Meijer S, Baas P, Hart AA, Rutgers EJ (2002) Long term survival of thoracoscopic metastasectomy vs metastasectomy by thoracotomy in patients with a solitary pulmonary lesion. Eur J Surg Oncol 28:864–868

Nakajima J, Takamoto S, Tanaka M, Takeuchi E, Murakawa T, Fukami T (2001) Thoracoscopic surgery and conventional open thoracotomy in metastatic lung cancer. Surg Endosc 15:849–853

Nakajima J, Murakawa T, Fukami T, Sano A, Sugiura M, Takamoto S (2007) Is finger palpation at operation indispensable for pulmonary metastasectomy in colorectal cancer? Ann Thorac Surg 84:1680–1684

Pastorino U, Valente M, Gasparini M, Azzarelli A, Santoro A, Alloisio M, Ongari M, Tavecchio L, Ravasi G (1989) Lung resection for metastatic sarcomas: total survival from primary treatment. J Surg Oncol 40:275–280

Pastorino U, Valente M, Gasparini M, Azzarelli A, Santoro A, Tavecchio L, Casali P, Ravasi G (1990) Median sternotomy and multiple lung resections for metastatic sarcomas. Eur J Cardiothorac Surg 4:477–481

Pastorino U, Veronesi G, Landoni C, Leon M, Picchio M, Solli PG, Leo F, Spaggiari L, Pelosi G, Bellomi M, Fazio F (2003) Fluorodeoxyglucose positron emission tomography improves preoperative staging of resectable lung metastasis. J Thorac Cardiovasc Surg 126:1906–1910

Pfannschmidt J, Klode J, Muley T, Dienemann H, Hoffmann H (2006a) Nodal involvement at the time of pulmonary metastasectomy: experiences in 245 patients. Ann Thorac Surg 81:448–454

Pfannschmidt J, Klode J, Muley T, Dienemann H, Hoffmann H (2006b) Pulmonary metastasectomy in patients with soft tissue sarcomas: experiences in 50 patients. Thorac Cardiovasc Surg 54:489–492

Potter DA, Kinsella T, Glatstein E, Wesley R, White DE, Seipp CA, Chang AE, Lack EE, Costa J, Rosenberg SA (1986) High-grade soft tissue sarcomas of the extremities. Cancer 58:190–205

Putnam JB (2000) Secondary tumors of the lung. In: Shields TW, Ponn RB (eds) General thoracic surgery. Philadelphia: Lippincott Williams and Wilkins, Philadelphia, pp 1311–1341

Putnam JB Jr (1998) Soft part sarcomas—metastases. Chest Surg Clin N Am 8:97–118

Putnam JB Jr, Roth JA, Wesley MN, Johnston MR, Rosenberg SA (1984) Analysis of prognostic factors in patients undergoing resection of pulmonary metastases from soft tissue sarcomas. J Thorac Cardiovasc Surg 87:260–268

Rehders A, Hosch SB, Scheunemann P, Stoecklein NH, Knoefel WT, Peiper M (2007) Benefit of surgical treatment of lung metastasis in soft tissue sarcoma. Arch Surg 142:70–75

Rolle A, Pereszlenyi A, Koch R, Richard M, Baier B (2006) Is surgery for multiple lung metastases reasonable? A total of 328 consecutive patients with multiple-laser metastasectomies with a new 1318-nm Nd:YAG laser. J Thorac Cardiovasc Surg 131:1236–1242

Roth JA, Pass HI, Wesley MN, White D, Putnam JB, Seipp C (1986) Comparison of median sternotomy and thoracotomy for resection of pulmonary metastases in patients with adult soft-tissue sarcomas. Ann Thorac Surg 42:134–138

Rusch VW (1995) Pulmonary metastasectomy. Current indications. Chest 107:322–331

Saito Y, Omiya H, Kohno K, Kobayashi T, Itoi K, Teramachi M, Sasaki M, Suzuki H, Takao H, Nakade M (2002) Pulmonary metastasectomy for 165 patients with colorectal carcinoma: a prognostic assessment. J Thorac Cardiovasc Surg 124:1007–1013

Sorensen JB (2004) Endobronchial metastases from extrapulmonary solid tumors. Acta Oncol 43:73–79

Thomford NR, Woolner LB, Clagett OT (1965) The surgical treatment of metastatic tumors in the lungs. J Thorac Cardiovasc Surg 49:357–363

van Geel AN, Pastorino U, Jauch KW, Judson IR, van Coevorden F, Buesa JM, Nielsen OS, Boudinet A, Tursz T, Schmitz PI (1996) Surgical treatment of lung metastases: The European Organization for Research and Treatment of Cancer-Soft Tissue and Bone Sarcoma Group study of 255 patients. Cancer 77:675–682

Virgo KS, Naunheim KS, Johnson FE (2006) Preoperative workup and postoperative surveillance for patients undergoing pulmonary metastasectomy. Thorac Surg Clin 16:125–131

Vogt-Moykopf I, Krysa S, Bulzebruck H, Schirren J (1994) Surgery for pulmonary metastases. The Heidelberg experience. Chest Surg Clin N Am 4:85–112

Watanabe M, Deguchi H, Sato M, Ozeki Y, Tanaka S, Izumi Y, Kobayashi K (1998) Midterm results of thoracoscopic surgery for pulmonary metastases especially from colorectal cancers. J Laparoendosc Adv Surg Tech A 8:195–200

Waters DJ, Coakley FV, Cohen MD, Davis MM, Karmazyn B, Gonin R, Hanna MP, Knapp DW, Heifetz SA (1998) The detection of pulmonary metastases by helical CT: a clinicopathologic study in dogs. J Comput Assist Tomogr 22:235–240

Webb W (1997) Magnetic resonance imaging of the thorax: clinical utility in comparison with CT. In: Freundlich IM, Bragg DG (eds) A radiologic approach to diseases of the chest, vol 2. Williams and Wilkens, Baltimore, pp 803–823

Weinlechner J (1882) Zur Kasuistik der Tumoren der Brustwand und deren Behandlung (Resektion der Rippen, Eröffnung der Brusthöhle, partielle Entfernung der Lunge). Wien Med Wochenschr 32:589–591, 624–628

Weiser MR, Downey RJ, Leung DH, Brennan MF (2000) Repeat resection of pulmonary metastases in patients with soft-tissue sarcoma. J Am Coll Surg 191:184–190

Younes RN, Gross JL, Deheinzelin D (2002) Surgical resection of unilateral lung metastases: is bilateral thoracotomy necessary? World J Surg 26:1112–1116

Part IV
Quality of Life Assessment

Quality of Life (QOL) in Patients with Osteosarcoma

Rajaram Nagarajan

Abstract Patients with osteosarcoma undergo extensive treatment using aggressive chemotherapy and surgery and this can have substantial acute and long-term effects on patients. In particular, quality of life (QOL) can be affected. It is important that QOL be examined to see how it is influenced. It is also important to determine who is at highest risk for impaired QOL and develop appropriate interventions. QOL is one of several outcomes that are influenced by the diagnosis and treatment of osteosarcoma. Other outcomes include function, disability, and body image. Currently, gaps exist in our knowledge of QOL in osteosarcoma patients and prospective studies are needed.

21.1
Osteosarcoma

According to Surveillance Epidemiology and End Results (SEER) program data, there are approximately 2,500 primary bone sarcomas

Rajaram Nagarajan (✉)
Cincinnati Children's Hospital Medical Center
Division of Hematology/Oncology
3333 Burnet Ave, MLC 7015, Cincinnati
OH 45229, USA
E-mail: Rajaram.nagarajan@cchc.org

diagnosed per year in the United States with 25%–30% of bone sarcomas occurring under the age of 21 years. The histology of the primary bone sarcomas vary across age groups. The most common bone tumor under the age of 21 years is osteosarcoma, which accounts for roughly 4% of all pediatric and young adult cancers and represents approximately 400 cases per year (Ries and Smith 1999). Osteosarcoma is thought to arise from primitive bone forming mesenchyme. In osteosarcoma, the most frequent site involvement is the long bones of the lower extremity (78%) with the central axis accounting for less than 10% (Ries and Smith 1999). The incidence of osteosarcoma varies within the pediatric age group. It is rather infrequent until about age 10, when the incidence rate markedly increases. The increase at age 10 years coincides with puberty and bone growth, which is reflected in the earlier peak incidence of osteosarcoma in females (Spector et al. 2006).

In older patients (over the age of 20 years) some of the most common malignant bone lesions are the hematopoietic tumors, namely multiple myeloma (most common malignant lesion) and lymphoma. After hematopoietic tumors, the next most common primary malignant bone tumors are sarcomas: osteosarcoma, followed by chondrosarcoma. Since there is quite a bit of heterogeneity in the older patient population, much of the discussion here refers to adolescents and young adults.

21.2
Treatment and Survival

Historically, treatment of osteosarcoma consisted primarily of amputation of the affected extremity. This led to only a 10%–20% survival rate (Wang and Schulz 1953; Friedman and Carter 1972). Effective multiagent chemotherapeutic regimens and improved imaging emerged in the 1970s and 1980s, altering the prognosis of individuals diagnosed with osteosarcoma (Link et al. 1986; Springfield 1991). Current survival of those with nonmetastatic disease now exceeds 60%. To avoid amputation, improve physical function, reduce disability, and enhance quality of life (QOL), oncological surgeons developed procedures (limb salvage/sparing procedures) to reconstruct large-segment bone and/or joint deficits created by limb-sparing tumor resections, which has led to the decline in the number of amputations (Springfield 1991).

For upper extremity tumors, there is little debate that the use of limb-sparing techniques is the preferred modality (Cheng and Gebhardt 1991; Aboulafia and Malawer 1993). In the lower extremity there continue to be two options for achieving local control: amputation and limb-sparing techniques. The benefits and drawbacks of both options have been debated in adult and pediatric patients. The issues are magnified in the pediatric population because of skeletal and/or psychological immaturity. Furthermore, the long-term outcomes of survivors of lower extremity bone tumors are becoming more important as we are curing more people with bone tumors, especially children who have long lifespans ahead of them.

Amputations in patients with lower extremity bone tumors are now infrequently seen and are being performed only when limb-sparing procedures would produce a less functional limb than an amputation or would compromise the curative intent of the surgery (inadequate margins). The best functional outcomes following an amputation are obtained when the amputation is performed at the lowest level possible, e.g., transtibial amputations fare better than transfemoral amputations. Amputations tend to have fewer complications and are typically related to stump healing/pain and phantom pain (Nagarajan et al. 2002).

There are a number of limb-sparing techniques currently being used, including endoprosthetic implants, allograft bone, composite endoprosthetic implants, expanding endoprostheses, arthrodesis, and rotationplasty (Nagarajan et al. 2002; Grimer 2005). The selected procedure is dependent on the site of the tumor, age of the patient, patient prognosis, and orthopedic surgeon expertise. Despite the preservation of the limb, the type and frequency of complications are much more common following the use of limb-sparing procedures than after amputation. Complications vary and are dependent on the type of surgery, site of the primary tumor, and size of the resection (Nagarajan et al. 2002). These complications can be debilitating and lead to subsequent amputations. The surgical complications are in addition to complications and issues seen with chemotherapy administration, which has acute (e.g., nausea, hair loss, neutropenia, missing school/work, etc.) and long-term effects (e.g., cardiomyopathy, infertility, second malignancy, etc.).

21.3
Quality of Life

Survivors of osteosarcoma represent a specific subgroup of cancer survivors whose QOL can be significantly impacted by cancer and treatment-related sequelae as described above. The potential impact of these treatments on QOL in children is further influenced by the emotional and skeletal maturity of the child at the time of diagnosis and treatment. QOL is defined broadly as an overall assessment of one's satisfaction with all the important aspects of life as compared to a self-perceived ideal. Also, most experts feel that QOL is a multidimensional measure with various domains, such as physical, psychological, and social well-being, spiritual health, and functional ability. Health-related QOL (HRQOL) is defined more narrowly and explicitly incorporates how one's disease and treatment influences QOL. Some consider HRQOL as an aspect of overall QOL, while others consider it a distinct concept (De Civita et al. 2005).

Multiple studies have attempted to quantify QOL, but they are small and have used a variety of measures; therefore, it has been difficult to make direct comparisons between various studies (Eiser and Grimer 1999; Nagarajan et al. 2002). In particular the differences in QOL of patients undergoing amputation and limb-sparing surgeries have been studied. The QOL of patients undergoing limb-sparing procedures was predicted to be superior to amputation; however, numerous studies have shown no improvement to only mild or moderate improvement in QOL. Sugarbaker et al. was one of the first to demonstrate no improvement in his review of 21 patients (9 with amputations and 12 with limb sparing surgery; Sugarbaker et al. 1982). Others have found similar results (Weddington et al. 1985; Rougraff et al. 1994; Hudson et al. 1998; Refaat et al. 2002), while some studies showed only a trend (no statistical significance) toward improvement in QOL in those with limb salvage (Postma et al. 1992; Marsden and Swanson 1997). Additionally, there are only a few studies with significant numbers of patients examining QOL measures, disability, and function (Davis et al. 1999; Marchese et al. 2004). In one of the larger studies from the Childhood Cancer Survivor Study (CCSS) (Robison et al. 2002), QOL of bone sarcomas survivors, which included Ewing's sarcoma, was examined. Survivors with and without an amputation did rather well in terms of QOL with no differences, but these were patients with an average of 21 years from diagnosis. Some predictors of poor QOL included older age, poor health, and female gender (Nagarajan et al. 2004). Other studies from the CCSS looked at health status and chronic health conditions and have found that bone sarcoma survivors continue to be a risk for poor outcomes when compared to other cancer survivors and to a sibling comparison group (Hudson et al. 2003; Oeffinger et al. 2006). This is significant in that these difficulties can lead to poor QOL.

Eiser and Grimer described the gaps in the QOL literature regarding bone tumors (Eiser and Grimer 1999). They concluded that body image and gender differences in QOL have not been adequately addressed in the literature. Additionally, most studies have looked at patients several years after treatment and have not explored the more immediate time frame, which would help reveal how one adapts to changes. Another area in which additional information is needed includes the impact on childhood survivors and their families.

21.4
Outcomes Model

QOL in osteosarcoma survivors can be looked at independently, but should also be examined in a larger framework of outcomes (see Fig. 21.1), since there are multiple outcomes that are influenced by the diagnosis and treatment of osteosarcoma. These include functional limitations, disability, and personal identity, in addition to QOL. These factors interact with each other and significantly influence on QOL. These interactions can be described by a modified disablement model proposed by Nagi (1976). Functional limitation in this model can be due to

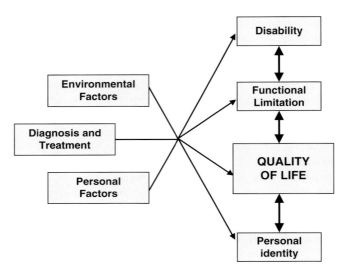

Fig. 21.1 Influences on QOL

an impairment of physical, mental, or emotional performance (e.g., inability to stand for long periods of time). Disability is defined as the limited ability or inability to perform actions, tasks, or activities required for self-care, home management, work, school, or leisure. Disability depends upon the sociocultural context of the individual and his environment; therefore, the same functional limitation in two individuals may results in disability for one, but not the other. QOL may suffer if there are significant functional limitations leading to disabilities that prevent one from participating in life's normal activities and daily cares. Without appropriate intervention or assistance this can further lead to depression and adjustment issues.

Another aspect that is significantly impacted by cancer treatment is personal identity, which includes body image and self-concept ("who am I"). In the past, body image focused on self-perception of one's body defined as "the picture we have in our minds of the size, shape, and form of our bodies." It is now clear that there is also a subjective component that is associated with the "feelings concerning these characteristics (size, shape, and form) and our constituent body parts." (White 2000). Body image is known to influence self-esteem, social anxiety, self-consciousness, and depressive symptoms, all of which are problems seen with cancer and cancer treatments and can influence QOL (White 2000). Although "self-concept" has been used and measured for quite some time, its definition has also not always been clear and has sometimes been interchanged with other self measures, such as self-esteem (Woodgate and McClement 1997). "Self-concept" refers to how a person defines and understands one's self ("who am I"), while self-esteem refers to how a person values one's self ("how do I feel about myself") (Woodgate and McClement 1997). Impairments in how one see oneself because of disabilities or limitations can lead to further impairments in how one value's oneself and to depression, all of which impacts QOL.

Personal and host factors include such qualities as gender, coping styles, emotional and physical maturity, and chemotherapy tolerance due to genetic polymorphisms in chemotherapy drug metabolism. These are significant factors in that they can influence all the factors in the model, but especially QOL. For example, there are gender-related differences in adaptation and coping styles (Znajda et al. 1999). Also emotional maturity (pre-adolescence vs adolescence) influences how one adapts to and processes body changes during therapy (hair loss, physical impairments from surgery and scars) (Kagan 1976; Ettinger and Heiney 1993; Felder-Puig et al. 1998). Physical maturity (+/− completion of bone growth) can dictate the type of surgical procedure that is needed, which affects the subsequent risk of complications. Genetic polymorphisms relating to chemotherapy metabolism and tolerance and its impact on QOL is unknown, but one can envision that those that suffer more severe side effects from chemotherapy can have impaired QOL, if only for the short term. Environmental influences on the outcomes include support from one's family and friends, as well as accommodations made by work and school. These are important factors in that these issues can help bring "normalcy" back into one's life and help provide support through the difficulties experienced during treatment.

When looking at osteosarcoma treatment, maximizing duration of life (survivorship) is generally the primary goal. However, survivorship can come with a price, for treatment can have a negative impact on the outcomes of the proposed model in some individuals. It is important that QOL and other measures are assessed prospectively to determine how these factors change over time and to determine predictors of poor outcome so that interventions can be developed.

References

Aboulafia A, Malawer M (1993) Surgical management of pelvic and extremity osteosarcoma. Cancer 71:3358–3366
Cheng E, Gebhardt M (1991) Allograft reconstruction of the shoulder after bone tumor resection. Orthop Clin North Am 22:37–48
Davis AM, Devlin M, Griffin AM, Wunder JS, Bell RS (1999) Functional outcome in amputation versus limb sparing of patients with lower extremity sarcoma: a matched case-control study. Arch Phys Med Rehabil 80:615–618
De Civita M, Regier D, Alamqir AH, Anis AH, Fitzgerald MJ, Marra CA (2005) Evaluating health-related quality-of-life studies in paediatric populations: some conceptual, methodological and developmental considerations and recent applications. Pharmacoeconomics 23:659–685
Eiser C, Grimer RJ (1999) Quality of life in survivors of a primary bone tumor: a systematic review. Sarcoma 4:183–190
Ettinger RS, Heiney SP (1993) Cancer in adolescents and young adults. Psychosocial concerns, coping strategies, and interventions. Cancer 71:3276–3280
Felder-Puig R, Formann AK, Mildner A, Bretschneider W, Bucher B, Windhager R, Zoubek A, Puig S, Topf R (1998) Quality of life and psychosocial adjustment of young patients after treatment of bone cancer. Cancer 83:69–75
Friedman MA, Carter SK (1972) The therapy of osteogenic sarcoma: current status and thoughts for the future. J Surg Oncol 4:482–510
Grimer RJ (2005) Surgical options for children with osteosarcoma. Lancet Oncol 6:85–92
Hudson M, Tyc V, Cremer LK, Luo X, Li H, Rao BN, Meyer WH, Crom DB, Pratt CB (1998) Patient satisfaction after limb sparing surgery and amputation for pediatric malignant bone tumors. J Pediatr Oncol Nurs 15:60–69
Hudson MM, Mertens AC, Yasui Y, Hobbie W, Chen H, Gurney JG, Yeazel M, Recklitis CJ, Marina N, Robison LR, Oeffinger KC; Childhood Cancer Survivor Study Investigators (2003) Health status of adult long-term survivors of childhood cancer: a report from the Childhood Cancer Survivor Study. JAMA 290:1583–1592
Kagan L (1976) Use of denial in adolescents with bone cancer. Health Social Work 1:70–87
Link MP, Goorin AM, Miser AW, Green AA, Pratt CB, Belasco JB, Pritchard J, Malpas JS, Baker AR, Kirkpatrick JA (1986) The effect of adjuvant chemotherapy on relapse-free survival in patients with osteosarcoma of the extremity. N Engl J Med 314:1600–1606
Marchese V, Ogle S, Womer RB, Dormans J, Ginsberg JP (2004) An examination of outcome measures to assess functional mobility in childhood survivors of osteosarcoma. Pediatr Blood Cancer 42:41–45
Marsden FW, Swanson CE (1997) Outcomes after multi-modality treatment of musculoskeletal

tumours. Acta Orthop Scand (Suppl) 273:101–105

Nagarajan R, Neglia JP, Clohisy DR, Robison LL (2002) Limb salvage and amputation in survivors of pediatric lower-extremity bone tumors: what are the long-term implications? J Clin Oncol 20:4493–4501

Nagarajan R, Clohisy DR, Neglia JP, Yasui Y, Mitby PA, Sklar C, Finklestein JZ, Greenberg M, Reaman GH, Zeltzer L, Robison LL (2004) Function and quality-of-life of survivors of pelvic and lower extremity osteosarcoma and Ewing's sarcoma: the Childhood Cancer Survivor Study. Br J Cancer 91:1858–1865

Nagi SZ (1976) An epidemiology of disability among adults in the United States. Milbank Mem Fund Q Health Soc 54:439–467

Oeffinger KC, Mertens AC, Sklar CA, Kawashima T, Hudson MM, Meadows AT, Friedman DL, Marina N, Hobbie W, Kadan-Lottick NS, Schwartz CL, Leisenring W, Robison LL; Childhood Cancer Survivor Study (2006) Chronic health conditions in adult survivors of childhood cancer. N Engl J Med 355:1572–1582

Postma A, Kingma A, De Ruiter JH, Schraffordt Koops H, Veth RP, Goëken LN, Kamps WA (1992) Quality of life in bone tumor patients comparing limb salvage and amputation of the lower extremity. J Surg Oncol 51:47–51

Refaat Y, Gunnoe J, Hornicek FJ, Mankin HJ (2002) Comparison of quality of life after amputation or limb salvage. Clin Orthop Relat Res 298–305

Ries LA, Smith MA (eds) (1999) Cancer incidence and survival among children and adolescents: United States SEER Program 1975–1995. National Cancer Institute, Bethesda

Robison LL, Mertens AC, Boice JD, Breslow NE, Donaldson SS, Green DM, Li FP, Meadows AT, Mulvihill JJ, Neglia JP, Nesbit ME, Packer RJ, Potter JD, Sklar CA, Smith MA, Stovall M, Strong LC, Yasui Y, Zeltzer LK (2002) Study design and cohort characteristics of the childhood cancer survivor study: a multi-institutional collaborative project. Med Pediatr Oncol 38:229–239

Rougraff BT, Simon MA, Kneisl JS, Greenberg DB, Mankin HJ (1994) Limb salvage compared with amputation for osteosarcoma of the distal end of the femur. A long-term oncological, functional, and quality-of-life study. J Bone Joint Surg 76:649–656

Spector L, Ross J, Nagarajan R (2006) Epidemiology of bone and soft tissue sarcomas. In: Pappo A (ed) Pediatric bone and soft tissue tumors. Springer-Veralg, Berlin Heidelberg New York, pp 1–11

Springfield DS (1991) Introduction to limb-salvage surgery for sarcomas. Orthop Clin North Am 22:1–5

Sugarbaker PH, Barofsky I, Rosenberg SA, Gianola FJ (1982) Quality of life assessment of patients in extremity sarcoma clinical trials. Surgery 91:17–23

Wang CC, Schulz MD (1953) A study of fifty cases treated at Massachusetts general hospital, 1930–1952 inclusive. N Engl J Med 248:571–576

Weddington WW Jr, Segraves KB, Simon MA (1985) Psychological outcome of extremity sarcoma survivors undergoing amputation or limb salvage. J Clin Oncol 3:1393–1399

White CA (2000) Body image dimensions and cancer: a heuristic cognitive behavioural model. Psychooncology 9:183–192

Woodgate R, McClement S (1997) Sense of self in children with cancer and in childhood cancer survivors: a critical review. J Pediatr Oncol Nurs 14:137–155

Znajda TL, Wunder JS, Bell RS, Davis AM (1999) Gender issues in patients with extremity soft-tissue sarcoma: a pilot study. Cancer Nurs 22:111–118

Clinical Trials in Osteosarcoma Treatment: Patients' Perspective Through Art

Lizzie Burns and Martha Perisoglou

Abstract Patients with osteosarcoma were encouraged to create artwork about their experiences of taking part in the EURAMOS 1 clinical trial. Art sessions allowed patients to express their feelings and talk openly about their condition and treatment. Each patient created artwork which reveals their experience through chemotherapy and surgery as well as their hopes for the future. Patients supported a positive focussed art activity which can help improve their quality of life during cancer treatment.

22.1 Introduction

Clinical trials depend on volunteers' participation to help advance medical treatments. While

Lizzie Burns and Martha Perisoglou (✉)
Artist-in-residence
The London Sarcoma Service
University College Hospital
Complementary Therapy Group
1st Floor Rosenheim Building
25 Grafton Way
London WC1E 6AU UK
E-mail: lizzie.burns@bioch.ox.ac.uk or
sciencetolife@yahoo.co.uk
www.londonsarcma.org

volunteers taking part in clinical trials understand their purpose, there is a more general need to communicate their importance to the public to ensure future generations continue to support medical research and clinical trials.

The UK Medical Research Council (MRC) is publicly funded to help improve human health through research across the biomedical spectrum, from fundamental lab-based science to clinical trials. There is a real challenge in finding ways to communicate the importance and relevance of clinical trials to the public. One example of an unusual project revealing the human stories behind the need for clinical trials is described in the following chapter. *Bringing Medicine to Life* was funded by the MRC and came about through the collaboration of scientist-turned-artist Dr. Lizzie Burns, with the MRC Clinical Trials Unit in London and paediatric oncologist Dr. Martha Perisoglou in the University College Hospital. The project shows the patients' perspective as seen through their artwork and comments, revealing an insight into their experience of osteosarcoma and their hopes about taking part in a clinical trial to help improve treatments for other patients in future. The artwork has been exhibited in hospitals to create an awareness of clinical trials and serves to highlight the beneficial role art can have in a therapeutic environment.

22.2 Patients with Osteosarcoma and the EURAMOS 1 Clinical Trial

Osteosarcoma is the most frequent bone cancer, accounting for half of all bone cancers in children. However, it is rare occurring in less than 5 per million children younger than 20 years of age. The incidence differs in different age groups. It is as low as 0.3 per million in children under the age of 5 years, 2.8 per million at the age of 5–9 years, 8.3 per million at the age of 10–14 years and 9.4 per million at the age of 15–19 years [1]. There is a second peak in older patients due to osteosarcomas arising in abnormal bones, such as those affected by Paget's disease or after radiotherapy.

Research into new ways of treating osteosarcoma is going on all the time and clinical trials are used to assess new treatments. These are particularly important for finding improvements in treatment for rare cancers such as osteosarcoma.

Currently, worldwide, the main clinical trial for osteosarcoma is the European and American Osteosarcoma (EURAMOS) 1 clinical trial. The EURAMOS 1 study is the culmination of collaboration between the North American Children's Oncology Group (COG), the German–Austrian–Swiss Cooperative Osteosarcoma Study Group (COSS), the European Osteosarcoma Intergroup (EOI) and the Scandinavian Sarcoma Group (SSG). The aim of the study is to evaluate whether it is possible to improve the outcome of both poor and good responders to pre-operative chemotherapy, by modification of post-operative chemotherapy. All patients receive pre-operative methotrexate, doxorubicin and cisplatin (MAP). Poor responders are randomised to receive MAP with or without ifosfamide and etoposide. Good responders will continue on MAP chemotherapy, and are randomised to maintenance pegylated interferon-α or observation (www.euramos.org).

22.3 Bringing Medicine to Life

Patients taking part in the EURAMOS 1 clinical trial were encouraged to create artwork about their experiences of osteosarcoma and participation in a clinical trial. Patients were approached initially by Dr. Perisoglou who explained that the project would involve at least one art session with pieces of artwork being used to create an exhibition. Where patients were under the age of 16 years, parents were approached about the possibility of them taking part in the project. Each patient received an information sheet outlining the project and highlighting that patients did not have to be artistic. Consent was obtained from all participants. Nine patients participated between April and November 2006, representing a significant number of EURAMOS 1 volunteers over that 7-month period.

Art sessions were co-ordinated by Dr. Perisoglou to ensure that patients were healthy enough to participate. Patients were then visited by artist Dr. Lizzie Burns who brought along a range of art materials including A3 sketchpads, coloured paper, oil and chalk pastels, paints, brushes, felt-tips and glitter glue. The session would start with an introduction to the project followed by a discussion about possible ideas for artwork based on their experiences or concerns. An interesting choice of arts materials helped get patients enthusiastic about the activity. In many cases they had not drawn or painted since childhood or did not consider themselves to be artistic. To encourage them to get started an emphasis was placed on there being no 'right' or 'wrong'. Patients were asked for permission for photographs to be taken while they created their artwork, and to record any comments they wanted to make about their pieces. They were able to choose which photographs and quotes were displayed to the public. In some cases, individuals did not want to be photographed but still wanted to contribute their artwork to the project.

Although the initial aim of the project was to communicate the experiences of patients taking part in a clinical trial to the wider public, it soon became apparent that the patients who took part enjoyed the opportunity to express themselves in hospital. Visits were an opportunity to talk about their experiences to someone outside the medical system. In many cases they became absorbed in the creative process, spending hours lost in concentration. It would be difficult and possibly inappropriate to attempt to quantify the benefits of such a subjective experience, but the effect of positive experiences in hospital is likely to be of emotional benefit to the person.

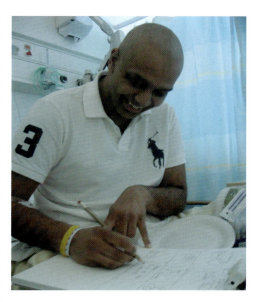

Fig. 22.1 Syed drawing his cancer story

22.4
The Patients' Perspective

Bringing medicine to life offers glimpses into the individual lives and experiences of nine patients living with osteosarcoma, the difficulties of diagnosis and treatment and, for older patients, their hopes about taking part in a clinical trial. Each individual, their experiences, outlook on life and artwork are unique and wherever possible their own words have been used to reveal their perspective.

22.4.1
Syed

Syed (Figs. 22.1, 22.2, 22.3, 22.4, and 22.5) was the oldest patient taking part in the project at the age of 34. He had not created art for many years and did not feel that he was particularly artistic. With some encouragement he soon developed

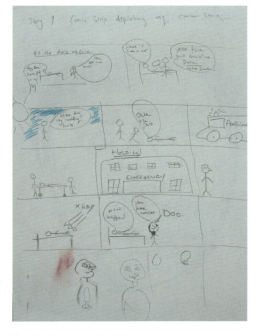

Fig. 22.2 Syed drawing his cancer story

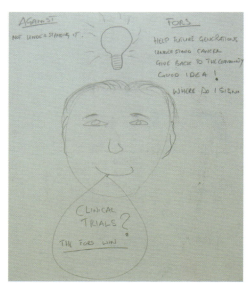

Fig. 22.3 Syed's drawing about taking part in a clinical trial

many ideas he wanted to communicate. He started with "my cancer story and I'm depicting what happened to me and all the events which led up to my cancer". Syed talked through his experiences while drawing a cartoon strip about his diagnosis:

- "I went to my doctor, and that's me being told by my doctor there's no problem."
- "There's me walking and my leg really hurt, I fell over and the ambulance came. I was conscious but in a lot of pain."
- "And then 'you have cancer'."
- "Actually I took it really well. They asked me, 'Do you have any questions?' and all I said was, 'How are you going to fix me?' "
- "I didn't ask anything else like, 'Am I going to die?' I just asked, 'What's going to happen?' "
- "The worst case scenario is you might die, the second best is they might chop your leg off and the best scenario is that you'll have a replacement leg and the chemo will start. Hopefully, fingers crossed, they are telling me I'll have a replacement leg, should be a good one, so I'm quite happy. I might come out of hospital saying 'no leg' but it doesn't matter, it's better than being dead."

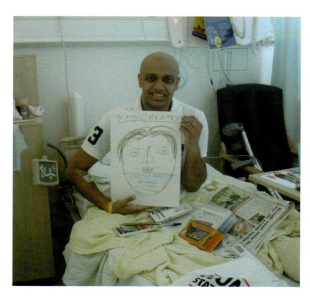

Fig. 22.4 Syed's dream

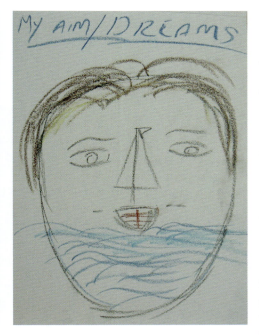

Fig. 22.5 Syed's dream

Syed drew a picture about deciding to take part in the clinical trial. He started by drawing a picture of himself asking the question, 'Clinical trials?' He drew a light bulb above his head to represent his thoughts and wrote a list of positive reasons for taking part which included "help future generations, understand cancer, give back to the community". He also talked about his doubts, which included "not understanding it" and the possibility a trial might not help to understand or identify better treatments. Syed looked at his list of pros and cons and then added "Good idea!" and "Where do I sign" before writing "the fors win".

During the session Syed explained how he made his decision:

- "When I came here the doctor said we're doing this EURAMOS trial on people with bone tumours. He gave me a couple of days to think about it." He talked about his personal reasons for taking part after speaking to his family and his perspective as the son of immigrant parents.
- "My uncle who is a doctor told me to go for it. He said that it's a good trial to go on."
- I said alright, nothing to lose and plus if it helps anyone, benefits anyone in the future, you can't be selfish all your life. You can give back something to society.
- The other way I look at is my parents are immigrants and there are countries out there you wouldn't have a chance. You'd die within a few years.
- As I said, I'm a very positive person and I like to look at things in a very positive light."

Syed drew a picture about his desire to get better and his aim to sail around the Greek islands later in the year. He drew a boat and was delighted to find he could transform this into part of his face which doubled up to show his dream to sail again. While working on *my aim/dream* he talked about his positive attitude towards life and cancer.

- "In everything I do, I'm very positive, and very competitive."
- "Everything I do, my business, my work, and when I play football, I like to win and even with this cancer I want to win. I don't want to let it get me down, get me depressed and ultimately, as I said, if I don't make it I don't make it but that's just life."
- "You never know tomorrow. When I leave hospital I could get hit by a bus and it all could be a waste of time but it's not. While you're living you try things."

Syed was able to talk about his experiences very openly while being creative and was very cheerful despite his circumstances. His remarkably positive outlook on life was obviously recognised by medical staff, with nurses sending other patients who were feeling depressed to spend time with him.

22.4.2
Omar

At 8 years old, Omar (Figs. 22.6 and 22.7) was one of the youngest patients to take part. In this case, he was too young to appreciate the significance of a trial but drew pictures about himself in hospital. His pastel drawings show him in hospital with a bed and the surrounding equipment. Despite not using a mirror, his self-portraits were very well observed showing his thinner hair after chemotherapy with a distinctive whorl of hair growing in strength at the

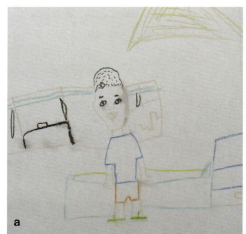

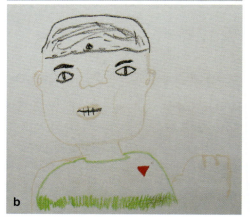

Fig. 22.7 Omar's drawing of himself in hospital

front of his hairline. Omar commented on the experience: "I enjoyed this art session".

22.4.3
Shane

At the age of 23, Shane (Figs. 22.8 and 22.9) approached a difficult stage in treatment with the possibility of an amputation to remove his tumour. At a relatively young age the prospect of losing a limb was obviously extremely distressing.

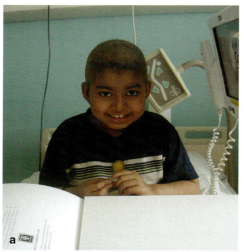

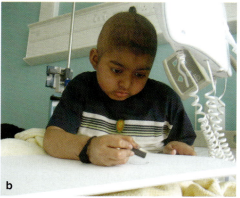

Fig. 22.6 Omar during the art session

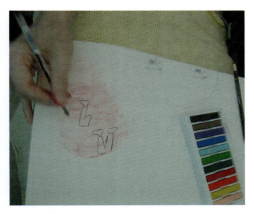

Fig. 22.8 Shane drawing *Walking on my mind*

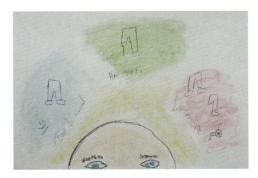

Fig. 22.9 Shane's *Walking on my mind*

Despite not considering himself to be artistic and finding talking about his experiences difficult, he still wanted to participate.

He decided to create a piece about his preoccupation with losing a leg and concern for walking again. He started by drawing the top of his head and drew his thoughts above about losing his leg and having to use a wheelchair. He then wrote about his desire for "learning to walk" and drew himself standing wearing an artificial limb and wrote "half way!". He then drew what appeared to be complete legs hidden by trousers and wrote "back to normal" and drew a smiling face.

Shane decided to add colour over his drawings to show how he felt about his leg and learning to walk with an artificial limb. He chose red for his immediate thoughts and emotions about an amputation while the future was shaded in calmer greens and blues. He drew a yellow cloud above his head to show where his thoughts had originated and to make the piece more visually striking. After completing the piece he decided to entitle it *walking on my mind* and wrote: "Shows me learning to walk and my feelings. This is the main thing on my mind."

22.4.4
Laura

Laura (Fig. 22.10) was undergoing chemotherapy at the age of 15 with the possibility of an amputation to remove her tumour. She felt shaky after taking painkillers and was unable to concentrate on drawing or painting. She wanted to participate by talking about her experiences and kept art materials to create artwork by herself.

During the visit Laura was accompanied by her mother and they talked together about her difficult experiences leading up to her diagnosis.

- "I found out in Accident and Emergency as I got so fed up with the pain for about 6 months. My grandparents took me as my parents were away on holiday. We went to A+E and waited there for 8 hours."
- "They felt my knee but didn't know what it was so they did an X-ray."
- "They found my knee to be abnormal and that it was probably cancer, but it was the way he blurted it out when they weren't even sure. They know it is now but what if it wasn't?"
- "When you find out something like that you just want someone to comfort you."

She then talked about her diagnosis:

- "I had a biopsy and went home but I broke my leg and was taken to hospital."

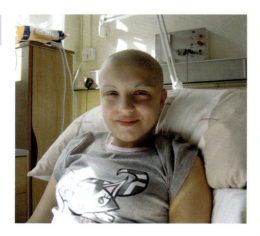

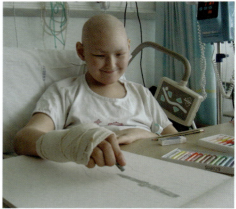

Fig. 22.10 Laura's *I want to live*

Fig. 22.11 Meg during the art session

- "I had a cast put on but no one would believe me that the cast was really digging into me."
- "When they finally listened they found there was a massive indentation where the tumour was getting bigger."
- "I am positive, but it's difficult to be with no good news."

Despite her distressing experiences, Laura was able to reflect on positive aspects of her life:

- "It has made me appreciate things more, I can't say how, but it has."
- "Like my hair for instance because I had to have my hair perfect."
- "The last photo I had taken when I had hair I thought it looked really ugly, but now I look back it looked really nice."
- "I really appreciate my hair now and it doesn't matter if it doesn't look 100% perfect."

She was able to simply state: "I want to live".

22.4.5
Meg

At 12 years old Meg (Figs. 22.11, 22.12, 22.13 and 22.14) was enthusiastic about art. She decided to create life-sized drawings showing how her leg had physically changed with the growth of a tumour and subsequent operations resulting in a bionic implant. While drawing, Meg talked about her leg and her experiences.

She started by drawing her leg "before when it was normal" and then drew her knee swollen and slightly bruised entitled *my leg with tumour*. She explained:

- "When it had the tumour in there it had stretched my leg. It felt really, really painful."
- "I went to the doctor and they gave me anti-inflammatories and they weren't working so my mum took me to the doctor again."
- "They X-rayed me and said I had a tumour in my knee."

She then drew her leg following her operation: "This is a picture of the scar where they took the tumour." She then drew "my bionic implant" and explained, "They then put in a metal implant, a bionic implant. When I grow I'll go into a magnetic field and it lengthens it. You can actually hear it. It feels fine."

Meg took part in another art session 4 months later during her final round of chemotherapy. She started by drawing a self-portrait in pencil but soon fell asleep due to the painkillers. While she slept her mother talked about her progress and hopes for the treatment coming to an end.

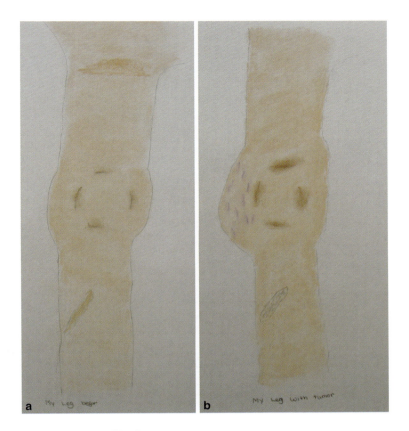

Fig. 22.12 a–d Meg's drawings of her leg

She broke her ankle after falling over. She was in plaster up to her knee and came out of that 3 or 4 weeks ago. She was having her last round of chemo and then she had a kidney problem and couldn't do this lot of chemo. This should have been 2 1/2 weeks ago and over and done by now. Her kidneys are OK now thankfully, so she came in and now she's fallen over and done her hip in! Her bones are very soft and practically see-through like an old lady. The tiniest little knock is all that's needed. We'll be in hospital for a few more weeks, but it's our last lot of chemo and then we've got more tests for her lung. She's got a little way to go but we're getting there.

22.4.6 Simon

Simon (Figs. 22.15) had completed his first found of chemotherapy at the age of 18 but was suffering from painful mouth ulcers following treatment with methotrexate. He found thinking and talking about his experiences difficult but wanted to create an abstract piece for the project. Simon did not want his artwork to be explained or analysed.

While drawing he talked about his situation and explained, "My friends don't know. I don't really want them to know. I've got too much to

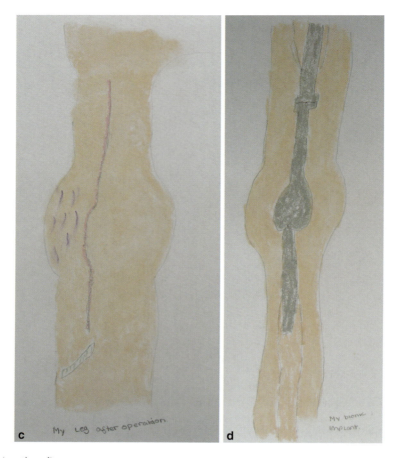

Fig. 22.12 (continued)

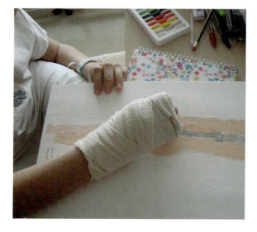

Fig. 22.13 Meg drawing *my bionic leg*

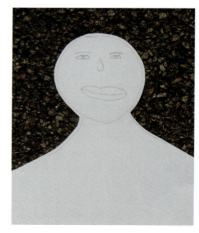

Fig. 22.14 Meg's self-portrait

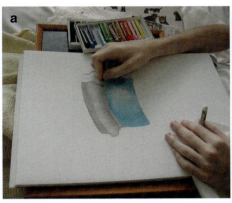 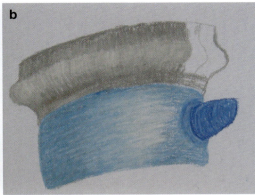

Fig. 22.15 Simon's drawing

deal with." Simon was able to concentrate on his drawing but found speaking very painful because of the mouth ulcers. He talked about his frustration and pain: "My knee doesn't hurt now but everything else does. I've traded one pain for another. I'd rather have my knee back."

Since talking was very difficult, Simon's mother spoke on his behalf about his decision to take part in the clinical trial. "As soon as we arrived they mentioned the trial straight away," she said. "He had to make the decision as to whether he would sign up for it or not." Simon decided to take part because "if the treatment in future can be improved and made better for other patients then it's something worth doing."

22.4.7 Bhavin

Bhavin (Figs. 22.16, 22.17, and 22.18) was the second oldest patient taking part in the project. At the age of 27 he had not drawn or painted since childhood but was enthusiastic about the opportunity and even started sketching ideas before the session.

He started by drawing a picture of himself in hospital and included his drip which he imagined to have a life of its own. "This is a very temperamental machine so don't mess with it." He enjoyed being creative and talked openly about his emotions and explained, "I have mixed feelings right now because the doctor has to cut my leg and at the same time my wife is expecting her first baby."

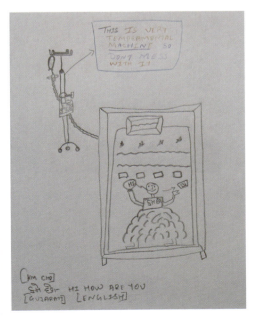

Fig. 22.16 Bhavin's drawing of himself in hospital

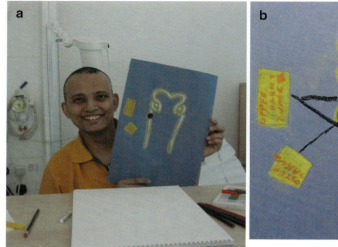
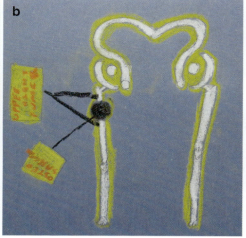

Fig. 22.17 Bhavin holding his drawing showing the inside of his legs

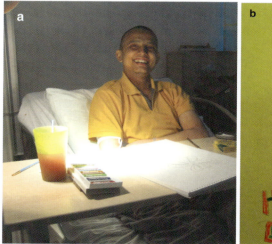
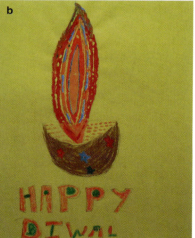

Fig. 22.18 Bhavin celebrating Diwali

He talked about his experiences in a very positive way and recalled how he reacted to his diagnosis:

- "When I was told my cancer was very rare, I told him I was never in a lucky draw and was never given a prize, but this was a surprise."

Bhavin talked about his decision to take part in the clinical trial:

- "I was explained how EURAMOS works and how it will help in the future."
- "It's a good cause so I just asked it won't affect my medicines."

- "My parents were a bit worried, but a friend who is a doctor told them it was a good thing and not to worry."

Bhavin wanted to show what was happening inside his body and what needed to be done to remove the tumour. He decided to create a colourful picture showing the inside of his legs with his tumour in black. While drawing he talked about how his doctor would be proud of the picture. He was able to indicate the location of the tumour and explained how six inches of bone would be removed and replaced by a metal implant. Bhavin commented on positive aspects of his condition and suggested, "If it was higher up I would have been in trouble. They would have to replace the hip and it would be a life-long problem of replacing it every 15 years." He surrounded his picture of bones with a yellow halo to make the image more visually striking. At the bottom he wrote positive statements: "Note:- this is a curable disease with help of chemotherapy and surgery", and also added in his own "motto:- just take it as it comes."

He then drew a piece to celebrate the coming of the Hindu Festival of light, Diwali. After drawing a candle he carefully painted the flame in vibrant colours and explained, "The picture symbolises bringing light, colour, happiness and prosperity to your life. In India each and every house is decorated with these candles. There would be lots of food and wherever you go you definitely have to eat something. I have a lot of hope for the future."

to express her feelings and explained she wanted to go out with her friends like any other teenager. On being asked how she came to a decision to take part in the trial, she replied, "I just thought why not basically. I made that decision myself."

Sam created a picture entitled *My life now"* and started by drawing herself wearing red pyjamas with her gold necklace and "no hair". She then drew a small picture of her leg in pencil showing "my scar" with another pencil drawing of "me being connected to her drip". She explained that she did not want to add colour to the drip as "it's not very interesting". Below the pencil drawings she drew a large picture of a car and carefully painted this in thick bright red paint. While painting, she explained the significance: "This is my brother's car because I want to get back in it when I can bend my leg again". She then drew her mobile phone which "I can't live without" and coloured it in with thick glitter glue to give texture and sparkle to this positive aspect of her life. To complete the portrait, she decided to convey her inner feelings. She drew a big ball of black, grey and red to express her feelings of frustration and anger about being unwell in hospital, her pain, and not being able to lead a normal life like her friends. Sam explained, "This is my anger". Despite not enjoying art previously, she spent hours absorbed in the creative process and was evidently proud of her achievement to have created a painting about her life and hopes for the future.

22.4.8
Sam

Sam (Figs. 22.19, 22.20 and 22.21) was on her sixth round of chemotherapy at the age of 17. Despite not enjoying art at school she was enthusiastic about the opportunity to create art and had lots of ideas for a piece about her experiences. Sam had not been able to find an outlet

22.4.9
Charlie

Charlie (Fig. 22.22) was the youngest patient. At the age of 5 he was angry and upset about his condition and did not welcome unfamiliar visitors. Charlie sought comfort from his mother and played with his toys and computer games.

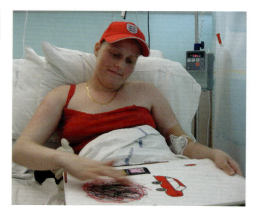

Fig. 22.19 Sam working on *My life now*

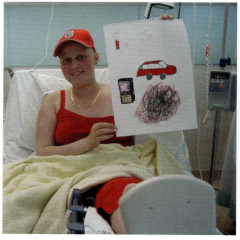

Fig. 22.21 Sam holding *My life now*

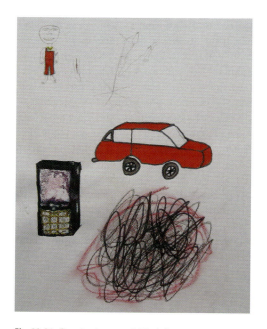

Fig. 22.20 Sam's picture of *My life now*

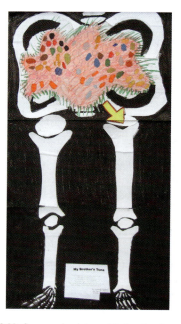

Fig. 22.22 Susanna's picture *My brother's tuna*

His mother talked on his behalf and explained:

- "His thoughts are, 'Why did I break my leg?' 'Why have I fallen over?' 'Why have I got the tumour?'"

- "And of course he's cross; he's a cross little 5-year-old and in the main he deals with it really well."
- "He gets cross with people poking him and prodding him. And why wouldn't he?"

His mother talked about her decision for taking part in the trial. She felt the trial was worthwhile but had to balance this with the need to protect him from additional contact with doctors. "We're only deciding to take part in the trial up to surgery at the moment. We thought it was a good thing and we are interested in participating. We'll see how we feel and how he is coping. It's quite a long trial and it could go on for quite a few years. He's only five. He's only little, so we're taking that into consideration and we have to decide if we want the extra 2 years."

Charlie was too young to create artwork about his experiences so his mother suggested her 10-year-old daughter might be more suitable. Susanna created a poignant, thoughtful and visually striking piece about her younger brother's cancer. She started by cutting out shapes of bones from white paper which she assembled into legs and added a colourful picture to represent her brother's tumour. She entitled the piece *My Brother's Tuna* and explained, "The reason why I named this piece of art MY BROTHER'S TUNA is because he said to my mum, 'Why have I got a fish in my leg?' The reason for this is because he is only 5 years old and he doesn't understand what a tumour is."

22.5
Art and Cancer

While the initial purpose of art sessions was to convey the importance of clinical trials, it soon became apparent that the opportunity for patients to express themselves was worthwhile and beneficial to the patients themselves. Art sessions were well received by patients who enjoyed the opportunity to be creative.

During treatment, patients can be in hospital for long periods of time and so art activities provide a welcome distraction from waiting. The project provided positive focussed activities to help patients express their emotions during treatment with the possibility of communicating this to a wider audience. Art sessions allowed patients to concentrate on an activity for themselves and to enjoy being creative and in control. An emphasis was placed on enjoying the creative process rather than feeling there was a 'right' or 'wrong'. Sessions allowed patients to talk openly about their feelings. One patient wanted to check that his artwork would not be analysed, which suggests part of the enjoyment and trust established during sessions may be due to a lack of psychological or artistic analysis.

During the diagnosis and treatment of cancer, patients face many emotional and physical difficulties such as pain, fatigue and anxiety. Several studies have suggested over 80% of cancer patients seek complementary therapy for their psychological well-being in addition to their standard medical treatments of surgery, chemotherapy and radiation [2]. A wide range of therapies such as relaxation, aromatherapy and massage have been found to help reduce symptoms and improve the patient's quality of life and ability to cope [3–6].

One such therapy is 'art therapy', which emerged in the 1940s as a form of psychotherapy. Art therapy is based on the belief that the creative process involved in the making of art is healing and life enhancing. A study by Nainis et al. found an hour-long art therapy session can significantly reduce eight symptoms associated with cancer including pain, tiredness, anxiety and depression [7]; 90% of patients found art activities to be a positive focussed distraction. While these results involved a trained art therapist, many of these observations were also observed in *"Bringing medicine to life"*. For example, despite undergoing chemotherapy, once patients started the creative process they were distracted for hours, which suggests feelings of tiredness were alleviated during art sessions. A control or comparison was not included in the Nainis et al.

paper. It could be speculated that any focussed activity would help distract patients from symptoms associated with cancer. However, art has the additional benefit of allowing patients to express their emotions and can help them talk more openly about their feelings. Also many patients may not be well enough to participate in more physically demanding activities while art activities require little effort and materials can easily be brought to a hospital bed.

The importance of art in helping people come to terms with tragedy is illustrated by Ahmed and Siddiqi's essay in *The Lancet* [8]. Following an earthquake in Pakistan in 2005 more than 100,000 people died and 75,000 were left injured. One of the many activities offered to help survivors were art sessions. From Ahmed and Siddiqi's experience (also shared by colleagues), the simple act of expression through art helped children come to terms with painful experiences by allowing them to convey their feelings and emotions. In this case, artwork was not explained by art therapists or psychologists but by the children themselves. Drawing and painting allowed children to talk openly about their experiences, which they could share with their family and friends. As was found in *Bringing medicine to life*, simply encouraging children or adults to create artwork about their feelings and events proved successful despite the absence of art therapy training.

Opportunities for cancer patients to create art in hospital can help distract from negative symptoms to improve their quality of life and well-being. Art can help patients express their emotions and feelings towards their condition. In some cases art sessions allowed patients to celebrate positive feelings about being alive as well as hopes and goals for the future. In other cases, patients were able to express difficult experiences and emotions such as frustration and anger about their condition and the emotional impact of losing a limb.

22.6 Conclusion

Patients taking part in a clinical trial revealed their unique perspective on their condition, treatment and hopes for the future. Art sessions allowed patients to express their feelings and talk openly to someone outside the medical system. They provided a positive focussed activity and brought a sense of playfulness to a hospital environment. Patients were proud of the work they produced and felt a sense of achievement. The project allowed patients to communicate their experiences to reveal the human stories behind the need for clinical trials.

Acknowledgements

Our special thanks to the inspiring people who took part in this project and our thanks to the UK Medical Research Council (MRC) who funded this project. Our thanks also to Prof. Janet Darbyshire and Prof. Max Parmar from the MRC Clinical Trials Unit and especially to **Dr. Jeremy Whelan** from the University College Hospital in London for his continued support.

References

1. Ries LAG, Smith MA, Gurney JG, et al (1999) Cancer Incidence and survival among children and adolescents: United States SEER program, 1975–1995. National Cancer Institute, SEER Program. NIH Pub No. 99-4649. National Cancer Institute, Bethesda
2. Richardson MA, Sanders T, Palmer JL, Greisinger A, Singletary SE (2000) Complementary/alternative medicine use in a comprehensive cancer centre and the implications for oncology. J Clin Oncol 18:2505–2514
3. Walker LG, Walker MB, Ogston K, Heys SD, Ah-See AK, Miller ID, Hutcheon AW, Sarkar TK, Eremin O (1999) Psychological, clinical and pathological effects of relaxation training and

guided imagery during primary chemotherapy. Br J Cancer 80:262–268
4. Speca M, Carlson LE, Goodey E, Angen M (2000) A randomized, wait-list controlled clinical trial: the effect of a mindfulness meditation-based stress reduction program on mood and symptoms of stress in cancer outpatients. Psychosom Med 62:613–622
5. Wilkinson S, Aldridge J, Salmon I, Cain E, Wilson B (1999) An evaluation of aromatherapy massage in palliative care. Palliat Med 13:409–417
6. Cassileth BR, Vickers AJ (2004) Massage therapy for symptom control: outcome study at a major cancer centre. J Pain Symptom Manage 28:244–249
7. Nainis N, Paice JA, Ratner J, Wirth JH, Lai J, Shott S (2006) Relieving symptoms in cancer: innovative use of art therapy. J Pain Symptom Manage 31:162–169
8. Ahmed SH, Siddiqi MN (2006) Essay: healing through art therapy in disaster settings. Lancet 368:S28–S29

Printing: Krips bv, Meppel, The Netherlands
Binding: Stürtz, Würzburg, Germany